GYNAECOLOGY
by Ten Teachers

First published in 1919 as 'Diseases of Women', *Gynaecology by Ten Teachers* is well established as a concise, yet comprehensive, guide within its field. The 21st Edition has been thoroughly updated by its latest team of 'teachers', integrating clinical material with the latest scientific developments that underpin patient care.

Each chapter is highly structured, with learning objectives, definitions, aetiology, clinical features, investigations, treatments and key point summaries and additional reading where appropriate. A key theme for this edition is 'professionalism' and information specific to this is threaded throughout the text.

Along with its companion *Obstetrics by Ten Teachers*, 21st Edition, the books continue to provide an accessible 'one stop shop' in gynaecology and for a new generation of doctors.

21st EDITION

GYNAECOLOGY
by Ten Teachers

Edited by

Emma J Crosbie
Professor of Gynaecological Oncology
Division of Cancer Sciences
University of Manchester
Consultant
Manchester University NHS Foundation Trust, UK

Louise C Kenny
Professor and Executive Pro-Vice Chancellor
Faculty of Health and Life Sciences
University of Liverpool, UK

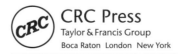

CRC Press
Taylor & Francis Group
Boca Raton London New York

CRC Press is an imprint of the
Taylor & Francis Group, an **informa** business

Designed cover image: From David A Litman via Shutterstock.com

Twenty-first edition published 2024
by CRC Press
2385 NW Executive Center Drive, Suite 320, Boca Raton, FL 33431

and by CRC Press
4 Park Square, Milton Park, Abingdon, Oxon, OX14 4RN

CRC Press is an imprint of Taylor & Francis Group, LLC

Within these twenty-first editions of *Gynaecology by Ten Teachers* terms such as woman/women, maternal, father, paternal, breastfeed, breastfeeding, breast fed and breast milk have been used throughout, but we wish to respectfully acknowledge that not all people who parent, are pregnant, give birth, need obstetric or gynaecological care, or are assigned biologically female or biologically male at birth, identify with these genders.

ISBN: 978-1-032-11007-3 (hbk)
ISBN: 978-1-032-11003-5 (pbk)
ISBN: 978-1-003-21803-6 (ebk)

DOI: 10.1201/9781003218036

Typeset in Palatino LT Std
by Evolution Design & Digital Ltd (Kent)

Access the Instructor and Student Resources: www.routledge.com/cw/crosbie

Printed in Great Britain by Bell and Bain Ltd, Glasgow

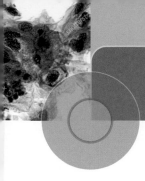

Dedication

This book is dedicated to our children
Susanna, Thomas and Louisa (EJC)
Conor and Eamon (LCK)

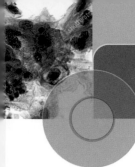

Contents

Additional resources for students and lecturers to accompany this textbook are available online.

Visit www.routledge.com/cw/crosbie for interactive SBAs and EMQs and figure slides.

Preface

Gynaecology by Ten Teachers was first published in 1919 as *Diseases of Women* and is one of the oldest, most respected and accessible texts on the subject. *Gynaecology by Ten Teachers* has informed generations of gynaecologists and now has a wide international audience. There is great responsibility in revising this, the 21st Edition to ensure its accessibility and relevance are maintained into the next century.

The 21st Edition has been written to reflect both changing undergraduate medical curricula and changing diagnostic and management protocols in gynaecology. The 'Ten Teachers' are all internationally renowned experts in their fields who are actively involved in the delivery of undergraduate and postgraduate teaching in the UK. This volume has been edited carefully to ensure consistency of structure, style and level of detail, in common with those of its sister text *Obstetrics by Ten Teachers*. The books can therefore be used together or independently as required. New self-assessment sections are presented consistently throughout, with detailed clinical scenarios for each subject in a structure similar to those used in most medical schools.

The global status of women's and girls' sexual and reproductive health and rights is disturbing. Millions of women have no access to contraception, undergo female genital mutilation and receive no gynaecological care. It is fitting, therefore, that the 21st Edition, published more than 100 years after the first, maintains a global aspect throughout.

The aim of the text now, as it was a century ago, is to prepare students for their undergraduate examinations and to continue to be useful afterwards in postgraduate studies and clinical practice. It is a text that the editors used as students, which inspired us to practise and teach in the specialty and which we still enjoy reading because it is concise yet comprehensive. We hope that, in addition to supporting medical students throughout their studies, general practitioners, trainees and allied healthcare professionals will find it useful in their work.

It has been a privilege and an honour to be the editors of this textbook. We echo a century of previous editors in hoping that this book will enthuse a new generation of doctors to become gynaecologists and work to improve the health and the safety of women through all reproductive ages.

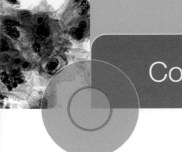

Contributors

Sharon Cameron
Professor
University of Edinburgh & NHS Lothian
Chalmers Centre, Edinburgh

Ying Cheong
Professor of Reproductive Medicine
Human Development and Health
Faculty of Medicine, University of Southampton
Medical Director, Complete Fertility

T Justin Clark
Consultant Gynaecologist
Birmingham Women's and Children Hospital
Honorary Professor of Gynaecology
University of Birmingham
Immediate Past President
British Society for Gynaecological Endoscopy

Emma J Crosbie
Professor of Gynaecological Oncology
Division of Cancer Sciences
University of Manchester
Consultant
Manchester University NHS Foundation Trust

Claudine Domoney
Consultant Obstetrician and Gynaecologist
College Tutor
Urogynaecology Lead

Leila Frodsham
Consultant Gynaecologist and Psychosexual Service
    Lead
Foundation Training Programme Director and
    Schwartz Round Medical Go Lead
Guy's and St Thomas' Hospital, London
Senior Clinical Lecturer and Women's Health Block
Co-Lead and Transition
King's College London
BMS Accredited Menopause Specialist

Dharani K Hapangama
Professor of Gynaecology/Deputy Head
Department of Women's and Children's Health
    Centre for Women's Health Research
Institute of Life Course and Medical Sciences
University of Liverpool
Consultant Gynaecologist
Liverpool Women's Hospital NHS Foundation Trust

Timothy Hillard
Consultant Gynaecologist
University Hospitals Dorset, Poole

Andrew Horne
Professor of Gynaecology and Reproductive Sciences
Centre for Reproductive Health | Institute for
    Regeneration and Repair
University of Edinburgh
Co-Director, EXPPECT Edinburgh
President-Elect, World Endometriosis Society
Specialty Advisor to the Chief Medical Officer for
    Obstetrics and Gynaecology
Scottish Government
Co-Editor-in-Chief, *Reproduction and Fertility*

Louise C Kenny
Professor and Executive Pro-Vice Chancellor
Faculty of Health and Life Sciences
University of Liverpool

Margaret Kingston
Consultant Physician
Professor
Director, Undergraduate Medical Studies
University of Manchester

Ranee Thakar
Consultant Urogynaecologist
Croydon University Hospital

Abbreviations

AFC	antral follicle count
AFP	α-fetoprotein
AIDS	acquired immune deficiency syndrome
AMH	anti-Müllerian hormone
APS	antiphospholipid syndrome
ART	assisted reproductive technology/antiretroviral therapy
AUB	abnormal uterine bleeding
AZF	azoospermic factor
BMD	bone mineral density
BMI	body mass index
BNF	British National Formulary
BOT	borderline ovarian tumour
BRCA	breast ovarian cancer syndrome
BSO	bilateral salpingo-oophorectomy
CAH	congenital adrenal hyperplasia
CAIS	complete androgen insensitivity syndrome
CBT	cognitive behavioural therapy
CHC	combined hormonal contraception
CIN	cervical intraepithelial neoplasia
CL	corpus luteum
COCP	combined oral contraceptive pill
CPP	chronic pelvic pain
CRP	C-reactive protein
CT	computed tomography
Cu-IUD	copper intrauterine device
CVD	cardiovascular disease
DHT	dihydrotestosterone
DNA	deoxyribonucleic acid
DSD	disorders of sexual development
E2	oestrogen
EC	emergency contraception
EIA	enzyme immunoassay
EMQ	extended matching question
EP	ectopic pregnancy
FBC	full blood count
FGM	female genital mutilation
FH	fetal heartbeat
FIGO	International Federation of Gynecology and Obstetrics
FSH	follicle-stimulating hormone
GnRH	gonadotrophin-releasing hormone
GP	general practitioner

HAART	highly active retroviral therapy
(β)hCG	(beta-)human chorionic gonadotrophin
HFEA	Human Fertilisation and Embryo Authority
HIFU	high-intensity focused ultrasound
HIV	human immunodeficiency virus
HMB	heavy menstrual bleeding
HPO	hypothalamic–pituitary–ovarian (axis)
HPV	human papillomavirus
HRT	hormone replacement therapy
HSG	hysterosalpingography
HSV	herpes simplex virus
HVS	high vaginal swab
HyCoSy	hysterocontrast synography
ICSI	intracytoplasmic sperm injection
Ig	immunoglobulin
IGF	insulin-like growth factor
IMB	intermenstrual bleeding
IUD	intrauterine device
IUI	intrauterine insemination
IUS	intrauterine releasing system
IVF	in vitro fertilization
LARC	long-acting reversible methods of contraception
LH	luteinizing hormone
LMP	last menstrual period
LMWH	low molecular weight heparin
LNG	levonorgestrel
LNG-IUD	levonorgestrel intrauterine device
LNG-IUS	levonorgestrel intrauterine system
MCV	mean corpuscular volume
MDT	multidisciplinary team
MEC	Medical Eligibility Criteria for Contraceptive Use
MMR	mismatch repair
MRI	magnetic resonance imaging
MRKH	Mayer–Rokitansky–Kuster–Hauser (syndrome)
MTCT	mother-to-child transmission
NAAT	nucleic acid amplification test
NICE	National Institute for Health and Care Excellence
NSAID	non-steroidal anti-inflammatory drug
OAB	overactive bladder
P4	progesterone
PAC	pre-assessment clinic
PARP	poly (ADP-ribose) polymerase
PCB	post-coital bleeding
PCOS	polycystic ovary syndrome
PCR	polymerase chain reaction
PFMT	pelvic floor muscle training
PG	prostaglandin
PGT	pre-implantation genetic testing

PID	pelvic inflammatory disease
PMB	postmenopausal bleeding
PMS	premenstrual syndrome
POF	premature ovarian failure
POI	premature ovarian insufficiency
POP	progestogen-only pill
PPH	post-partum haemorrhage
PUL	pregnancy of unknown location
RCOG	Royal College of Obstetricians and Gynaecologists
RNA	ribonucleic acid
RR	relative risk
SBA	single best answer
SCJ	squamocolumnar junction
SFA	semen fluid analysis
SIS	saline infusion sonography
SRY	sex-determining region of the Y chromosome
STI	sexually transmitted infection
TED	thromboembolic deterrent (stockings)
TVUSS	transvaginal ultrasound scan
UAE	umbilical/uterine artery embolization
UPA	ulipristal acetate
USS	ultrasound scan
VL	viral load
VTE	venous thromboembolism
WHI	Women's Health Initiative
WHO	World Health Organization

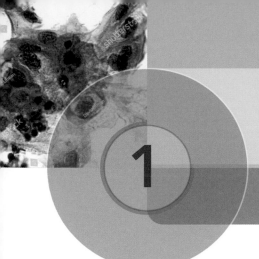

Development and anatomy of the female sexual organs and pelvis

YING CHEONG

Learning Objectives
- Understand that sexual differentiation and development begin in early embryonic life.
- Understand the embryonic development and the anatomy of the perineum, vagina, cervix, uterus, ovaries, bladder and ureters.
- Describe the blood supply and lymphatics of the perineum and pelvis.
- Understand the innervation of the perineum and pelvis.
- Understand the vulnerability of certain structures in gynaecological surgery.
- Describe the structural anomalies resulting from Müllerian tract disorders.

SEXUAL DIFFERENTIATION OF THE FETUS AND DEVELOPMENT OF SEXUAL ORGANS

There are four main phases of genital development: the indifferent gonadal phase at 4–6 weeks' gestation, the gonadal differentiation phase at about 7 weeks' gestation, ductal differentiation at 9–11 weeks and external genitalia differentiation at 10–12 weeks.

The gonadal rudiments appear as the 'genital ridge' overlying the embryonic kidney in the intermediate mesoderm during the fourth week of embryonic life, and they remain sexually indifferent until the seventh week (**Figure 1.1**). The undifferentiated gonad has the potential to become either a testis or an ovary – and hence is termed bipotential – and the chromosomal complement of the zygote determines its fate. The development of either the testis or the ovary is an active gene-directed process. In the male, the activity of the sex-determining region of the Y chromosome (*SRY*) gene causes the gonad to begin development into a testis. In the past, ovarian development was considered a 'default' development due solely to the absence of *SRY*; however, in the last 10 years, ovarian-determining genes have also been found that actively lead to the development of a female gonad.

At ductal differentiation phase, the fetus has two sets of structures called the Müllerian (or paramesonephric) ducts and Wolffian (or mesonephric) ducts, which have the potential to develop into female or male, respectively, internal and external genitalia.

10.1201/9781003218036-1

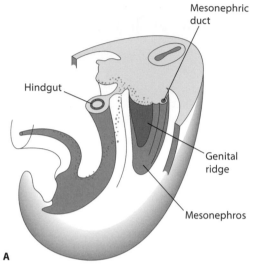

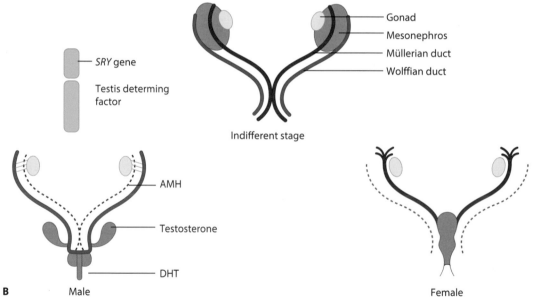

Figure 1.1 (**A**) Cross-section diagram of the posterior abdominal wall showing the genital ridge. (**B**) Diagrammatic representation of the embryological pathways of male and female development. (AMH, anti-Müllerian hormone; DHT, dihydrotestosterone; SRY, sex-determining region of the Y chromosome.)

DEVELOPMENT OF THE MALE SEXUAL ORGANS

As the gonad develops into a testis, it differentiates into two cell types. The Sertoli cells produce anti-Müllerian hormone (AMH) and the Leydig cells produce testosterone. AMH suppresses further development of the Müllerian ducts, whereas testosterone stimulates the Wolffian ducts to develop into the vas deferens, epididymis and seminal vesicles. In addition, in the external genital skin, testosterone is converted by the enzyme 5-alpha-reductase into dihydrotestosterone (DHT). This acts to virilize the external genitalia. The genital tubercle becomes the penis and the labioscrotal folds fuse to form the scrotum. The urogenital folds fuse along the ventral surface of the penis and enclose the urethra so that it opens at the tip of the penis.

DEVELOPMENT OF THE FEMALE SEXUAL ORGANS

In the primitive ovary, granulosa cells – derived from the proliferating coelomic epithelium – surround the germ cells and form primordial follicles. Each primordial follicle consists of an oocyte within a single layer of granulosa cells. Theca cells develop from the proliferating coelomic epithelium and are separated from the granulosa cells by a basal lamina. The maximum number of primordial follicles is reached at 20 weeks' gestation, when there are six to seven million primordial follicles present. The numbers of these reduce by atresia and at birth only one to two million remain. Atresia continues throughout life and, by menarche, only 300,000–400,000 are present and, by the menopause, there are none.

The development of an oocyte within a primordial follicle is arrested at the prophase of its first meiotic division. It remains in that state until it undergoes atresia or enters the meiotic process preceding ovulation.

In the female, the absence of testicular AMH allows the Müllerian structures to develop, and the female reproductive tract derives from these paired

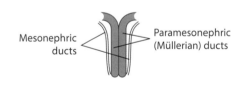

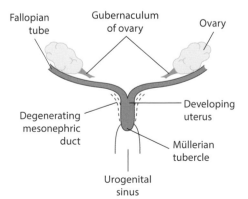

Figure 1.2 Caudal parts of the paramesonephric ducts (top) fuse to form the uterus and fallopian tubes.

ducts. At 9–11 weeks, the proximal two-thirds of the vagina develop from the paired Müllerian ducts, which grow in a caudal and medial direction and fuse in the midline (formation of septum). The midline fusion of these structures produces the uterus, cervix and upper two-thirds of the vagina, and the unfused caudal segments form the fallopian tubes, as shown in **Figure 1.2**.

Cells proliferate from the upper portion of the urogenital sinus to form structures called the sinovaginal bulbs. The caudal extension of the Müllerian ducts projects into the posterior wall of the urogenital sinus as the Müllerian tubercle. The Müllerian tubercles and the urogenital sinus fuse to form the vaginal plate, which extends from the Müllerian ducts to the urogenital sinus. This plate begins to canalize, starting at the hymen and proceeding upwards to the cervix in the sixth embryonic month. At 5 months, Müllerian organogenesis is complete with uterine septal resorption/canalization.

EXTERNAL FEMALE GENITALIA

The external genitalia do not virilize in the absence of testosterone. Between the fifth and seventh weeks of life, the cloacal folds, which are a pair of swellings adjacent to the cloacal membrane, fuse anteriorly to become the genital tubercle. This will become the clitoris. The perineum develops and divides the cloacal membrane into an anterior urogenital membrane and a posterior anal membrane. The cloacal folds anteriorly are called the urethral folds, which form the labia minora. Another pair of folds within the cloacal membrane form the labioscrotal folds that eventually become the labia majora. The urogenital sinus becomes the vestibule of the vagina. The external genitalia are recognizably female by the end of the 12th embryonic week.

FEMALE ANATOMY

EXTERNAL GENITALIA

The external genitalia are commonly called the vulva and include the mons pubis, the labia majora and minora, the vaginal vestibule, the clitoris and the greater vestibular glands (**Figure 1.3**). The mons pubis is a fibro-fatty pad covered by hair-bearing skin that covers the bony pubic ramus.

The labia majora are two folds of skin with underlying adipose tissue lying either side of the vaginal opening. They contain sebaceous and sweat glands and a few specialized apocrine glands. In the deepest part of each labium is a core of fatty tissue continuous with that of the inguinal canal and the fibres of the round ligament, which terminate here.

The labia minora are two thin folds of skin that lie between the labia majora. These vary in size and may protrude beyond the labia majora where they are visible, but may also be concealed by the labia majora. Anteriorly, they divide in two to form the prepuce and frenulum of the clitoris (clitoral hood). Posteriorly, they divide to form a fold of skin called the fourchette at the back of the vaginal introitus. They contain sebaceous glands, but have no adipose tissue. They are not well developed before puberty and they atrophy after the menopause. Both the labia minora and the labia majora become engorged during sexual arousal.

The clitoris is an erectile structure measuring approximately 0.5–3.5 cm in length. The body of the clitoris is the main part of the visible clitoris and is made up of paired columns of erectile tissue and vascular tissue called the corpora cavernosa. These become the crura at the bottom of the clitoris and run deeper and laterally. The vestibule is the cleft between the labia minora. It contains openings of the urethra, the Bartholin's glands and the vagina. The vagina is surrounded by two bulbs of erectile and vascular tissue that are extensive and almost completely cover the distal vaginal wall. These have traditionally been named the bulb of the vaginal vestibule, although recent work on both dissection and magnetic resonance imaging (MRI) suggests that they may be part of the clitoris and should be

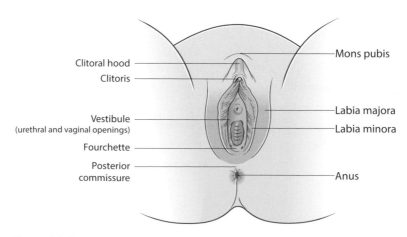

Clitoral hood
Clitoris
Vestibule (urethral and vaginal openings)
Fourchette
Posterior commissure
Mons pubis
Labia majora
Labia minora
Anus

Figure 1.3 Anatomy of the external genitalia.

renamed 'clitoral bulbs'. Their function is unknown but they probably add support to the distal vaginal wall to enhance its rigidity during penetration.

The Bartholin's glands are bilateral and about the size of a pea. They open via a 2 cm duct into the vestibule below the hymen and contribute to lubrication during intercourse.

The hymen is a thin covering of mucous membrane across the entrance to the vagina. It is usually perforated, which allows menstruation. The hymen is ruptured during intercourse and any remaining tags are called carunculae myrtiformes.

FEMALE INTERNAL REPRODUCTIVE ORGANS

VAGINA

The vagina is a fibromuscular canal lined with stratified squamous epithelium that leads from the uterus to the vulva. It is longer in the posterior wall (approximately 9 cm) than in the anterior wall (approximately 7 cm). The vaginal walls are normally in apposition, except at the vault where they are separated by the cervix. The vault of the vagina is divided into four fornices: posterior, anterior and two lateral (**Figure 1.4**).

The mid-vagina is a transverse slit while the lower vagina is an H-shape in transverse section. The vaginal walls are lined with transverse folds. The vagina has no glands and is kept moist by secretions from the uterine and cervical glands and by transudation from its epithelial lining. The epithelium is thick and rich in glycogen, which increases in the post-ovulatory phase of the cycle. However, before puberty and after the menopause, the vagina is devoid of glycogen due to the lack of oestrogen. Doderlein's bacillus is a normal commensal of the vaginal flora and breaks down glycogen to form lactic acid, producing a pH of around 4.5. This plays a protective role for the vagina in decreasing the growth of pathogenic bacteria.

The upper posterior wall forms the anterior peritoneal reflection of the pouch of Douglas. The

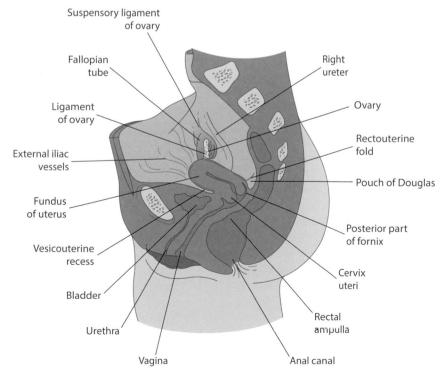

Figure 1.4 Sagittal section of the female pelvis.

middle third is separated from the rectum by the pelvic fascia and the lower third abuts the perineal body. Anteriorly, the vagina is in direct contact with the base of the bladder, while the urethra runs down the lower half in the midline to open into the vestibule. Its muscles fuse with the anterior vagina wall. Laterally, at the fornices, the vagina is related to the cardinal ligaments. Below this are the levator ani muscles and the ischiorectal fossae. The cardinal ligaments and the uterosacral ligaments, which form posteriorly from the parametrium, support the upper part of the vagina.

At birth, the vagina is under the influence of maternal oestrogens, so the epithelium is well developed. After a couple of weeks, the effects of the oestrogen disappear, and the pH rises to 7 and the epithelium atrophies. At puberty, the reverse occurs and, finally, at the menopause, the vagina tends to shrink and the epithelium atrophies once again.

UTERUS

The uterus is shaped like an inverted pear tapering inferiorly to the cervix and in its non-pregnant state is situated entirely within the pelvis. It is hollow and has thick, muscular walls. Its maximum external dimensions are approximately 7.5 cm long, 5 cm wide and 3 cm thick. An adult uterus weighs approximately 70 g. In the upper part, the uterus is termed the body or corpus. The area of insertion of each fallopian tube is termed the cornu, and that part of the body above the cornu is called the fundus. The uterus tapers to a small constricted area (the isthmus) and below this is the cervix, which projects obliquely into the vagina. The longitudinal axis of the uterus is approximately at right angles to the vagina and normally tilts forwards. This is called anteversion. In addition, the long axis of the cervix is rarely the same as the long axis of the uterus. The uterus is also usually flexed forwards on itself at the isthmus, called antiflexion. However, in around 20% of cases, the uterus is tilted backwards, or retroverted and retroflexed. This has no pathological significance, although retroversion that is fixed and immobile may be associated with endometriosis. This has relevance in gynaecological surgery and is referred to again in **Chapter 2**.

The cavity of the uterus is the shape of an inverted triangle and when sectioned coronally the fallopian tubes open at lateral angles. The constriction at the isthmus where the corpus joins the cervix is the anatomical os. Seen microscopically, the site of the histological internal os is where the mucous membrane of the isthmus becomes that of the cervix.

The uterus consists of three layers: the outer serous layer (peritoneum), the middle muscular layer (myometrium) and the inner mucous layer (endometrium). The peritoneum covers the body of the uterus and posteriorly it covers the supravaginal part of the cervix. The peritoneum is intimately attached to a subserous fibrous layer, except laterally where it spreads out to form the leaves of the broad ligament.

The muscular myometrium forms the main bulk of the uterus and is made up of interlacing smooth muscle fibres intermingling with areolar tissue, blood vessels, nerves and lymphatics. Externally, the muscle fibres are mostly longitudinal, but the thicker intermediate layer has interlacing longitudinal, oblique and transverse fibres. Internally, they are mainly longitudinal and circular.

The inner endometrial layer has tubular glands that dip into the myometrium. The endometrial layer is covered by a single layer of columnar epithelium. The luminal and glandular epithelia are ciliated. The mechanistic function of the cilia is largely unknown, although recent studies have indicated a role in implantation and reproduction. The endometrium undergoes cyclical changes during menstruation, as described in **Chapter 3**, and varies in thickness.

CERVIX

The cervix is narrower than the body of the uterus and is approximately 2.5 cm in length. Lateral to the cervix lies cellular connective tissue called the parametrium. The ureter runs about 1 cm laterally to the supravaginal cervix within the parametrium. The posterior aspect of the cervix is covered by the peritoneum of the pouch of Douglas.

The upper part of the cervix mostly consists of involuntary muscle, whereas the lower part is mainly fibrous connective tissue. The mucous membrane of the cervical canal (endocervix) has anterior and posterior columns from which folds radiate out – these are the arbour vitae. The mucous membrane has numerous deep glandular follicles that secrete clear alkaline mucus, the main component of physiological vaginal discharge. The epithelium of the endocervix is columnar and is also ciliated in its upper two-thirds. This changes to stratified squamous epithelium around the region of the external os and the junction of these two types of epithelium is called the squamocolumnar junction.

Age changes to anatomy

The disappearance of maternal oestrogens from the circulation after birth causes the uterus to decrease in length by around one-third and in weight by around one-half. The cervix is then twice the length of the uterus. During childhood, the uterus grows slowly in length, in parallel with height and age. The average longitudinal diameter ranges from 2.5 cm at the age of 2 years to 3.5 cm at 10 years. After the onset of puberty, the anteroposterior and transverse diameters of the uterus start to increase, leading to a sharper rise in the volume of the uterus. The increase in uterine volume continues well after menarche, and the uterus reaches its adult size and configuration by the late teenage years. After the menopause, the uterus atrophies, the mucosa becomes very thin, the glands almost disappear and the wall becomes relatively less muscular.

FALLOPIAN TUBES

The fallopian tube extends outwards from the uterine cornu to end near the ovary. At the abdominal ostium, the tube opens into the peritoneal cavity, which is therefore in communication with the exterior of the body via the uterus and the vagina. This is essential to allow the sperm and egg to meet. The fallopian tubes convey the ovum from the ovary towards the uterus and promote oxygenation and nutrition for the sperm, ovum and zygote should fertilization occur.

The fallopian tube runs in the upper margin of the broad ligament, known as the mesosalpinx, which encloses the tube so that it is completely covered with peritoneum except for a narrow strip along this inferior aspect. Each tube is about 10 cm long and is described in four parts:

1. the interstitial portion
2. the isthmus
3. the ampulla
4. the infundibulum or fimbrial portion

The interstitial portion lies within the wall of the uterus, while the isthmus is the narrow portion adjoining the uterus. This passes into the widest and longest portion, the ampulla. This, in turn, terminates in the extremity known as the infundibulum. The opening of the tube into the peritoneal cavity is surrounded by finger-like processes, known as fimbria, into which the muscle coat does not extend. The inner surfaces of the fimbriae are covered by ciliated epithelium that is similar to the lining of the fallopian tube itself. One of these fimbria is longer than the others and extends to, and partially embraces, the ovary. The muscular fibres of the wall of the tube are arranged in an inner circular layer and an outer longitudinal layer.

The tubal epithelium forms a number of branched folds or plicae that run longitudinally; the lumen of the ampulla is almost filled with these folds. The folds have a cellular stroma, but at their bases the epithelium is separated from the muscle by only a very scanty amount of stroma. There is no submucosa and there are no glands. The epithelium of the fallopian tubes contains two functioning cell types: the ciliated cells, which act to produce a constant current of fluid in the direction of the uterus, and the secretory cells, which contribute to the volume of tubal fluid. Changes occur under the influence of the menstrual cycle, but there is no cell shedding during menstruation.

OVARIES

The size and appearance of the ovaries depend on both age and stage of the menstrual cycle. In a child, the ovaries are small structures approximately 1.5 cm long; however, they increase to adult size in puberty due to proliferation of stromal cells and commencing maturation of the ovarian follicles. In the young adult, they are almond-shaped and measure approximately 3 cm long, 1.5 cm wide and 1 cm thick. After the menopause, no active follicles are present and the ovary becomes smaller with a wrinkled surface. The ovary is the only intra-abdominal structure not to be covered by peritoneum. Each ovary is attached to the cornu of the uterus by the ovarian ligament and at the hilum to the broad ligament by the mesovarium, which contains its supply of nerves and blood vessels. The ovary has a dual blood supply, namely from the ovarian and uterine arteries. The ovarian artery is a direct branch from the abdominal aorta and supplies blood to the ovary via the suspensory ligament. The uterine artery contributes to the blood supply through the ovarian ligament. Laterally, each ovary is attached to the suspensory ligament of the ovary by folds of peritoneum that become continuous with the peritoneum of the overlying psoas major.

Anterior to the ovaries lie the fallopian tubes, the superior portion of the bladder and the uterovesical pouch. Posterior to the ovary lies the ureter, which runs downwards and forwards in front of the internal iliac artery.

Structure of the ovary

The ovary has a central vascular medulla consisting of loose connective tissue containing many elastin fibres and non-striated muscle cells. The ovary also has an outer, thicker cortex that is denser than the medulla, consisting of networks of reticular fibres and fusiform cells, although there is no clear-cut demarcation between the two (the medulla and the cortex). The surface of the ovaries is covered by a single layer of cuboidal cells, the germinal epithelium. Beneath this is an ill-defined layer of condensed connective tissue called the tunica albuginea, which increases in density with age. At birth, numerous primordial follicles are found, mostly in the cortex, but some are found in the medulla. With puberty, some form each month into the Graafian follicles under gonadotrophic control, to ovulate and subsequently form corpus lutea and ultimately the atretic follicles, the corpora albicans.

BLADDER, URETHRA AND URETER

Bladder

The bladder wall is made up of involuntary muscle arranged in an inner longitudinal layer, a middle circular layer and an outer longitudinal layer. It is lined with transitional epithelium and has an average capacity of 400 mL.

The ureters open into the base of the bladder after running medially for about 1 cm through the bladder wall. The urethra leaves the bladder below the ureteric orifices. The triangular area lying between the ureteric orifices and the internal meatus of the urethra is known as the trigone. At the internal meatus,

the middle layer of muscle forms anterior and posterior loops around the neck of the bladder, with some fibres of the loops being continuous with the circular muscle of the urethra.

The base of the bladder is adjacent to the cervix, with only a thin layer of tissue intervening. It is separated from the anterior vaginal wall below by the pubocervical fascia that stretches from the pubis to the cervix.

Urethra

The female urethra is about 3.5 cm long and is lined with transitional epithelium. It has a slight posterior angulation at the junction of its lower and middle thirds. The smooth muscle of its wall is arranged in outer longitudinal and inner circular layers. As the urethra passes through the two layers of the urogenital diaphragm, it is embraced by the striated fibres of the deep transverse perineal muscle (also known as the compressor urethrae) and some of the striated fibres of this muscle form a loop on the urethra. Between the muscular coat and the epithelium is a plexus of veins. There are a number of tubular mucous glands and in the lower part a number of crypts that occasionally become infected. In its upper two-thirds, the urethra is separated from the symphysis by loose connective tissue, but in its lower third it is attached to the pubic ramus on each side by strong bands of fibrous tissue called the pubourethral tissue. Posteriorly, it is firmly attached in its lower two-thirds to the anterior vaginal wall. This means that the upper part of the urethra is mobile, but the lower part is relatively fixed.

Medial fibres of the pubococcygeus of the levator ani muscles are inserted into the urethra and vaginal wall. When they contract, they pull the anterior vaginal wall and the upper part of the urethra forwards, forming an angle of about 100° between the posterior wall of the urethra and the bladder base. On voluntary voiding of urine, the base of the bladder and the upper part of the urethra descend and the posterior angle disappears so that the base of the bladder and the posterior wall of the urethra come to lie in a straight line.

Ureter

As the ureter crosses the pelvic brim, it lies in front of the bifurcation of the common iliac artery. It runs downwards and forwards on the lateral wall of the

Because of its close relationship to the cervix, the vault of the vagina and the uterine artery, the ureter may be damaged during hysterectomy. Apart from being cut or tied, in radical procedures the ureter may undergo necrosis because of interference with its blood supply. It may be displaced by scar tissue or by fibromyomata or cysts that are growing between the layers of the broad ligament and may suffer injury if its position is not noticed at surgery.

BOX 1.2: Ovarian blood supply damage during salpingectomy

Due to the proximity of the ovarian blood supply to the fallopian tube, the blood supply to the ovary can be easily compromised during surgical procedure to remove the fallopian tube (salpingectomy). Damage to the blood supply of the ovary can in due course have an impact on the viability of oocytes and diminish its ovarian reserve (see **Chapter 7**).

pelvis to reach the pelvic floor and then passes inwards and forwards attached to the peritoneum of the back of the broad ligament to pass beneath the uterine artery. It next passes forwards through a fibrous tunnel – the ureteric canal – in the upper part of the cardinal ligament. Finally, it runs close to the lateral vaginal fornix to enter the trigone of the bladder.

Its blood supply is derived from small branches of the ovarian artery, from a small vessel arising near the iliac bifurcation, from a branch of the uterine artery where it crosses beneath it and from small branches of the vesical artery.

RECTUM

The rectum extends from the level of the third sacral vertebra to a point about 2.5 cm in front of the coccyx, where it passes through the pelvic floor to become continuous with the anal canal. Its direction follows the curve of the sacrum and is about 11 cm in length. The front and sides are covered by the peritoneum of the rectovaginal pouch. In the middle third, only the front is covered by peritoneum. In the lower third, there is no peritoneal covering and the rectum is separated from the posterior wall of the vagina by the rectovaginal fascial septum. Lateral to the rectum are the uterosacral ligaments, beside which run some of the lymphatics draining the cervix and vagina.

PELVIC MUSCLES, LIGAMENTS AND FASCIA

The pelvic diaphragm is formed by the levator ani muscles, which are broad, flat muscles whose fibres pass downwards and inwards (**Figure 1.5**). The two

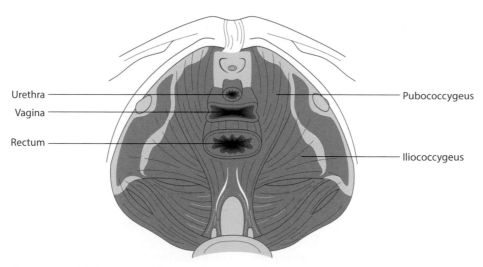

Figure 1.5 Pelvic floor musculature.

Urethra

Vagina

Rectum

Pubococcygeus

Iliococcygeus

muscles, one on either side, constitute the pelvic diaphragm. The muscles arise by linear origin from the following points:

- the lower part of the body of the os pubis
- the internal surface of the parietal pelvic fascia along the 'white line'
- the pelvic surface of the ischial spine

The levator ani muscles are inserted into the following points:

- the preanal raphe and the central point of the perineum, where one muscle meets the other on the opposite side
- the wall of the anal canal, where the fibres blend with the deep external sphincter muscle
- the postanal or anococcygeal raphe, where again one muscle meets the other on the opposite side
- the lower part of the coccyx

The muscle is described in two parts:

1. the pubococcygeus, which arises from the pubic bone and the anterior part of the tendinous arch of the pelvic fascia (the 'white line')
2. the iliococcygeus, which arises from the posterior part of the tendinous arch and the ischial spine

The medial borders of the pubococcygeus muscle pass on either side from the pubic bone to the preanal raphe. They thus embrace the vagina and on contraction have some sphincteric action. The nerve supply is from the third and fourth sacral nerves. The pubococcygeus muscles support the pelvic and abdominal viscera, including the bladder. The medial edge passes beneath the bladder and runs laterally to the urethra, into which some of its fibres are inserted. Together with the fibres from the opposite muscle, they form a loop that maintains the angle between the posterior aspect of the urethra and the bladder base. During micturition, this loop relaxes to allow the bladder neck and upper urethra to open and descend.

Urogenital diaphragm

The urogenital diaphragm (also known as the triangular ligament) is made up of two layers of pelvic fascia that fill the gap between the descending pubic rami and lies beneath the levator ani muscles. The deep transverse perineal muscles (compressor urethrae) lie between the two layers and the diaphragm is pierced by the urethra and vagina.

Perineal body

This is a mass of muscular tissue that lies between the anal canal and the lower third of the vagina. Its apex is at the lower end of the rectovaginal septum at the point where the rectum and posterior vaginal walls come into contact. Its base is covered with skin and extends from the fourchette to the anus. It is the point of insertion of the superficial perineal muscles and is bounded above by the levator ani muscles where they come into contact in the midline between the posterior vaginal wall and the rectum.

Pelvic peritoneum

The peritoneum is reflected from the lateral borders of the uterus to form, on either side, a double fold of peritoneum – the broad ligament. Despite the name, this is not a ligament but a peritoneal fold and it does not support the uterus. The fallopian tube runs in the upper free edge of the broad ligament as far as the point at which the tube opens into the peritoneal cavity. The part of the broad ligament that is lateral to the opening is called the infundibulopelvic fold and in it the ovarian vessels and nerves pass from the side wall of the pelvis to lie between the two layers of the broad ligament (**Figure 1.6A**). The mesosalpinx, the portion of the broad ligament that lies above the ovary, is layered; between its layers, any Wolffian remnants that may remain can be found. Below the ovary, the base of the broad ligament widens out and contains a considerable amount of loose connective tissue called the parametrium. The ureter is attached to the posterior leaf of the broad ligament at this point.

The ovary is attached to the posterior layer of the broad ligament by a short mesentery (the mesovarium) through which the ovarian vessels and nerves enter the hilum.

The ovarian ligament lies beneath the posterior layer of the broad ligament and passes from the medial pole of the ovary to the uterus just below the point of entry of the fallopian tube. The round ligament is the continuation of the same structure and runs forwards under the anterior leaf of peritoneum to enter the inguinal canal, ending in the subcutaneous tissue of the labium major.

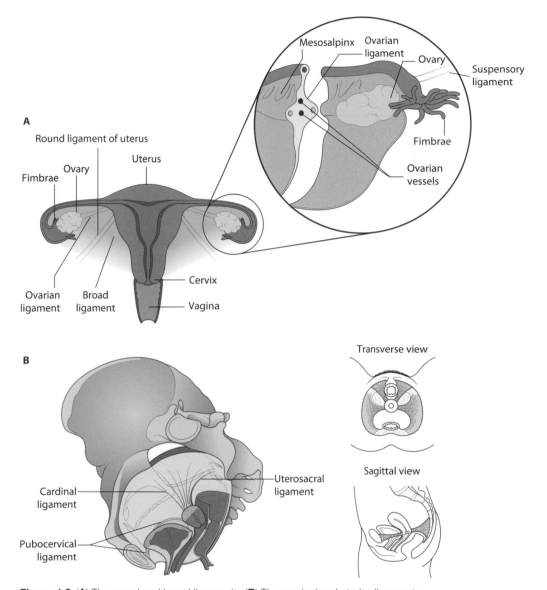

Figure 1.6 (**A**) The round and broad ligaments. (**B**) The cervical and uterine ligaments.

Connective tissue fills the irregular spaces between the various pelvic organs. Much of it is loose cellular tissue, but in some places it is condensed to form strong ligaments that contain some smooth muscle fibres and form the fascial sheaths that enclose the various viscera. The pelvic arteries, veins, lymphatics, nerves and ureters run through it. The cellular tissue is continuous above with the extraperitoneal tissue of the abdominal wall, but below it is cut off from the ischiorectal fossa by the pelvic fascia and the levator ani muscles. The pelvic fascia may be regarded as a specialized part of this connective tissue and has parietal and visceral components.

The parietal pelvic fascia lines the wall of the pelvic cavity covering the obturator and pyramidalis muscles. The thickened tendinous arch (known as the white line) lies on the side wall of the pelvis. It is here that the levator ani muscle arises and the cardinal ligament gains its lateral attachment. Where the parietal pelvic fascia encounters bone, such as in the pubic region, it blends with the periosteum. It also forms the upper layer of the urogenital diaphragm.

Each viscus has a fascial sheath that is dense in the case of the vagina and cervix and at the base of the bladder, but is tenuous or absent over the body of the uterus and the dome of the bladder. From the point of view of the gynaecologist, certain parts of the visceral fascia are important, as follows:

- The cardinal ligaments (transverse cervical ligaments) provide the essential support of the uterus and vaginal vault. These are two strong fan-shaped fibromuscular bands that pass from the cervix and vaginal vault to the side wall of the pelvis on either side.
- The uterosacral ligaments run from the cervix and vaginal vault to the sacrum. In the erect position, they are almost vertical in direction and support the cervix.
- The bladder is supported laterally by condensations of the vesical pelvic fascia, one each side, and by a sheet of pubocervical fascia, which lies beneath it anteriorly.

Arteries supplying the pelvic organs

Because the ovary develops on the posterior abdominal wall and later migrates down into the pelvis, it carries its blood supply with it directly from the abdominal aorta. The ovarian artery arises from the aorta just below the renal artery and runs downwards on the surface of the psoas muscle to the pelvic brim, where it crosses in front of the ureter and then passes into the infundibulopelvic fold of the broad ligament. The artery divides into branches that supply the ovary and fallopian tube and then run on to reach the uterus, where they anastomose with the terminal branches of the uterine artery.

Internal iliac (hypogastric) artery

This vessel is about 4 cm in length and begins at the bifurcation of the common iliac artery in front of the sacroiliac joint. It soon divides into anterior and posterior branches; the branches that supply the pelvic organs are all from the anterior division and are as follows:

- The uterine artery provides the main blood supply to the uterus. The artery first runs downwards on the lateral wall of the pelvis,

in the same direction as the ureter. It then turns inwards and forwards, lying in the base of the broad ligament. On reaching the wall of the uterus, the artery turns upwards to run tortuously to the upper part of the uterus, where it anastomoses with the ovarian artery. In this part of its course, it sends many branches into the substance of the uterus. The uterine artery supplies a branch to the ureter as it crosses it and shortly afterwards another branch is given off to supply the cervix and upper vagina.
- The vaginal artery runs at a lower level to supply the vagina.
- The vesical arteries are variable in number and supply the bladder and terminal ureter. One usually runs in the roof of the ureteric canal.
- The middle rectal artery often arises in common with the lowest vesical artery.
- The pudendal artery leaves the pelvic cavity through the sciatic foramen and, after winding round the ischial spine, enters the ischiorectal fossa where it gives off the inferior rectal artery. It terminates in the perineal and vulval arteries, supplying the erectile tissue of the vestibular bulbs and clitoris.
- The superior rectal artery is the continuation of the inferior mesenteric artery and descends in the base of the mesocolon. It divides into two branches that run on either side of the rectum and supply numerous branches to it.

Pelvic veins

The veins around the bladder, uterus, vagina and rectum form plexuses that intercommunicate freely. Venous drainage from the uterine, vaginal and vesical plexus is chiefly into the internal iliac veins. Venous drainage from the rectal plexus is via the superior rectal veins to the inferior mesenteric veins, and via the middle and inferior rectal veins to the internal pudendal veins and so to the iliac veins.

The ovarian veins on each side begin in the pampiniform plexus, which lies between the layers of the broad ligament. At first, there are two veins on each side accompanying the corresponding ovarian artery. Higher up, the vein becomes single, with that on the right ending in the inferior vena cava and that on the left ending in the left renal vein.

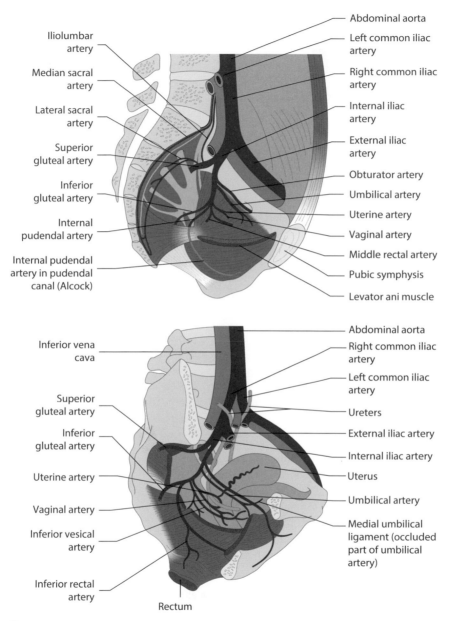

Iliolumbar artery
Median sacral artery
Lateral sacral artery
Superior gluteal artery
Inferior gluteal artery
Internal pudendal artery
Internal pudendal artery in pudendal canal (Alcock)

Abdominal aorta
Left common iliac artery
Right common iliac artery
Internal iliac artery
External iliac artery
Obturator artery
Umbilical artery
Uterine artery
Vaginal artery
Middle rectal artery
Pubic symphysis
Levator ani muscle

Inferior vena cava
Superior gluteal artery
Inferior gluteal artery
Uterine artery
Vaginal artery
Inferior vesical artery
Inferior rectal artery
Rectum

Abdominal aorta
Right common iliac artery
Left common iliac artery
Ureters
External iliac artery
Internal iliac artery
Uterus
Umbilical artery
Medial umbilical ligament (occluded part of umbilical artery)

Figure 1.7 Blood supply of the pelvis and perineum.

LYMPHATICS

Lymph draining from all the lower extremities and the vulva and perineal regions is all filtered through the inguinal and superficial femoral nodes before continuing along the deep pathways on the side wall of the pelvis. One deep chain passes upwards laterally to the major blood vessels, forming in turn the external iliac, common iliac and para-aortic groups of nodes.

Medially, another chain of vessels passes from the deep femoral nodes through the femoral canal to the obturator and internal iliac groups of nodes. These last nodes are interspersed among the origins of the branches of the internal iliac artery receiving lymph directly from the organs supplied by this

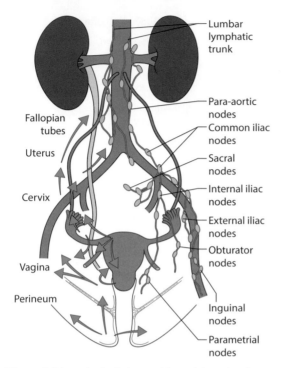

Figure 1.8 Lymphatic drainage of the pelvis and perineum.

Labels on figure:
- Lumbar lymphatic trunk
- Para-aortic nodes
- Common iliac nodes
- Sacral nodes
- Internal iliac nodes
- External iliac nodes
- Obturator nodes
- Inguinal nodes
- Parametrial nodes
- Fallopian tubes
- Uterus
- Cervix
- Vagina
- Perineum

artery, including the upper vagina, cervix and body of the uterus.

From the internal iliac and common iliac nodes, afferent vessels pass up the para-aortic chains, and finally all lymphatic drainage from the legs and pelvis flows into the lumbar lymphatic trunks and cisterna chyli at the level of the second lumbar vertebra. From here, all the lymph is carried by the thoracic duct through the thorax with no intervening nodes to empty into the junction of the left subclavian and internal jugular veins.

Tumour cells that penetrate or bypass the pelvic and para-aortic nodes are rapidly disseminated via the great veins at the root of the neck.

Lymphatic drainage from the genital tract

The lymph vessel from individual parts of the genital tract drain into this system of pelvic lymph nodes in the following manner:

- The vulva and perineum medial to the labiocrural skin folds contain superficial lymphatics that pass upwards towards the mons pubis, then curve laterally to the superficial and inguinal nodes. Drainage from these is through the fossa ovalis into the deep femoral nodes. The largest of these, lying in the upper part of the femoral canal, is known as the node of Cloquet.
- The lymphatics of the lower third of the vagina follow the vulval drainage to the superficial lymph nodes, whereas those from the upper two-thirds pass upwards to join the lymphatic vessels of the cervix.
- The lymphatics of the cervix pass either laterally in the base of the broad ligament or posteriorly along the uterosacral ligaments to reach the side wall of the pelvis. Most of the vessels drain to the internal iliac obturator and external iliac nodes, but vessels also pass directly to the common iliac and lower para-aortic nodes. Radical surgery for carcinoma of the cervix should include removal of all these node groups on both sides of the pelvis.
- Most of the lymphatic vessels of the body of the uterus join those of the cervix and therefore reach similar groups of nodes. A few vessels at the fundus follow the ovarian channels and there is an inconsistent pathway along the round ligament to the inguinal nodes.
- The ovary and fallopian tube have a plexus of vessels that drain along the infundibulopelvic fold to the para-aortic nodes on both sides of the midline. On the left, these are found around the left renal pedicle, while on the right there may only be one node intervening before the lymph flows into the thoracic duct, thus accounting for the rapid early spread of metastatic carcinoma to distant sites such as the lungs.
- The lymphatic drainage of the bladder and upper urethra is to the iliac nodes, while those of the lower part of the urethra follow those of the vulva.
- Lymphatics from the lower anal canal drain to the superficial inguinal nodes and the remainder of the rectal drainage follows pararectal channels accompanying the blood vessels to both the internal iliac nodes (middle rectal artery) and the para-aortic nodes and the origin of the inferior mesenteric artery.

Nerve supply of the vulva and perineum

The pudendal nerve arises from the second, third and fourth sacral nerves. As it passes along the outer wall of the ischiorectal fossa, it gives off an inferior rectal branch and divides into the perineal nerve and dorsal nerve of the clitoris. The perineal nerve gives the sensory supply to the vulva and also innervates the anterior part of the external anal canal and the levator ani and the superficial perineal muscles. The dorsal nerve of the clitoris is sensory. Sensory fibres from the mons and labia also pass in the ilioinguinal and genitofemoral nerves to the first lumbar root. The posterior femoral cutaneous nerve carries sensation from the perineum to the small sciatic nerve and thus to the first, second and third sacral nerves. The main nerve supply of the levator ani muscles comes from the third and fourth sacral nerves.

Nerve supply of the pelvic viscera

The innervation of the pelvic viscera is complex and not well understood. All pelvic viscera receive dual innervation (i.e. both sympathetic and parasympathetic). Nerve fibres of the preaortic plexus of the sympathetic nervous system are continuous with those of the superior hypogastric plexus, which lies in front of the last lumber vertebra and is wrongly called the 'presacral nerve'. Below this, the superior hypogastric plexus divides and, on each side, its fibres are continuous with fibres passing beside the rectum to join the uterovaginal plexus (inferior hypogastric plexus or plexus of Frankenhauser). This plexus lies in the loose cellular tissue posterolateral to the cervix, below the uterosacral folds of peritoneum. Parasympathetic fibres from the second, third and fourth sacral nerves join the uterovaginal plexus. Fibres from (or to) the bladder, uterus, vagina and rectum join the plexus. The uterovaginal plexus contains a few ganglion cells, so it is likely that a few motor cells also have their relay stations there and then pass onwards with the blood vessels onto the viscera.

The ovary is not innervated by the nerves already described, but from the ovarian plexus that surrounds the ovarian vessels and joins the preaortic plexus high up.

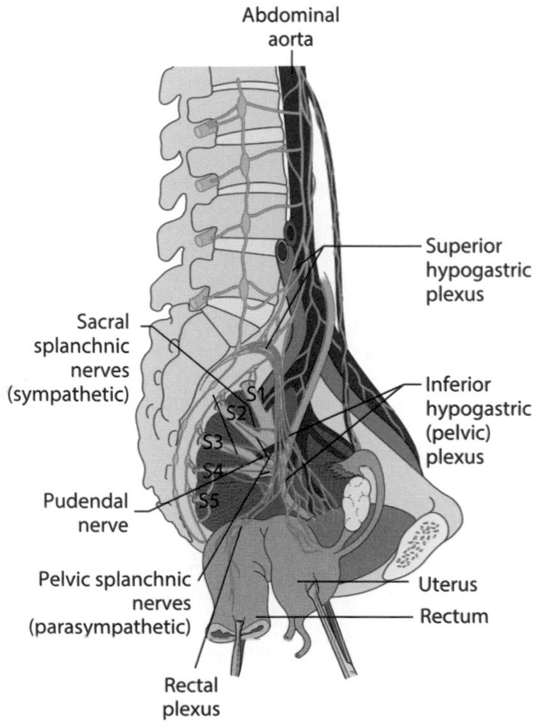

Figure 1.9 Nerve supply of the pelvis and perineum.

Labels: Abdominal aorta; Superior hypogastric plexus; Sacral splanchnic nerves (sympathetic); Inferior hypogastric (pelvic) plexus; S1, S2, S3, S4, S5; Pudendal nerve; Pelvic splanchnic nerves (parasympathetic); Uterus; Rectum; Rectal plexus

---

🔑 KEY LEARNING POINTS

- An adult uterus consists of three layers: the peritoneum, myometrium and endometrium.
- The cervix is narrower than the body of the uterus and is approximately 2.5 cm in length. The ureter runs about 1 cm lateral to the cervix.
- The ovary is the only intraperitoneal structure not covered by peritoneum.
- The main supports to the pelvic floor are the connective tissue and levator ani muscles. The main supports of the uterus are the uterosacral and cardinal ligaments, which are condensations of connective tissue.
- The ovarian arteries arise directly from the aorta, while the right ovarian vein drains into the vena cava and the left drains into the left renal vein.
- The major nerve supply of the pelvis comes from the pudendal nerves, which arise from the second, third and fourth sacral nerves.

STRUCTURAL ABNORMALITIES OF PELVIC ORGANS

MÜLLERIAN ANOMALIES

In various phases of Müllerian development, anomalies can lead to structural abnormalities (**Table 1.1**). Müllerian anomalies are common, occurring in up to 6% of the female population, and may be asymptomatic. The aetiology is unknown, although associated renal anomalies are present in up to 30%. Several classifications are used that are relevant to clinical management. **Figure 1.10** illustrates the classification used in Europe. Müllerian anomalies can be associated with infertility, recurrent pregnancy loss and poorer reproductive outcomes. Current evidence does not support routine surgical correction and each patient's clinical situation must be personalized.

Table 1.1 Clinical significance of Müllerian development anomalies

Müllerian development	Clinical significance
Organogenesis	Defects lead to agenesis or hypoplasia (unicornuate or absent uterus)
Fusion of Müllerian ducts	Horizontal fusion/unification defects: • partial – bicournuate uterus • complete – uterus didelphys • vertical fusion (imperferate hymen, transverse vaginal septum)
Septal defects	Canalization defects: • complete or partial septate uterus • arcuate uterus

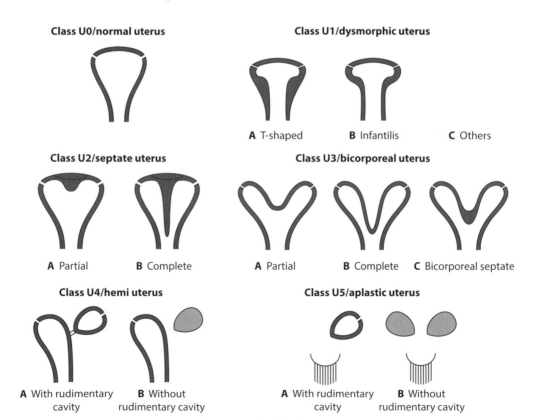

Class U0/normal uterus

Class U1/dysmorphic uterus
A T-shaped **B** Infantilis **C** Others

Class U2/septate uterus
A Partial **B** Complete

Class U3/bicorporeal uterus
A Partial **B** Complete **C** Bicorporeal septate

Class U4/hemi uterus
A With rudimentary cavity **B** Without rudimentary cavity

Class U5/aplastic uterus
A With rudimentary cavity **B** Without rudimentary cavity

Class U6/unclassified cases

Figure 1.10 Müllerian structural abnormalities.

MÜLLERIAN OBSTRUCTION

Failure of complete canalization of the Müllerian structures can lead to menstrual obstruction. The obstruction most commonly occurs at the junction of the lower third of the vagina at the level of the hymen, although more proximal obstruction can occur. Presentation with an imperforate hymen is usually with increasing abdominal pain in a girl in early adolescence. The retained menstrual blood stretches the vagina, causing a haematocolpos. This can cause a large pelvic mass and can usually be seen as a bulging membrane at the vaginal entrance. Treatment is simple with a surgical incision of the hymen and drainage of the retained blood.

MÜLLERIAN DUPLICATION

Duplication of the Müllerian system can occur, resulting in a wide range of anomalies. It may be a complete duplication of the uterus, cervix and vagina, but it may also simply be a midline uterine septum in otherwise normal internal genitalia. Second uterine horns may also occur and can be rudimentary or functional.

MÜLLERIAN AGENESIS

In approximately 1 in 5,000 to 1 in 40,000 girls, the Müllerian system does not develop, resulting in an absent or rudimentary uterus and upper vagina. This condition is known as Rokitansky syndrome or Mayer–Rokitansky–Kuster–Hauser (MRKH) syndrome. The ovaries function normally and so the most common presentation is with primary amenorrhoea in the presence of otherwise normal pubertal development. The aetiology of this condition is not known, although possible factors include environmental, genetic, hormonal and receptor factors. On examination, the vagina will be blind ending and is likely to be shortened in length. An ultrasound scan will confirm the presence of ovaries, but no functioning uterus will be present.

Treatment options focus on psychological support and on the creation of a vagina comfortable for penetrative intercourse, as discussed in **Chapter 3**. Individuals with MRKH syndrome may have their own genetic children, using ovum retrieval, assisted conception techniques and a surrogate for the pregnancy. In the future, they may be candidates for uterine transplantation, and there is extensive ongoing research being undertaken in this area.

VESTIGIAL STRUCTURES

Vestigial remains of the mesonephric duct and tubules are always present in young children, but are variable structures in adults. The epoophoron, a series of parallel blind tubules, lies in the broad ligament between the mesovarium and the fallopian tube. The tubules run to the rudimentary duct of the epoophoron, which runs parallel to the lateral fallopian tube. Situated in the broad ligament between the epoophoron and the uterus, a few rudimentary tubules are occasionally seen – the paroophoron. In a few individuals, the caudal part of the mesonephric duct is well developed, running alongside the uterus to the internal os. This is the duct of Gartner.

FURTHER READING

Netter FH (2011). *Atlas of Human Anatomy*. Saunders/Elsevier.

Setchell M, Hudson CN (2013). *Shaw's Textbook of Operative Gynaecology*. Elsevier.

SELF-ASSESSMENT

For interactive SBAs and EMQs relating to this chapter, visit www.routledge.com/cw/crosbie.

CASE HISTORY 1

A 15-year-old girl was seen in the gynaecology clinic with her mother. She had not yet started her periods. She described breast development at age 12 and pubic hair development. All her friends had started their periods and she wondered what was wrong.

She also described abdominal pain that had started a couple of years ago. Initially she had ignored it but now it was interfering with sport. It was intermittent and, on questioning, she wondered if it was coming about monthly. It was a cramping lower abdominal pain. She had a boyfriend but was not sexually active. Medically, there were no problems, no previous operations and no allergies. Socially, she was doing well at school. On examination, there was normal breast development and distribution of pubic hair. There was a hard swelling in the lower abdomen that was quite tender. On observation of the genitalia, a blue swelling at the level of the hymen was seen.

A What is the most likely diagnosis?
B Which investigations(s) should be performed and what is the differential diagnosis?

ANSWERS

A The most likely diagnosis is a haematocolpos from an imperforate hymen. Menstrual fluid had been collecting above the hymen, as it could not escape. Over time, this had distended the vagina and filled the uterine cavity. This was causing the swelling and the cyclical pain.

B An ultrasound should be performed to confirm the diagnosis and exclude any Müllerian structural alterations. The important differential is obstruction due to a horizontal vaginal plate at a higher level. In this case, the ultrasound would not show blood filling the vagina down to the introitus because the site of an imperforate plate is higher in the vagina and is due to imperforate urogenital sinus. The additional finding of the blue vaginal swelling also points to the hymen being the level of obstruction.

The girl was admitted for day case surgery. An incision was made in the hymen under general anaesthetic and 700 mL of old blood was evacuated. She made a good recovery and her periods commenced shortly afterwards.

CASE HISTORY 2

A 34-year-old woman was seen in the gynaecology clinic with a history of three recurrent pregnancy losses. She described having heavy but regular periods. Her GP arranged an ultrasound, which showed a partition within her uterus that extended from the uterine fundus to her cervix. On her pelvic examination, she was found to have a normal vulva, vagina and cervix.

A What is the diagnosis?
B What investigation should be arranged?

ANSWERS

A The diagnosis is complete uterine septum.
B An ultrasound of her kidneys should be performed. In various phases of Müllerian development, anomalies of development can lead to structural abnormalities. Müllerian anomalies are common, occurring in up to 6% of the female population, and may be asymptomatic. The aetiology is unknown, although associated renal anomalies are present in up to 30%. Several classifications are used that are relevant to clinical management. Müllerian anomalies can be associated with infertility, recurrent pregnancy loss and poorer reproductive outcomes. Current evidence does not support routine surgical correction and each patient's clinical situation must be personalized.

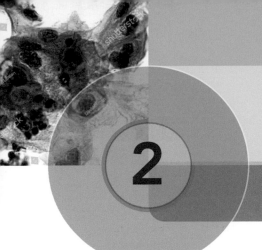

Gynaecological history, examination and investigations

2

CLAUDINE DOMONEY

Learning Objectives
- Understand that a detailed and structured gynaecological history is vital for making a diagnosis and will place the patient's symptoms in their social context.
- Understand that the gynaecological examination will be customised by the history to elucidate causes of symptoms and/or direct investigations.
- Understand when ultrasound, magnetic resonance imaging (MRI) or computed tomography (CT) scanning is indicated in gynaecology.
- Understand how biochemical, haematological and microbiological investigations are guided by gynaecological history and examination findings.

HISTORY

The gynaecological consultation should ideally be held in a closed room with adequate facilities and privacy. Some patients will feel anxious about the consultation, so it is important that the student or doctor establishes an initial rapport and endeavours to put them at ease. The practitioner should introduce themselves by name and status, and check the patient's details. Ideally, there should be no more than one other person in the room, but any student or attending nurse should be introduced by name and their role briefly explained.

It is important to be aware of different attitudes to gynaecological issues in a culturally diverse population. Respect and sensitivity should always be shown and stereotypical assumptions should never be

BOX 2.1: Support during the consultation

Some patients will attend the consultation with another person. This could include their partner, a family member, their child or a friend. As long as the patient consents, this person can be included during the initial consultation, but this is usually limited to one person. In some instances, the additional person can provide support during the consultation. When English is not the patient's first language, an independent interpreter should always be used to ensure that the patient's views are being communicated. It is important that a part of the consultation, including the examination, should be conducted with the patient alone to allow for privacy and a safe space to discuss sensitive topics and answer specific queries.

10.1201/9781003218036-2

made. Enough time should be allowed for the patient to express themselves, and the doctor's manner, including body language, should be one of interest while they guide the consultation with appropriate opening questions and leave pauses. A history that is taken with sensitivity will often allow the patient to reveal their true concerns and expectations, which can help direct management. While there are a number of specialist terms used in gynaecology (see **Box 2.2** 'Glossary of gynaecological terms'), care should be taken to avoid medicalized language and to use lay terms or the patient's own words where possible, clarifying meaning when required.

A history-taking template can be used to ensure that a complete and relevant gynaecological history is taken and may prevent the omission of important points (see **Box 2.3** 'Template for gynaecological history taking in suggested order'). Some gynaecology clinics will use a template routinely to standardise the consultation, particularly with electronic records, but there should be additional allowance for the patient's concerns and expectations to be heard.

SOCIAL HISTORY

Sensitive enquiry should be made about the patient's social situation, including details of their occupation, who they live with, their housing and whether or not they are in a stable (and sexual) relationship. A history regarding smoking and alcohol intake should also be obtained. Any pertinent family or other relevant social problems should be briefly discussed. If the patient has sexual issues, it is important to enquire if this has had an impact on their relationship. When admission and surgery are being contemplated, it is necessary to establish what support they have at home, particularly if they are elderly or frail.

Specific gynaecological problems require more focused history taking, and the issues that need to be discussed in more detail are set out in the following sections.

ABNORMAL UTERINE BLEEDING (see **Chapter 4**)

- Length of time of problem
- Amount of blood loss
- Timing of bleeding related to sex and menstrual cycle or to the last menstrual bleed in the case of postmenopausal bleeding
- For HMB, objective measurement is difficult (see **Box 2.4** 'How to quantify heavy menstrual bleeding')

BOX 2.2: Glossary of gynaecological terms

Menarche	Start of menstruation
Last menstrual period (LMP)	Date of the first day of the last menstrual bleed
Amenorrhoea	Absence of bleeds for more than 6 months in someone of reproductive age (see **Chapter 3**)
Oligomenorrhoea	Infrequent menstrual bleeds more than 35 days apart (see **Chapter 3**)
Dysmenorrhoea	Painful menstrual bleeding (primary or secondary) (see **Chapter 4**)
Menorrhagia	Now called heavy menstrual bleeding (HMB) (see **Chapter 4**)
Abnormal uterine bleeding	Includes post-coital bleeding (PCB) and intermenstrual bleeding (IMB) (see **Chapter 4**)
Dyspareunia	Painful intercourse (superficial or deep) (see **Chapter 13**)
Incontinence	Involuntary loss of urine (stress, urge or mixed) (see **Chapter 10**), flatal or faecal control
Prolapse	Feeling of something coming down in the vagina/bulge/heaviness (see **Chapter 10**)

BOX 2.3: Template for gynaecological history taking in suggested order

1 General
- Name, age and occupation
- A brief statement of the general nature and duration of the main complaints (try to use the patient's own words rather than medical terms at this stage)

2 History of presenting complaint
This section should focus on the presenting complaint (e.g. menstrual problems, pain, subfertility, urinary incontinence, etc.)

3 Menstrual history
This will be explored in all patients except those who are postmenopausal (for whom, instead, the last period and/or use of hormone replacement therapy (HRT) will be required).
- Usual duration of each period and length of full cycle (how many days from day 1 of bleed to day 1 of next bleed)
- First day of LMP
- Pattern of bleeding (regular or irregular)
- Amount of blood loss (patients will have different ideas as to what constitutes 'normal' or a 'heavy period')

4 Cervical screening
This will be explored in all patients.
- Date of last screening (and whether it was compliant with the current screening programme), its outcome and any previous abnormalities, colposcopy or treatments
- History of human papillomavirus (HPV) vaccination, if age appropriate

5 Sexual and contraceptive history
- Present partner(s), sexual orientation (to be determined with sensitivity)
- Contraceptive method or needs (hormonal and barrier)

6 Other gynaecological symptoms
The following questions should be asked, with a brief exploration of the answers. The areas in which more detailed questions need to be asked are set out later in this chapter.
- Any irregular bleeding?
- Any abnormal vaginal discharge?
- Any HMB, IMB or PCB?

- Any pelvic pain? If yes, where from, how often, for how long and is it related to the menstrual cycle?
- Are you currently in a sexual relationship? If yes, do have any sexual issues? Do you have pain?
- Any fertility issues and/or plans?
- Any problems with urinary, flatal or faecal continence? That is, do you have any leakage?
- What is your menopausal history and have you used HRT?

7 Previous gynaecological history
This section should include any previous gynaecological treatments or surgery.
- Previous obstetric history: How many pregnancies have you had?
- Number of children with ages and birth weights, mode of delivery and any complications
- Number of miscarriages and gestation at which they occurred
- Any terminations of pregnancy, with method, gestational age and any complications (to be discussed sensitively)

8 Previous medical history
- Any serious illnesses or operations, with dates
- Any general skin conditions if complaining of genital irritation

9 Medication and allergies
- Allergies, including to what and the reaction
- Current/previous medications tried

10 Family history
- Significant autoimmune disease, any cancers (particularly breast ovarian cancer syndrome (BRCA)-related cancers), thrombophilias or vascular disease

11 Systems enquiry (only if relevant)
- Appetite, weight loss, weight gain
- Bowel function (if urogynaecological complaint, more detail may be required)
- Bladder function (if urogynaecological complaint, more detail may be required)

NB: Gender: not all people seen in a gynaecology clinic identify as women – trans men, non-binary people and other people have gynaecological issues. Trans women may also be seen in a gynaecology service. Although specialist clinics provide more comprehensive support, this is not available to all. It is important to refer to all patients according to their preference and use the right pronouns (she/her, he/him, they/them).

- Is the bleeding more or less than usual?
- Do you use tampons, towels/sanitary pads or both?
- How often does soaked sanitary wear need to be changed? Do you change during the night?
- Are clots present?
- Do you experience flooding – 'like turning on a tap'?
- Is the bleeding so heavy (flooding) that it spills over your towel/tampon and onto your pants, clothes or bedding?
- Have you had to take any time off work due to this bleeding?
- Do you ever find you are confined to your house when the bleeding is at its worst?
- Do you feel dizzy or short of breath, particularly after a period, or find it hard to climb stairs?
- Does it limit/restrict your lifestyle?

EARLY PREGNANCY PROBLEMS (see **Chapter 5**)

- Date of LMP, whether it was normal and the regularity of the cycle – used to establish likely gestation
- Whether contraception is being used and whether the patient plans to proceed with pregnancy if unintended

PREGNANCY SYMPTOMS

- Episodes of bleeding or pain in this pregnancy
- Whether a scan has already been performed to establish viability and site of the pregnancy
- Whether there are risk factors for an ectopic pregnancy (sexually transmitted infection [STI], delayed conception, progesterone only contraception, previous ectopics)
- Previous history of miscarriages, the gestation and their management/complications (surgical, medical, conservative)

CONTRACEPTION AND EMERGENCY CONTRACEPTION (see **Chapter 6**)

- LMP
- Exact timing of unprotected intercourse(s), if the patient requires emergency contraception
- Contraindications to oestrogen-based contraception (thromboembolism, obesity, smoking, age, migraines with aura)
- Regular or multiple partners
- Previous sexual health screening
- Other gynaecological/menstrual problems (which may be improved with certain forms of contraception)

FERTILITY (see **Chapter 7**)

- Length of time in present relationship using no contraception
- Length of time 'trying for pregnancy'
- Frequency of intercourse
- Previous tests performed, both male and female (and male partner previous fertility)
- Previous STIs
- Previous fertility treatments attempted
- Particular attention to length and regularity of menstrual cycle
- Evidence of uterine problems (HMB, scanty periods, previous surgery, abdominal fullness)
- Evidence of polycystic ovary syndrome (oligomenorrhoea, hirsutism, excess weight, acne)
- Evidence of endocrine problems such as thyroid signs and symptoms (exophthalmos, heat sensitivity, weight change, tremor) and prolactinomas (galactorrhoea, visual field disturbance, headaches)

MENOPAUSE (see **Chapter 8**)

- Date of last natural menstrual period if known (may not if taking HRT or the combined oral contraceptive pill or has an intrauterine system)
- Postmenopausal bleeding
- Evidence of any menopausal symptoms (such as hot flushes, sleep disturbance, emotional or

psychological issues, sexual problems, vaginal dryness)
- Any HRT taken now or previously and any specific cautions such as breast cancer, thromboembolic events, cardio/cerebrovascular disease

UROGYNAECOLOGY (see **Chapter 10**)

- Number of times passing urine during the day/ at night, frequency/nocturia
- Urgent need to pass urine and loss of urine with urge, urgency/urge leak
- Uncontrolled passage of urine on coughing or straining (stress incontinence)
- Difficulty in passing urine (either initiation or complete emptying/poor flow)
- Daily fluid intake and timing
- Exacerbating factors such as alcohol, caffeine
- Extent to which affects general life, such as fluid restricting or planning routes around toilet facilities
- Incontinence of flatus or faeces
- Incontinence during sexual intercourse
- Feeling of something coming down/bulge/ heaviness in vagina
- Risk factors such as number of pregnancies and vaginal and instrumental births
- Evidence of abdominal masses such as fibroids
- Menopausal status and HRT

SEXUAL HEALTH (see **Chapter 9**)

- Whether the patient is in a sexual relationship and, if so, any problems or pain
- Regular sexual partner or not and other partners
- Vaginal/anal/oral sex (to be asked delicately depending on history) – asking about the need for contraception can be a sensitive way of asking about penetrative sex in someone of reproductive age if heterosexual

CONTRACEPTION

- Previous contraception (including side effects)
- Previous sexual health screening/STIs

- Symptoms of abnormal vaginal discharge, its colour and odour
- Vaginal and perineal discomfort or itching or lesions

PELVIC PAIN (see **Chapter 11**)

- Site of pain, its nature and severity, its frequency and duration
- Factors that aggravate or relieve pain – specifically enquire about temporal relationship to menstrual cycle and intercourse
- Whether the pain radiates anywhere or is associated with bowel or bladder function – ask about bowel activity
- If there is pain during intercourse – deep or superficial, associated sexual dysfunction (see **Chapter 13**)

SUMMARY

The history should be summarised in one to two sentences before proceeding to the examination to focus the problem and alert the examiner to the salient features (see **Box 2.5** 'Sample history').

- Privacy and confidentiality are essential in gynaecological history taking.
- It is important to avoid medical language.

BOX 2.5: Sample history

This 32-year-old Afro-Caribbean woman has presented to the gynaecology clinic with heavy regular periods. She uses eight towels a day and floods at night. She has symptoms of anaemia. Her periods became heavier 3 years ago. There is no abnormal pain. She has also noted abdominal fullness and frequency of urine during the day.

Her last cervical screening test was 2 years ago and was normal. She has had two full-term normal deliveries; her children are aged 6 and 10. She uses condoms with her regular partner for contraception. She would like more children in a few years' time. She has had no STIs. She has had no previous surgery and is fit and well, takes no medication and has no allergies.

- The symptoms experienced by the patient and the relevance in their lives are both important.
- A systematic and thorough gynaecological history should be taken at each consultation.
- Specific areas of the history should then be explored.

EXAMINATION

Initial general examination is part of overall assessment. Important information about the patient can be obtained by watching them walk into the examination room. Poor mobility may affect decisions regarding surgery or future management. Body mass index (BMI) and blood pressure measurements before consultation may be helpful.

Any examination should always be carried out with the patient's consent and with appropriate privacy and sensitivity. Check and explain that the door is closed and check the patient's comfort (e.g. is an elderly patient comfortable with the head position and are they warm enough) before proceeding. Indicate there is a chair to place her clothes on and a modesty sheet to cover herself when laying down. A female chaperone must be present throughout the examination.

It is good practice to perform a general examination, which should include examining the hands and mucous membranes for evidence of anaemia. The supraclavicular area should be palpated for the presence of nodes, particularly on the left side where, in cases of abdominal malignancy, one might palpate the enlarged Virchow's node (this is also known as the Troisier sign). The thyroid gland can be palpated or observed. The breasts should be examined as part of the examination if indicated by the history or pelvic examination; this is particularly relevant if there is a suspected ovarian mass, as there may be a breast tumour with secondaries in the ovaries known as Krukenburg tumours. In addition, a pleural effusion may be elicited as a consequence of abdominal ascites.

ABDOMINAL EXAMINATION

The patient should empty their bladder before the abdominal examination for comfort (unless demonstration of urinary leakage may be helpful). If a

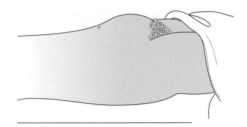

Figure 2.1 A patient in the correct position for abdominal examination, showing obvious abdominal distension.

urine infection or pregnancy is suspected, a sample should be tested. The patient should be comfortable and lying semi-recumbent with a sheet covering them from the waist down, but the area from the xiphisternum to the symphysis pubis should be left exposed (**Figure 2.1**). Palpation is traditionally performed while standing on the right-hand side of the patient using the right hand. Abdominal examination comprises inspection, palpation, percussion and, if appropriate, auscultation.

INSPECTION

The contour of the abdomen should be inspected and noted. There may be an obvious distension or mass. The presence of surgical scars, dilated veins or striae gravidarum (stretch marks) should be noted. It is important specifically to examine the umbilicus for laparoscopy scars and just above the symphysis pubis for Pfannenstiel scars (used for caesarean section, hysterectomy, etc.). The patient should be asked to raise their head or cough and any hernias or divarication of the rectus muscles will be evident.

PALPATION

First, if the patient has any abdominal pain, they should be asked to point to the site – the area should not be examined until the end of palpation. Palpation is performed by examining the left lower quadrant and proceeding in a total of four steps to the right lower quadrant of the abdomen. Palpation should include examination for masses, the liver, spleen and kidneys. If a mass is present but one can palpate below it, then it is more likely to be an abdominal mass than a pelvic mass. It is important to remember that one of the characteristics of a pelvic mass is that it arises from the pelvis, hence one cannot palpate below it. If the patient has pain, their abdomen should be palpated gently and the examiner should look for signs of peritonism (i.e. guarding and rebound tenderness). The patient should also be examined for inguinal hernias and lymph nodes.

PERCUSSION

Percussion is particularly useful if free fluid is suspected. In the recumbent position, ascitic fluid will settle down into a horseshoe shape and dullness in the flanks can be demonstrated. As the patient moves over to their side, the dullness will move to their lowermost side. This is known as 'shifting dullness'. A fluid thrill can also be elicited. An enlarged bladder due to urinary retention will also be dull to percussion but is likely to be very uncomfortable.

AUSCULTATION

This method is not specifically useful for a routine gynaecological examination. However, a patient will sometimes present with an acute abdomen, a bowel obstruction or a post-operative ileus and, in this situation, listening for bowel sounds will be important.

PELVIC EXAMINATION

Before proceeding to a vaginal examination, the patient's verbal consent should be obtained and a female chaperone should be present for any intimate examination. It is good practice (and common in most UK medical schools) for a student to have written consent. This is mandatory if the patient will be under anaesthetic for the examination. Non-sterile gloves can be used for the examination unless the patient is pregnant, in which case sterile gloves should be worn. There are three components to the pelvic examination: inspection, speculum examination and bimanual examination.

INSPECTION

The external genitalia and surrounding skin, including the perianal area, are first inspected under a good light with the patient in the dorsal position, the hips flexed and abducted and the knees flexed

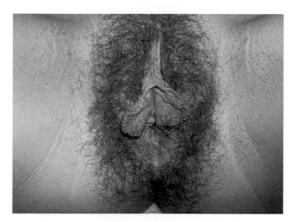

Figure 2.2 The normal vulva.

(**Figure 2.2**). Although the 'frog-leg' position is frequently employed, the author prefers feet apart for all except children. The patient is asked to cough or bear down to demonstrate any signs of a prolapse or stress incontinence. Abnormal signs such as skin discolouration, lumps, scars from previous episiotomy, deficient perineum or prolapse (see **Chapter 10**) are noted. Female genital mutilation (FGM) (see **Chapter 13**) should be described.

SPECULUM EXAMINATION

A sterile speculum is an instrument that is inserted into the vagina to obtain a clearer view of the vagina, cervix and descent of pelvic organs. There are two principal types in widespread use. The first is a bivalve or Cusco's speculum (**Figure 2.3A**), which holds back the anterior and posterior walls of the vagina and allows visualization of the cervix when opened out (**Figure 2.3B**). It has a retaining screw that can be tightened to allow the speculum to stay in place during a procedure or cervical sampling (e.g. screening or swab). There are different sizes – most sexually active individuals will accommodate a medium size. A small speculum is more appropriate for those who are postmenopausal but, on occasion, a 'virgin' speculum can be used. Internal examinations on patients who have not been sexually active must be considered carefully depending on circumstances and the patient's wishes. A Sim's speculum (**Figure 2.4A**) may also be used for examination of prolapse, as it allows inspection of the vaginal walls. It is used in the left lateral position (**Figure 2.4B**).

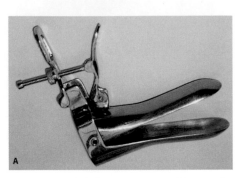

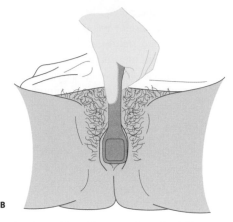

Figure 2.3 (**A**) Cusco's speculum. (**B**) Cusco's speculum in position. The speculum should be inserted at about 45° to the vertical and rotated to the vertical as it is introduced. Once it is fully inserted, the blades should be opened up to visualize the cervix.

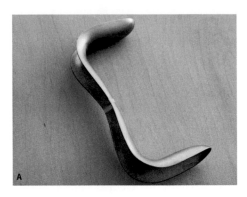

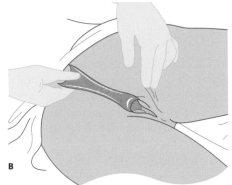

Figure 2.4 (**A**) Sim's speculum. (**B**) Sim's speculum inserted with the patient in the left lateral position. The speculum is used to hold back the posterior vaginal walls to allow inspection of the anterior wall and vault. The speculum can be rotated 180° or withdrawn slowly to visualize the posterior wall. A Valsalva manoeuvre (bearing down) may be needed to demonstrate prolapse.

The choice of speculum will depend on the patient's presenting problem or both may be used.

Excessive lubrication should be avoided and, if a cervical screening sample is being taken, lubrication with water should be considered, as lubricant may interfere with cytological analysis. Microbiology swabs are taken from the vaginal fornices and endocervix. Endocervical swabs for chlamydia and gonorrhoea may be taken from the endocervical canal (see **Chapter 9**), although urine tests are also available. Swabs can also be directed to areas of purulent/significant discharge. Cervical screening samples are taken according to specific guidance.

BIMANUAL EXAMINATION

This is usually performed after the speculum examination (although initial digital examination in individuals who are significantly anxious may be preferred) and is performed to assess the pelvic organs. It is a technique that requires practice. There are a variety of 'model pelvises' that can be used to train the student in the basics of the examination. Some UK medical schools employ gynaecology teaching associates, who are trained in teaching communication about pelvic examination and use their own bodies to teach the examination

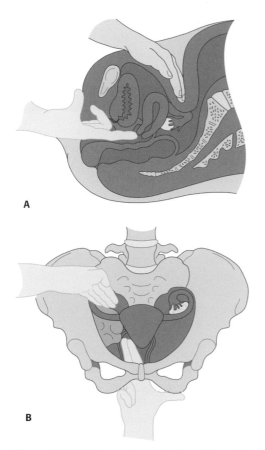

A

B

Figure 2.5 (A) Bimanual examination of the pelvis assessing the uterine position and size. **(B)** Bimanual examination of the lateral fornix.

process and give feedback. It is customary to use the left hand to part the labia and expose the vestibule and then insert one or two fingers of the right hand into the vagina. The fingers are passed upwards and backwards to reach the cervix (**Figure 2.5A**). The cervix is palpated and any irregularity, hardness or tenderness is noted. The left hand is now placed on the abdomen above the pubic symphysis and pressed down into the pelvis to palpate the fundus of the uterus. The size, shape, position, mobility, consistency and tenderness are noted. The normal uterus is pear-shaped and about 9 cm in length. It is usually anteverted with the angle of the axis falling forwards (see **Chapter 1**) and is normally freely mobile and non-tender. The tips of the fingers are then placed into each lateral fornix to palpate the

adnexa (tubes and ovaries) on each side. The fingers are pushed backwards and upwards, while at the same time pushing down in the corresponding area with the fingers of the abdominal hand. It is unusual to be able to feel normal ovaries. Any swelling or tenderness is noted (**Figure 2.5B**). The posterior fornix should also be palpated to identify the uterosacral ligaments, which may be tender or scarred in individuals with endometriosis.

BOX 2.6: Version and flexion of the uterus

The position and the size of the uterus are important, particularly in any patient requiring any type of intra-uterine instrumentation (intrauterine device/system insertion, hysteroscopy, laparoscopy). The reason for this is that the instrument will be guided into the uterus along its axis. It takes some experience to get this correct. If an acutely retroflexed uterus is missed, perforation through the anterior wall with surgical instruments is more likely. If an acutely anteverted uterus is missed, posterior perforation is possible.

The size of an enlarged uterus is described in terms of the size of the uterus in weeks of gestation, for example a '6-week sized uterus' is a non-pregnant uterus of the size associated with 6 weeks' pregnancy, about the size of a small orange. For very large uteri, it can be useful to describe by abdominal landmarks, for example to umbilicus or xiphisternum or according to expected pregnant uterine size (e.g. halfway to umbilicus = 16 weeks' size).

Pelvic floor tone may be assessed during the bimanual examination by asking the patient to contract their pelvic floor.

RECTAL EXAMINATION

In some situations, a rectal examination with specific additional consent can be useful in addition to a vaginal examination to assess the anal sphincter or a prolapse or to palpate the uterosacral ligaments more thoroughly. Occasionally, a rectovaginal examination (index finger in the vagina and middle finger in the rectum) may be useful to identify a lesion in the rectovaginal septum.

BOX 2.7: Global context

A rectal examination can be used as an alternative to a vaginal examination in children and in adults who have never had sex, if ultrasound is not available as an investigation. It is less sensitive than a vaginal examination and can be quite uncomfortable, but it will help pick up a pelvic mass.

FGM may be encountered in girls and women of sub-Saharan origin. The presence and type must be recorded. In some cases, this will make vaginal examination impossible. The presence of FGM must be recorded in the case notes as a legal requirement.

Some cultures would prohibit examination by a male practitioner, except in cases of emergency.

BOX 2.8: Professionalism

- Pelvic examination is classed by the Royal College of Obstetricians and Gynaecologists (RCOG) as an 'intimate examination' and, as such, should be taught initially by simulation, and thereafter with consent.
- Written consent by a student should be taken prior to examination under anaesthetic for teaching practice.
- An explanation of the necessity and procedure of vaginal examination should be given.
- A female chaperone must be present.

SUMMARY

- The size and consistency of the pelvic organs may indicate the diagnosis and need for further investigations.
- Accurate determination of anteversion or retroversion of the uterus is paramount immediately prior to procedures that require dilation of the uterine cervix to reduce the chance of perforation. This takes experience.
- Extreme reluctance to a vaginal examination, even with a qualified female doctor, should alert the practitioner to psychological issues that should be explored.
- Some patients will be reluctant to be examined while bleeding. They should be reassured and encouraged if this is part of the presenting complaint. Some patients will prefer to return when not bleeding.

INVESTIGATIONS

Once the examination is complete, the patient should be given the opportunity to dress in privacy and come back into the consultation room to sit down and discuss the findings. You should now be able to give a summary of the whole case and formulate a differential diagnosis. This will then determine the appropriate further investigations needed (if any). Swabs and cervical and urine samples will have been taken earlier in the examination. The urine should be kept and checked for beta-human chorionic gonadotrophin (hCG) in premenopausal patients if intrauterine examination is required. This section outlines further tests.

IMAGING

Ultrasound imaging in gynaecology has become uniformly available in the UK. Basic competence in gynaecological ultrasound is part of the RCOG curriculum for training doctors. Ultrasound imaging of the uterus and adnexa is part of the investigations of nearly all gynaecological problems, perhaps with the exception of contraception and sexual health screening in asymptomatic individuals and hormonal management such as menopause and premenstrual syndrome.

Pelvic ultrasound using a transvaginal ultrasound scan (TVUSS) is performed is the investigation of choice for many gynaecological problems in adults. The probe is cleaned in the presence of the patient and covered with a probe cover (or commonly a latex-free condom), containing ultrasound gel on the inside and outside. The probe is inserted into the vagina while the images are viewed on a screen. The images can be shared with the patient, if appropriate, once the correct image has been determined. The presence of pain and the correlation with images can be useful diagnostically. The resolution of TVUSS is high, particularly if the organ lies close to the probe, and the depth of images visible is around 12 cm. Excellent images of the uterus and adnexa, including the internal architecture of the myometrium, endometrium, fallopian tubes *when abnormal* and ovaries are achievable (**Figure 2.6A–D**), as well as images of early intra-uterine pregnancies. For those who have not been sexually active, children and teenagers, and some elderly patients, an abdominal ultrasound is more

BOX 2.9: Clinical context

- Ultrasound imaging of the pelvic organs has become part of routine assessment in gynaecology in the UK, but does not replace pelvic examination.
- TVUSS has excellent resolution and is inexpensive – it can enable accurate and instant diagnosis of many gynaecological problems, including acute and early pregnancy problems.
- The availability of ultrasound before or during a gynaecological consultation can often avoid the need for a patient to return to see the practitioner.
- Uterine and ovarian pathologies have specific appearances and can be diagnosed with accuracy.
- More expensive tests such as MRI are usually not needed in gynaecology. Increasingly, 3D ultrasound is used to diagnose uterine and adnexal abnormalities.
- Increased BMI can cause difficulty in visualization of pelvic structures on TVUSS.

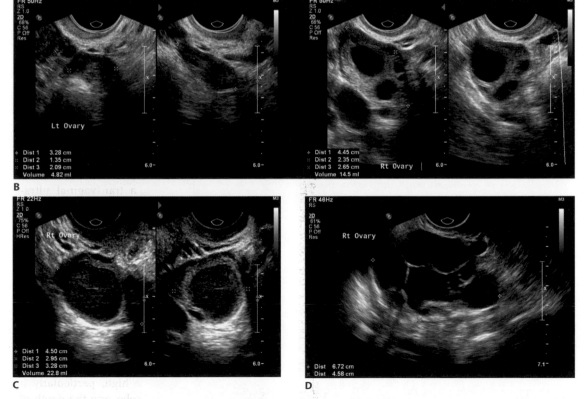

Figure 2.6 (**A**) Transvaginal ultrasound scan (TVUSS) of normal uterus. (**B**) TVUSS of left and right ovaries. (**C**) TVUSS of haemorrhagic cyst. (**D**) TVUSS of multiseptated cyst.

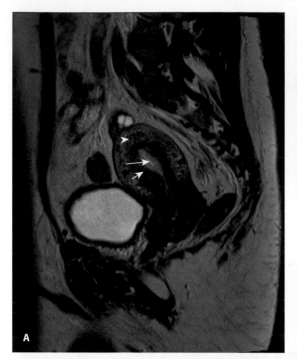

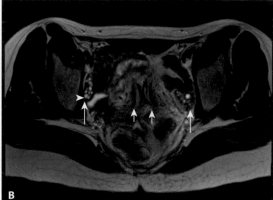

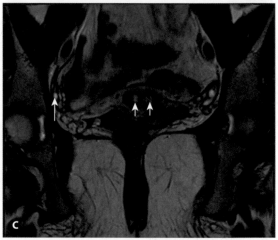

Figure 2.7 (**A**) Magnetic resonance imaging (MRI) of normal pelvis (long arrow, endometrium; short arrow, inner myometrium and cervix; arrowhead, outer myometrium). (**B**) Axial MRI of pelvis in a patient with uterus didelphys and double cervices (long arrows, ovaries; short arrows, cervices; arrowhead, follicle). (**C**) Coronal MRI in a patient with uterus didelphys (long arrow, right ovary; short arrows, cervices). (Images courtesy of Dr Sarah Natas, Consultant Radiologist.)

appropriate. In some patients with a large pelvic mass, both types of ultrasound may be utilized.

Instillation of saline through the cervix (saline instillation sonography) allows distension of the cavity of the uterus to enable the detection of abnormalities such as endometrial polyps and submucosal fibroids. 3D TVUSS improves the ability to diagnose structural abnormalities in the uterus.

T2-weighted MRI, although expensive, may be requested to distinguish fibroid change from adenomyosis and to delineate ovarian cysts and assess malignancy. It can also be used to identify structural abnormalities in the genital tract (**Figure 2.7A–C**). Increasingly, expert 3D TVUSS is used as a cheaper alternative. When malignancy has been identified, CT may be indicated to determine the stage of the disease.

ENDOMETRIAL BIOPSY

Biopsy of the endometrium can be performed without anaesthetic in most patients, and is indicated for those over 45 with menstrual symptoms, including HMB and PCB, after ensuring that the patient is not pregnant (see **Chapter 4**) (**Figure 2.8**). Endometrial

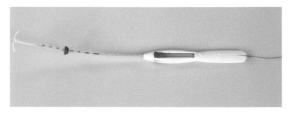

Figure 2.8 Endometrial sampler.

biopsy is complemented by TVUSS and outpatient or inpatient hysteroscopy and guided biopsy, where indicated.

In addition to imaging and histology, there are a number of investigations that are common in gynaecology (**Table 2.1**).

Table 2.1 Common investigations in gynaecology

Investigation	Relevant condition	Result
FBC and haematinics in anaemic patients	Suspected anaemia from heavy bleeding Pre-operative assessment	Low haemoglobin, low MCV and low iron stores
FSH/LH/E2 should be taken during early follicular phase (further described in **Chapter 3**)	Irregular menstrual cycle, menopausal symptoms	Raised gonadotrophins in ovarian failure Low E2 and raised FSH in ovarian failure High LH in PCOS (but can capture ovulatn) Low FSH/LH/E2 in hypogonadotrophic hypogonadism
Progesterone (further described in **Chapter 7**)	Mid-luteal phase progesterone, day 21 in a 28-day cycle, 7 days before menstruation in a longer cycle	Confirmation of ovulation
HVS for microbiology, NAAT taken as a vulvovaginal swab for chlamydia (further described in **Chapter 9**)	Vaginal discharge or risk of STI	Culture positive
Endocrine tests (further described in **Chapter 3**)	Irregular bleeds with systemic symptoms	Abnormal thyroid function, raised prolactin and raised androgens may indicate endocrine disturbance
AMH (further described in **Chapter 7**)	Ovarian reserve	Indicates high, medium or low fertility potential
Beta-hCG (further described in **Chapter 5**)	Pregnancy	May be used in cases of pregnancy of unknown location

AMH, anti-Müllerian hormone; E2, oestrogen; FBC, full blood count; FSH, follicle-stimulating hormone; HIV, human immunodeficiency virus; hCG, human chorionic gonadotrophin; HVS, high vaginal swab; LH, luteinizing hormone; MCV, mean corpuscular volume; PCOS, polycystic ovary syndrome; STI, sexually transmitted infection.

⊙⟳ KEY LEARNING POINTS

- The consultation should be performed in a private environment and in a sensitive fashion.
- The practitioner should introduce themselves, be courteous and explain what is about to happen and why.
- The practitioner should be familiar with the history template and use it regularly to avoid omissions.
- Remember to summarize the history to the patient before proceeding to the examination.

- A female chaperone should always be present for an intimate examination.
- The practitioner should be sensitive to the patient's needs and anxiety and respect the patient's privacy and dignity.
- The examination should begin with a general assessment of the patient.
- The patient should be asked to inform the practitioner if the examination is uncomfortable.

(Contd.)

(Contd.)

Positioning and acknowledgement of anxiety are key to successful examinations.

- The practitioner should reassure the patient during the examination and give feedback about what is being done. Sensitive observations can be made to check (dis)comfort, sensation and correlation with reported symptoms.
- After the examination, the practitioner should make sure that the patient is comfortable and allow them to get dressed in privacy.
- The practitioner should explain the findings to the patient in suitable language and give them the opportunity to ask questions.

- Prepare a differential diagnosis and order any appropriate investigations.
- TVUSS is inexpensive and is an accurate aid for the diagnosis of most gynaecological conditions.
- Further imaging modalities may be used to aid more complex diagnoses.
- Biochemistry and haematology may complete these findings, plus cervical screening/swabs/urine.
- Histological specimens from endometrium or superficial biopsy may be required.

FURTHER READING

RCOG Training in Ultrasound. https://www.rcog.org.uk/en/careers-training.

SELF-ASSESSMENT

For interactive SBAs and EMQs relating to this chapter, visit www.routledge.com/cw/crosbie.

CASE HISTORY 1

A 32-year-old Afro-Caribbean teacher has come to the clinic to see you. She has had increasingly heavy periods over the last 18 months. Her periods are regular and there is no IMB or PCB; bleeding is for 5 days every 28 days. On the second and third day of bleeding, she uses tampons and towels together, which get soaked in blood within 1 hour. In classes, she has had to run out when she had flooding, and she has passed clots about 4 cm in size. This is really embarrassing with the school children and she has taken to wearing nappies just in case. She is avoiding classroom teaching while she has a period but cannot explain why to her male head teacher. When her period finishes, she feels 'washed out' and easily gets short of breath when exercising. She has not tried any treatment so far.

She has never been pregnant and hoped to get pregnant soon after her marriage last year, but nothing has happened in the last 8 months. She has never had an STI, is in her only and stable sexual relationship and has no abnormal vaginal discharge, and her cervical screening history is normal; the last screen was 2 years ago.

On questioning, she admits to feeling full in the abdomen when she lies on her stomach. There is no pain as such and sex is not painful. She has never had surgery, has a healthy lifestyle, does not smoke or drink much alcohol and has no medical conditions. There is no family history of illnesses. She is not allergic to any prescribed medicines.

On examination, the abdomen is distended by a hard mass rising from the pelvis and coming halfway between the pubic symphysis and umbilicus. It is not tender. Cusco's speculum shows that the cervix is normal. Bimanual examination reveals the anteverted uterus to be enlarged to the size of a melon (about 16 weeks' size for a pregnant uterus).

A What are the important parts of the history?
B Which investigations should be commenced?
C What treatment would you suggest?

ANSWERS

A The important parts of the history here are a clear history of menstrual disturbance and the timescale over which it occurred. There are three issues: heavy embarrassing periods, likely symptoms of anaemia and the desire to get pregnant so far without success. The healthy lifestyle and lack of previous surgery are important in case surgery is required. The lack of drug allergies is very important to know for medications.

B Investigations should include the following:
- Full blood count to exclude anaemia. Without a personal or family history of thyroid disease, biochemical thyroid function is not indicated.

As the cycle is regular, no other hormonal tests are indicated at this stage.
- TVUSS. The scan shows that the uterus is enlarged with fibroids. There are three fibroids of which the largest is 6 cm × 8 cm at the fundus. There is a 2 cm × 2.5 cm submucosal fibroid in the uterine cavity.
- Cervical screening and swabs are not required, as there are no symptoms of discharge or IMB and she has a normal cervical screening history.

C Treatments should be discussed with the patient as described in later chapters. This patient will benefit from a transcervical resection of her submucosal fibroid, which is probably causing both her heavy menstrual bleeding and also her subfertility.

CASE HISTORY 2

A 32-year-old woman presents with infrequent periods for many years. She has never had cervical screening and has just started her first sexual relationship. Her BMI is 29 but she has recently lost a lot of weight. Otherwise, she is fit and healthy and is a non-smoker with minimal alcohol intake. There is a family history of bowel cancer. A previous encounter with a gynaecologist caused great anxiety.

A What is the gynaecological term to describe her periods?

B What gynaecological concerns might she have?

C She is worried about the risk of cancer due to her non-attendance at invitations to have a cervical smear and family history. How might you reassure her?

D On examination, what particular signs might you specifically look for?

E Would an intimate examination be appropriate?

F What initial tests would you recommend?

ANSWERS

A Oligomenorrhoea is the term for periods that are fewer than 35 days apart or fewer than four to eight periods a year.

B She may be concerned about the impact this has on fertility and whether she needs contraception, in addition to the impact on her general health.

C You should offer her cervical screening after explaining what it involves. Now that she has become sexually active, it may be easier. It was not indicated before she became sexually active, as she would not have been exposed to HPV, which is the cause of cervical cell changes; therefore, she has not missed the opportunity to screen for this. You should reassure her that cervical cancer is not hereditary or related to bowel cancer. If she has a close family history of other cancers including endometrial cancer, she may have a hereditary syndrome such as Lynch syndrome, but this is uncommon.

D You would examine for signs of polycystic ovary syndrome with hyperandrogenism such as hirsutism and acne, other endocrine disorders such as abdominal striae, moon face and other skin changes.

E Intimate examination may be appropriate and should be offered sensitively, acknowledging that she has had a difficult experience previously. If she declines, a pelvic scan even with a vaginal probe may be acceptable with a skilled and experienced person after adequate explanation. However, a transabdominal scan may also reveal enough to make a diagnosis. She should not be made to feel inadequate or guilty about her choices – she may be more confident at a future appointment if she is allowed to control what she is comfortable with.

F She should have a hormone profile and a pelvic scan. If she declines a transvaginal scan and the transabdominal scan is limited due to body habitus, an MRI may, in some circumstances, be indicated.

CASE HISTORY 3

Michael, a 28-year-old transgender man, attends his GP with signs and symptoms of hay fever. During the consultation, the GP asks if Michael has attended the clinic for cervical screening. Michael had a bilateral mastectomy the previous year but still has a uterus and cervix. He received an invitation to attend for cervical screening shortly after his 25th birthday, but he did not feel comfortable attending the clinic. He has been living as a man since he transitioned shortly after his 18th birthday.

A   Does Michael require cervical screening?
B   What barriers might affect Michael in accessing healthcare?
C   What other issues should the GP raise with Michael?

ANSWERS

A   Michael is a transgender man. This means he was assigned female at birth but now identifies and lives as a man. Cisgender is a term used for people whose gender identity matches their sex assigned at birth. A transgender man assigned female at birth, who has not had surgery to remove the cervix, is recommended to undertake cervical screening with the same frequency as a ciswoman. However, there is evidence to suggest that cervical screening rates within the trans community are generally lower than in the cisgender community.
B   There are numerous barriers to accessing cervical screening for a transgender man with a cervix.
  • Invitations to cervical screenings from the national call/recall system are only sent to patients registered as 'female' with their GP practice or clinic. This means that a transgender man with a cervix who is registered as 'male' will not be invited to participate. Furthermore, a transgender man may not have disclosed his sex as assigned at birth to their GP practice or clinic, which means that the clinic staff may be unaware the patient is eligible for screening.
  • Following cervical screening, rates of recall for transgender men with a cervix are high due to labelling issues on the sample, which can result in the screening sample being rejected by the laboratory. This is distressing for the patient, as well as being a waste of time and money.
  • Although significant progress has been made, prejudice and discrimination against transgender people can still occur within healthcare settings in the form of transphobia, misgendering and microaggressions, which means that some transgender men will be too afraid to attend screening.
C   As Michael still has his cervix and uterus, he may require contraception and sexual health screening. Similar barriers to access exist for these services. The key requirement as a health provider is to be sensitive and aware of these issues so that members of the trans community can easily access healthcare when they need it most and feel comfortable disclosing their sexual orientation or gender identity so that they get the best possible care. Further information about screening and the trans community can be found here: https://www.gov.uk/government/publications/nhs-population-screening-information-for-transgender-people/nhs-population-screening-information-for-trans-people.

CASE HISTORY 4

A 45-year-old woman is referred to a gynaecology clinic complaining of frequent heavy bleeds with no regular pattern. She has a new partner and, having had three children, is wanting to get pregnant again. She reports having multiple non-specific symptoms, including joint and muscle pains, increased headaches before her period, irritable mood and feeling tired all the time. She has also recently had an increase in discharge and generalized pain. An ultrasound scan organised by her GP has reported multiple small fibroids and her hormone profile is normal.

A   What other tests might be offered?
B   What will you tell her about her fertility status?
C   How might you manage her period problems?
D   What are your differential diagnoses?

ANSWERS

A   She should have a full blood count to determine whether she is anaemic, a thyroid function profile to assess whether this has had an impact on her menstrual cycle, and you should consider a further hormone profile on days 2–5 of the menstrual cycle to assess her menopausal status, although in a perimenopausal woman the hormone profile may be normal, as the hormones are unpredictably fluctuant. Early in the menstrual cycle, raised follicle-stimulating hormone may indicate a perimenopausal picture. Anti-Müllerian hormone level gives an indication of ovarian reserve, but will not reliably rule out an inability to conceive. The reporting of pain and discharge should always suggest a possibility of an STI, so a sensitive approach to infection screening should be taken.

B   You may suggest that her fertility will be reduced due to age and that the chances of miscarriage will be higher due to increased chromosomal abnormalities. However, if she was to decide against conceiving again, she still needs contraception.

C   The most effective ways of managing period problems are generally contraceptive, as they control the menstrual cycle. Recommending tranexamic and mefenamic acid during the period itself does not have an impact on her chances of conceiving.

D   She may be perimenopausal, leading to reduced ovulation, as the ovaries have fewer eggs to release, which disrupts the phases of the menstrual cycle; she may have dysfunctional uterine bleeding, although the presence of fibroids indicates a reason for abnormal bleeding (dysfunctional uterine bleeding is a diagnosis of exclusion); she may have anaemia secondary to heavy menstrual bleeding due to fibroids; or she may have disordered bleeding due to endocrine problems (e.g. thyroid problems – hypo- or hyperthyroidism (more commonly hypothyroidism in this age group)). She may also have endometrial hyperplasia or an endometrial polyp, so if the scan was some time ago, this may be repeated. Premenstrual syndrome frequently increases towards the menopause and a past history of premenstrual syndrome in addition to a history of postnatal depression should be documented.

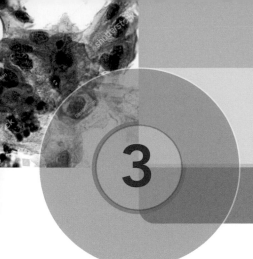

Hormonal control of the menstrual cycle and hormonal disorders

3

DHARANI K HAPANGAMA

Learning Objectives
- Describe the features of the ovarian and endometrial changes relevant to the normal menstrual cycle.
- Describe puberty and the accompanying normal secondary sexual differentiation.
- Understand the classification and causes of abnormal puberty and disorders of sexual development.
- Describe the causes and investigation of primary and secondary amenorrhoea and oligomenorrhoea.
- Understand the epidemiology and effects of polycystic ovary syndrome, as well as its diagnosis and management.
- Describe the common effects and management of premenstrual syndrome.
- Describe the premature cessation of periods.

INTRODUCTION

This chapter considers the hormonal control of the menstrual cycle and the abnormalities that may affect its physiological initiation, regulation and cessation.

PHYSIOLOGY OF THE MENSTRUAL CYCLE

The main function of the female reproductive tract is to achieve and nurture a pregnancy until birth. The external manifestation of a normal menstrual cycle is the presence of regular monthly vaginal bleeding, or menstruation. This occurs as a result of the shedding of the endometrial lining following failure of fertilization of the oocyte or failure of implantation. The cycle depends on changes occurring after puberty within the ovaries and fluctuation in ovarian hormone levels, which are themselves controlled by the pituitary gland and hypothalamus within the hypothalamic–pituitary–ovarian (HPO) axis. In situations of disorders of sexual development (DSD) or hormonal abnormalities, menstruation may not begin.

HYPOTHALAMUS

The hypothalamus in the forebrain secretes the peptide hormone gonadotrophin-releasing hormone (GnRH), which in turn controls pituitary hormone secretion. GnRH must be released in a pulsatile fashion to stimulate pituitary secretion of luteinizing hormone (LH) and follicle-stimulating hormone (FSH).

10.1201/9781003218036-3

PITUITARY GLAND

GnRH stimulation of the basophil cells in the anterior pituitary gland causes them to synthesize and release the gonadotrophic hormones FSH and LH. This process is modulated by the ovarian sex steroid hormones oestrogen and progesterone. Low levels of oestrogen have an inhibitory effect on LH production (negative feedback), whereas high levels of oestrogen will increase LH production (positive feedback). The mechanism of action for the positive feedback effect of oestrogen involves an increase in pituitary GnRH receptor concentrations, through direct stimulation of GnRH neurons by kissipeptin. The high levels of circulating oestrogen in the late follicular phase of the cycle therefore act via the positive-feedback mechanism on the HPO axis to generate a periovulatory LH surge from the pituitary gland.

The clinical relevance of these mechanisms is seen in the use of the combined oral contraceptive pill, which artificially creates a constant serum oestrogen level in the negative-feedback range, inducing a correspondingly low level of gonadotrophin hormone release.

Unlike oestrogen, low levels of progesterone have a positive-feedback effect on pituitary LH and FSH secretion (as seen immediately prior to ovulation) and contribute to the LH and FSH surge. High levels of progesterone, as seen in the luteal phase, inhibit pituitary LH and FSH production. Positive-feedback effects of low progesterone levels occur via increasing sensitivity to GnRH in the pituitary gland, while its negative-feedback effects are generated through both decreasing GnRH production from the hypothalamus and decreasing sensitivity to GnRH in the pituitary gland. These effects of progesterone on gonadotropic hormone release require prior priming by oestrogen (**Figure 3.1**).

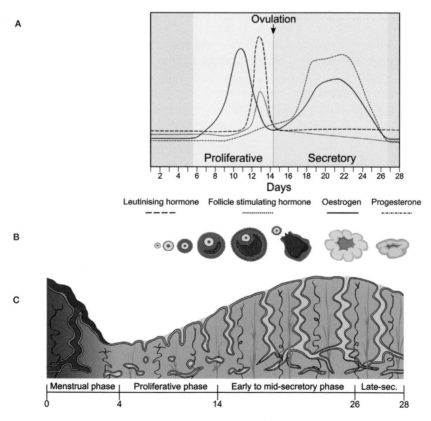

Figure 3.1 Changes in hormone levels of the hypothalamic–pituitary–ovarian axis (**A**), ovarian follicular activity (**B**) and endometrium (**C**), during the menstrual cycle.

OVARY

Starting at menarche, the primordial follicles containing oocytes, which are arrested at the first prophase step in meiotic division, will start to activate and grow in a cyclical fashion. This results in ovulation and subsequent menstruation in the event of non-fertilization. In the course of a normal menstrual cycle, the ovary will go through three phases: the follicular, ovulatory and luteal phases.

FOLLICULAR PHASE

The initial stages of follicular development are independent of hormone stimulation. However, if the pituitary hormones LH and FSH are absent, follicular development will fail at the preantral stage, and follicular atresia will ensue.

FSH levels rise in the first days of the menstrual cycle, when oestrogen, progesterone and inhibin levels are low. This stimulates a cohort of small antral follicles on the ovaries to grow. Within the follicles, there are two cell types that are involved in the processing of steroids, including oestrogen and progesterone. These are the theca and the granulosa cells, which respond to LH and FSH stimulation, respectively. LH stimulates the production of androgens from cholesterol within theca cells. These androgens are converted into oestrogens by the process of aromatization in granulosa cells, under the influence of FSH.

As the follicles grow and oestrogen secretion increases, there is negative feedback on the pituitary gland to decrease FSH secretion. This assists in the selection of one follicle (usually the one with the highest oestrogen-producing capacity) to continue in its development towards ovulation – the dominant follicle. Therefore, the follicle that has the most efficient aromatase activity and the highest concentration of FSH-induced LH receptors will survive as FSH levels drop, while smaller follicles will undergo atresia.

There are other autocrine and paracrine mediators playing a role in the follicular phase of the menstrual cycle. These include inhibin and activin. Inhibin is secreted by the granulosa cells within the ovaries. It participates in providing feedback to the pituitary gland to downregulate FSH release and also appears to enhance ongoing androgen synthesis. Activin is structurally similar to inhibin, but has an opposite action. Activin is produced in granulosa cells and in the pituitary gland, and acts to increase FSH binding on the follicles.

Insulin-like growth factors (IGF-I, IGF-II) act as paracrine regulators. Circulating levels do not change during the menstrual cycle, but follicular fluid levels increase towards ovulation, with the highest level found in the dominant follicle.

Kisspeptins are proteins that have more recently been found to play a role in the regulation of the HPO axis, via the mediation of the metabolic hormone leptin's effect on the hypothalamus. Leptin is thought to be key in the relationship between energy production, weight and reproductive health. Mutations in kisspeptin receptor 1 are associated with delayed or absent puberty, probably due to a reduction in leptin-linked triggers for gonadotrophin release.

OVULATORY PHASE

By the end of the follicular phase, which lasts an average of 14 days, the dominant follicle has grown to approximately 20 mm in diameter. As the follicle matures, FSH induces LH receptors on the granulosa cells to compensate for lower FSH levels and prepare for the signal for ovulation. The production of oestrogen increases until it reaches the necessary threshold to exert a positive-feedback effort on the hypothalamus and the pituitary gland, to cause the LH surge. This occurs over 24–36 hours, during which time the LH-induced luteinization of granulosa cells in the dominant follicle causes progesterone to be produced, adding further to the positive feedback for LH secretion and causing a small periovulatory rise in FSH. Androgens, synthesized in the theca cells, also rise around the time of ovulation, and this is thought to have an important role in stimulating libido, ensuring that sexual activity is likely to occur at the time of greatest fertility.

The LH surge is one of the best predictors of imminent ovulation, and this is the hormone detected in urine by most over-the-counter 'ovulation predictor' tests. The LH surge has another function in stimulating the resumption of meiosis in the oocyte just prior to its release. The physical release of the oocyte occurs after breakdown of the follicular wall, takes place under the influence of LH, FSH and proteolytic enzymes, such as plasminogen activators and prostaglandins (PGs). Studies have shown that inhibition of PG production may result in failure of ovulation. Thus, individuals wishing to become pregnant should be advised to avoid taking PG synthetase inhibitors, such as aspirin and ibuprofen, which may inhibit oocyte release.

LUTEAL PHASE

After the release of the oocyte, the remaining granulosa and theca cells on the ovary form the corpus luteum (CL). The granulosa cells have a vacuolated appearance with accumulated yellow pigment, hence the name CL (meaning 'yellow body'). The CL undergoes extensive vascularization in order to supply granulosa cells with a rich blood supply for continued steroidogenesis. This is aided by local production of vascular endothelial growth factor.

Ongoing pituitary LH secretion and granulosa cell activity ensure a supply of progesterone, which stabilizes and differentiates the endometrium in preparation for pregnancy. Progesterone levels are at their highest in the cycle during the luteal phase. This also has the effect of suppressing FSH and LH secretion to a level that will not support further follicular growth in the ovary during that cycle.

The luteal phase lasts 14 days in most people, without great variation. In the absence of beta-human chorionic gonadotrophin (βhCG) being produced from an implanting embryo, the CL will regress in a process known as luteolysis, forming the corpus albicans. The mature CL becomes less sensitive to LH, produces less progesterone and will gradually disappear from the ovary. The withdrawal of progesterone causes the shedding of the endometrial functionalis layer and thus menstruation. The reduction in the levels of progesterone, oestrogen and inhibin feeding back to the pituitary gland causes increased secretion of gonadotrophic hormones, particularly FSH. New preantral follicles begin to be stimulated and the cycle begins anew.

ENDOMETRIUM

The hormone changes brought about by the HPO axis during the menstrual cycle will occur whether the uterus is present or not. However, the specific

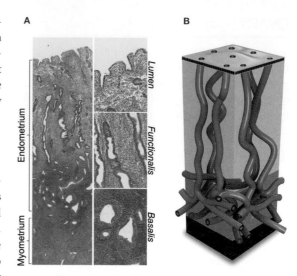

Figure 3.2 Uterine wall. Full thickness normal endometrium demonstrating basalis and functionalis (**A**) and schematic of the unique endometrial glandular organisation in women (**B**). (Modified from Tempest *et al.* (2022). Novel microarchitecture of human endometrial glands: implications in endometrial regeneration and pathologies. *Human Reproduction Update*, 28(2): 153–171.)

secondary changes in the uterine endometrium give the most obvious external sign of regular cycles, menstruation (**Figure 3.2**).

Human endometrium is organized into two functionally very different layers: (1) the superficial functionalis, which only appears after puberty and disappears after menopause, and (2) the deeper basalis overlying the uterine muscle (myometrium), which is present throughout a person's life. The classical cyclical changes in the endometrium occur in the functionalis layer, while the basalis – consisting of a complex network of mycelium-like, interconnected horizontal basalis glands and dense stroma – is less proliferative, less sensitive to hormones, structurally stable and the permanent mucosal compartment of the uterus (**Figure 3.2**).

PROLIFERATIVE PHASE

After menstruation, the endometrium enters the proliferative phase, when glandular and stromal growth begins. The current understanding is that endometrial stem cells located in the basalis layer are retained after menstrual sloughing and they are responsible for regenerating a new functionalis layer. During this phase, the epithelium lining the endometrial glands changes from a single layer of columnar cells to a pseudostratified epithelium with frequent mitoses. Endometrial thickness increases rapidly, from 0.2 mm at menstruation to 3.5–5 mm at the end of the proliferative phase. Gland-specific rapid proliferation causes glands to lengthen and coil.

SECRETORY PHASE

After ovulation (generally around day 14), there is a period of endometrial glandular secretory activity. Following the LH surge, the subsequent increase in progesterone causes an inhibition of oestrogen-induced cellular proliferation and the endometrium does not thicken any further. The endometrial glands become more tortuous, spiral arteries grow and fluid is secreted into glandular lumen and into the uterine cavity, providing a source of nutrients, growth factors and cytokines to support embryo implantation and early pregnancy establishment. Later in the secretory phase, progesterone further induces differentiation of the endometrial stroma to form a temporary layer, known as the decidua. The decidualized stromal cells release several cytokines and chemokines, instigating the recruitment of leucocytes and vascular growth (angiogenesis). Stromal cells show increased mitotic activity, nuclear enlargement and the generation of a basement membrane (**Figure 3.3**).

Apical membrane projections of the endometrial epithelial cells, known as pinopodes, appear around days 19–21 and appear to be a progesterone-dependent process in making the endometrium receptive for embryo implantation (**Figure 3.4**). The

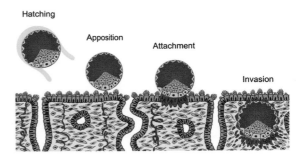

Figure 3.4 The three steps of human embryo implantation: apposition, attachment and invasion.

endometrial functionalis is primed for successful embryo implantation only for a short period in every menstrual cycle, called the 'window of implantation'.

MENSTRUATION

Approximately 14 days after ovulation, in the absence of an embryo producing (β)hCG, the CL demises and the consequent fall in circulating levels of oestrogen and progesterone initiates vasoconstriction of spiral arterioles and ischaemia, prompting an acute inflammatory reaction, immune cell infiltration and the launch of the inflammatory cascade. This is associated with an increase in proinflammatory cytokines, PGs and destructive enzymes of the extracellular matrix. It also activates the endometrial stem cells that are responsible for regeneration. Although the functionalis layer is shed over 1–3 days, menstrual bleeding continues until days 5 or 6 of the cycle, when the endometrium regenerates. Endometrial haemostasis, which is responsible for cessation of menstrual bleeding, involves platelet aggregation, fibrin deposition and thrombus formation, while myometrial contractions are responsible for period 'cramps'. Uterine contractions support the expulsion of menstrual debris and cause haemostasis through a pressure effect on the vasculature.

The effects of oestrogen and progesterone on the endometrium are reproduced artificially in patients taking the combined oral contraceptive pill or hormone replacement therapy (HRT), who experience a withdrawal bleed during their pill-free week each month. Progesterone withdrawal increases endometrial PG synthesis and decreases its metabolism, and high PG levels are reported in patients with heavy

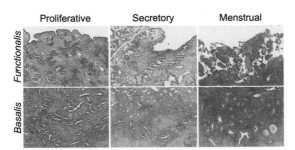

Figure 3.3 Tissue sections of normal endometrium during proliferative, secretory and menstrual phases of the menstrual cycle.

menstrual bleeding. The cyclooxygenase-2 enzyme is involved in PG synthesis and this is the target of non-steroidal anti-inflammatory drugs that are used for the treatment of heavy and painful periods.

PUBERTY AND SECONDARY SEXUAL DEVELOPMENT

NORMAL PUBERTY

Puberty is a period of maturation during which body growth and sexual development change a child into an adult. During childhood, the HPO axis is suppressed and levels of GnRH, FSH and LH are very low. From the age of 8–9 years, GnRH is secreted in pulsations of increasing amplitude and frequency. These are initially sleep related, but, as puberty progresses, they extend throughout the day. This stimulates the secretion of FSH and LH by the pituitary gland, which in turn triggers follicular growth and steroidogenesis in the ovary. The oestrogen produced by the ovary then initiates the physical changes of puberty, which are further influenced by many factors including race, heredity, body weight

and exercise. Kisspeptin and many other puberty-activating/inhibitor genes are involved in the onset of puberty.

The physical changes occurring in puberty are breast development (thelarche), pubic and axillary hair growth (adrenarche), growth spurt and onset of menstruation (menarche).

The first physical sign of puberty is breast budding and this occurs 2–3 years before menarche. The appearance of pubic hair is dependent on the secretion of adrenal androgens and usually happens after thelarche. In addition to increasing levels of adrenal and gonadal hormones, growth hormone secretion also increases at adolescence, leading to a pubertal growth spurt. The mean age of menarche is 12.8 years but it may take over 3 years before the menstrual cycle establishes a regular pattern. Initial cycles are usually anovulatory and can be unpredictable and irregular. The absence of menstruation is called amenorrhoea, which may be primary or secondary (see **Box 3.2** 'Amenorrhoea' later in this chapter). Pubertal development was described by Tanner, and the stages of breast and pubic hair development are often referred to as Tanner stages 1–5 (**Figure 3.5, Table 3.1**).

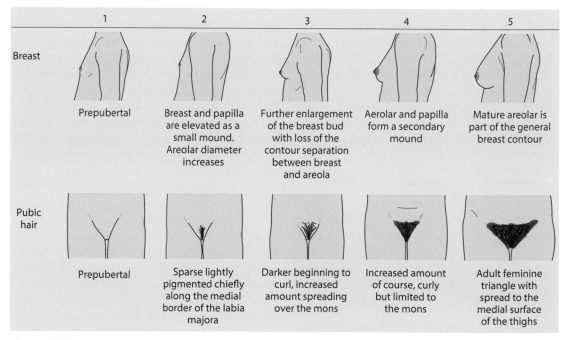

Figure 3.5 Tanner staging.

Table 3.1 Tanner staging

Stage	Pubic hair scale	Breast development
Stage 1	No hair	No glandular breast tissue palpable
Stage 2	Downy hair	Breast bud palpable under the areola (first pubertal sign in females)
Stage 3	Scant terminal hair	Breast tissue palpable outside areola; no areolar development
Stage 4	Terminal hair that fills the entire triangle overlying the pubic region	Areola elevated above the contour of the breast, forming a 'double scoop' appearance
Stage 5	Terminal hair that extends beyond the inguinal crease onto the thigh	Areolar mound recedes into single breast contour with areolar hyperpigmentation, papillae development and nipple protrusion

BOX 3.1: Hypo- and hypergonadotrophic hypogonadism

*Hypo*gonadotrophic hypogonadism
- This is central and may be constitutional, but other causes must be excluded. These include anorexia nervosa, excessive exercise and chronic illness, such as diabetes or renal failure. Rarer causes include a pituitary tumour and Kallmann syndrome.
- It is associated with delayed puberty and primary amenorrhoea.

*Hyper*gonadotrophic hypogonadism
- This is caused by gonadal failure.
- The gonad does not function, despite high gonadotrophins.
- It is associated with Turner syndrome and XX gonadal dysgenesis.
- Premature ovarian failure can occur at any age, including prior to pubertal age, and may be idiopathic, but can also be part of an autoimmune or metabolic disorder or following chemo- or radiotherapy for childhood cancer.
- It is associated with delayed puberty and primary amenorrhoea.
- It can also occur later in life and will cause secondary amenorrhoea after normal sexual development.

PRECOCIOUS PUBERTY

Precocious puberty is defined as the onset of puberty before the age of 8 years in a girl or 9 years in a boy. It is classified as either central or peripheral. Central precocious puberty is gonadotrophin dependent. The aetiology is often unknown, although up to 25% of cases are due to central nervous system malformations or brain tumours. Peripheral precocious puberty, which is gonadotrophin independent, is always pathological and can be caused by oestrogen secretion, such as exogenous ingestion or a hormone-producing tumour.

DELAYED PUBERTY

When there are no signs of secondary sexual characteristics by the age of 14 years, this is termed delayed puberty. It is due to either a central defect (hypogonadotrophic hypogonadism) or a failure of gonadal function (hypergonadotrophic hypogonadism), which are described in **Box 3.1** 'Hypo- and hypergonadotrophic hypogonadism'.

DISORDERS OF SEXUAL DEVELOPMENT

DSDs are conditions in which the sequence of events described earlier in this chapter does not happen. The clinical consequences of this depend on where within the sequence the variation occurs. DSDs may be diagnosed at birth with ambiguous or abnormal genitalia, but may also be seen at puberty in girls who present with primary amenorrhoea or increasing virilization.

There has been a change in the terminology used to refer to these conditions over the last 10 years. Older terms, such as 'hermaphrodite' and 'intersex', are confusing to both the clinician and patients, and in addition can be hurtful. The accepted terminology, according to the 2006 Chicago consensus statement (Hughes *et al.*, 2006), is summarized in **Table 3.2**.

Table 3.2 Summary of terminology for disorders of sex development (DSDs) according to the 2006 Chicago consensus statement

Previous terms	Accepted revised terms
Intersex	DSD
Male pseudohermaphrodite	46,XY DSD
Undervirilization of XY male	
Undermasculinization of XY male	
Female pseudohermaphrodite	46,XX DSD
Overvirilization of an XX female	
Masculinization of an XX female	
True hermaphrodite	Ovotesticular DSD
XX male or XX sex reversal	46,XX testicular DSD
XY sex reversal	46,XY complete gonadal dysgenesis

Source: Hughes *et al.* (2006).

NON-STRUCTURAL CAUSES OF DISORDERS OF SEXUAL DEVELOPMENT

TURNER SYNDROME

The total complement of chromosomes is 45 in Turner syndrome, which results from a complete or partial absence of one X chromosome (45,XO). Turner syndrome is the most common chromosomal anomaly in females, occurring in 1 in 2,500 live female births. A mosaic karyotype is not uncommon, leading to a variable presentation. Although there can be variations, the most typical clinical features include short stature, webbing of the neck and a wide carrying angle. Associated medical conditions include coarctation of the aorta, inflammatory bowel disease, sensorineural and conduction deafness, renal anomalies and endocrine dysfunction, such as autoimmune thyroid disease.

In this condition, the ovary does not complete its normal development and only the stroma is present at birth. The gonads are called 'streak gonads' and do not function to produce oestrogen or oocytes. Diagnosis is usually made at birth or in early childhood from the clinical appearance of the baby or due to short stature during childhood. However, in about 10% of cases, the diagnosis is not made until adolescence with delayed puberty. The ovaries do not produce oestrogen, so the normal physical changes of puberty cannot happen. In childhood, treatment is focused on growth, but, in adolescence, treatment focuses on the induction of puberty. Pregnancy is possible only with ovum donation. Psychological input and support is important. In those with mosaicism, the clinical picture can vary and normal puberty and menstruation can occur, although with early cessation of periods.

46,XY GONADAL DYSGENESIS

In this situation, the gonads do not develop into a testis, despite the presence of an XY karyotype. In about 15% of cases, this is due to a mutation in the sex-determining region of the Y chromosome (*SRY*) gene, but in most cases the cause is unknown. In complete gonadal dysgenesis (Swyer syndrome), the gonad remains as a streak gonad and does not produce any hormones. In the absence of anti-Müllerian hormone (AMH), the Müllerian structures do not regress and the uterus, vagina and fallopian tubes develop normally. The absence of testosterone means the fetus does not virilize. The baby is phenotypically female, although with an XY karyotype. The gonads do not function, and presentation is usually at adolescence with delayed puberty. The dysgenetic gonad has a high malignancy risk and should be removed when the diagnosis is made. This is usually performed laparoscopically. Puberty must be induced with oestrogen and pregnancies have been reported with a donor oocyte. Full disclosure of the diagnosis including the XY karyotype is essential, although this can be devastating and, thus, specialized psychological input is crucial.

Mixed gonadal dysgenesis is a more complex condition. The karyotype may be 46,XX, but XX/XY mosaicism is present in up to 20%. In this situation, both functioning ovarian and testicular tissue can be present and, if so, this condition is known as ovotesticular DSD. The anatomical findings vary depending on the function of the gonads. For example, if the testis is functional, then the baby will virilize and have ambiguous or normal male genitalia. The Müllerian structures are usually absent on the side of the functioning testis, but a unicornuate uterus may be present if there is an ovary or streak gonad.

46,XY DISORDER OF SEXUAL DEVELOPMENT

The most common cause of 46,XY DSD – complete androgen insensitivity syndrome (CAIS) – occurs in individuals in whom virilization of the external genitalia does not occur, due to a partial or complete inability of the androgen receptor to respond to androgen stimulation. In the fetus with CAIS, testes form normally due to the action of the *SRY* gene. At the appropriate time, these testes secrete AMH, leading to the regression of the Müllerian ducts. Hence, individuals with CAIS do not have a uterus. Testosterone is also produced at the appropriate time; however, due to the inability of the androgen receptor to respond, the external genitalia do not virilize and instead undergo female development. The baby is born with normal female external genitalia, an absent uterus and testes that are found somewhere in their line of descent through the abdomen from the pelvis to the inguinal canal. Presentation is usually at puberty with primary amenorrhoea, although if the testes are in the inguinal canal they can cause a hernia in a younger individual. Once the diagnosis is made, initial management is psychological, with full disclosure of the XY karyotype and the information that the patient will be infertile.

Gonadectomy is recommended because of the small long-term risk of testicular malignancy, although this can be deferred until after puberty. Once the gonads are removed, long-term HRT will be required. The vagina is usually shortened and treatment will be required to create a vagina suitable for penetrative intercourse. Vaginal dilation is the most effective method of improving vaginal length and entails the insertion of vaginal moulds of gradually increasing length and width for at least 30 minutes a day. Surgical vaginal reconstruction operations are reserved for patients who have not responded to a dilation treatment programme.

In cases of partial androgen insensitivity, the androgen receptor has limited responsiveness with limited virilization. The child is usually diagnosed at birth with ambiguous genitalia.

5-ALPHA-REDUCTASE DEFICIENCY

In this condition, the fetus has an XY karyotype and normal functioning testes that produce both testosterone and AMH. However, the fetus is unable to convert testosterone to dihydrotestosterone in the peripheral tissues and so cannot virilize normally. Presentation is usually with ambiguous genitalia at birth, but can also be with increasing virilization at puberty of a female child, due to the large increase in circulating testosterone with the onset of puberty. In the Western world, the child is usually assigned a female sex, but there have been descriptions of a few communities where transition from female to male gender at puberty is accepted.

46,XX DISORDER OF SEXUAL DEVELOPMENT

The most common cause of 46,XX DSD – congenital adrenal hyperplasia (CAH) – leads to virilization of a female fetus. It is due to an enzyme deficiency in the corticosteroid production pathway in the adrenal gland, with over 90% being a deficiency in 21-hydroxylase, which converts progesterone to deoxycorticosterone and 17-hydroxyprogesterone to deoxycortisol. The reduced levels of cortisol being produced drive the negative-feedback loop, resulting in hyperplasia of the adrenal glands. This leads to an excess of androgen precursors and then to elevated testosterone production. Raised androgen levels in a female fetus will lead to virilization of the external genitalia. The clitoris is enlarged and the labia are fused and scrotal in appearance. The upper vagina joins the urethra and opens as one common channel onto the perineum. In addition, two-thirds of children with 21-hydroxylase CAH will have a 'salt-losing' variety, which also affects the ability to produce aldosterone. This represents a life-threatening situation, and those children who are salt losing often become dangerously unwell within a few days of birth. Affected individuals require lifelong steroid replacement, such as hydrocortisone, along with fludrocortisone for those who are salt losing. Once the infant is well and stabilized on their steroid regime, surgical treatment of the genitalia is considered. Traditionally, all female infants with CAH underwent feminizing genital surgery within the first year of life. This management is now controversial, as adult patients with CAH are very dissatisfied with the outcome of their surgery and argue that surgery should have been deferred until they were old enough to have a choice. Surgery certainly leaves scarring and may reduce sexual sensitivity, but the alternative of leaving the genitalia virilized throughout childhood can be difficult for parents to consider. At present, cases are managed individually by a multidisciplinary team involving surgeons, endocrinologists and psychologists.

DISORDERS OF MENSTRUAL REGULARITY

AMENORRHOEA AND OLIGOMENORRHOEA

Amenorrhoea is defined as the absence of menstruation for more than 6 months in the absence of pregnancy in a person of reproductive age, and oligomenorrhoea is defined as irregular periods at intervals of more than 35 days, with only four to nine periods a year.

BOX 3.2: Amenorrhoea

- Primary amenorrhoea is when menstruation has not commenced by 16 years of age.
- Secondary amenorrhoea is the absence of menstruation for more than 6 months in a healthy individual of reproductive age that is not due to pregnancy, lactation or the menopause.

HYPOTHALAMIC DISORDERS

Hypothalamic disorders will give rise to hypogonadotrophic hypogonadism, with the following causes:

- excessive exercise, weight loss and stress
- hypothalamic lesions (craniopharyngioma, glioma), which can compress hypothalamic tissue or block dopamine
- head injuries
- Kallmann syndrome (X-linked recessive condition resulting in deficiency in GnRH causing underdeveloped genitalia)

- systemic disorders including sarcoidosis and tuberculosis resulting in an infiltrative process in the hypothalamic–hypophyseal region
- drugs: progestogens, HRT or dopamine antagonists

PITUITARY DISORDERS

Pituitary disorders will also give rise to hypogonadotrophic hypogonadism, with the following causes:

- adenomas, of which prolactinoma is most common
- pituitary necrosis (e.g. Sheehan syndrome, due to prolonged hypotension following major obstetric haemorrhage)
- iatrogenic damage (surgery or radiotherapy)
- congenital failure of pituitary development

OVARIAN DISORDERS

Anovulation is often due to polycystic ovary syndrome (PCOS), described later in this chapter. Ovarian failure is the cause of hypergonadotrophic hypogonadism. Premature ovarian failure (POF) is defined as cessation of periods before 40 years of age and is described in **Chapter 8**.

ENDOMETRIAL DISORDERS

Primary amenorrhoea may result from Müllerian defects in the genital tract, including an absent uterus or outflow tract abnormalities, leading to a haematocolpos. Secondary amenorrhoea may result from scarring of the endometrium called Asherman syndrome and is described further in **Chapter 4**.

Findings from the history should guide the examination (**Table 3.3**). A general inspection of the patient should be carried out to assess body mass index, secondary sexual characteristics (hair growth and breast development using Tanner scores) and signs of endocrine abnormalities (hirsutism, acne, abdominal striae, moon face and skin changes). If the history is suggestive of a pituitary lesion, an assessment of visual fields is indicated. External genitalia and a vaginal examination should be performed to detect structural outflow abnormalities or demonstrate atrophic changes consistent with hypo-oestrogenism.

Table 3.3 History and examination of patients with amenorrhoea/oligomenorrhoea

Information required	Relevant factors	Possible diagnoses
Developmental history including menarche	Delayed/incomplete puberty	Congenital malformation or chromosomal abnormality
Menstrual history	Oligomenorrhoea	PCOS
	Secondary amenorrhoea	POF
Reproductive history	Infertility	PCOS
		Congenital malformation
Cyclical symptoms	Cyclical pain without menstruation	Congenital malformation
		Imperforate hymen
Hair growth	Hirsutism, androgenic alopecia	PCOS
	Hair loss	Hypothyroidism
Weight	Dramatic weight loss	Hypothalamic malfunction, hormone producing malignancy
	Difficulty losing weight	PCOS, hypothyroidism
Lifestyle	Exercise, stress	Hypothalamic malfunction
Past medical history	Systemic diseases (e.g. sarcoidosis)	Hypothalamic malfunction
Past surgical history	Evacuation of uterus	Asherman syndrome, cervical stenosis
Drug history	Dopamine agonists, HRT	Hypothalamic malfunction
	Past chemotherapy	POF
Headache, visual disturbance		Pituitary adenoma
Galactorrhoea		Prolactinoma

HRT, hormone replacement therapy; PCOS, polycystic ovary syndrome; POF, premature ovarian failure.

INVESTIGATION OF AMENORRHOEA/ OLIGOMENORRHOEA

Findings from the history and examination should guide the choice and order of investigations. A pregnancy test should be carried out if the patient is sexually active. Blood can be taken for LH, FSH and testosterone: raised LH or raised testosterone could be suggestive of PCOS, while raised FSH may be suggestive of POF. A raised prolactin level may indicate a prolactinoma. Thyroid function should be checked if clinically indicated. An ultrasound scan can be useful in detecting the classical appearances of polycystic ovaries (see **Figure 3.6**) and magnetic

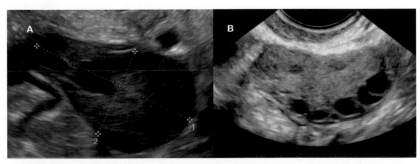

Figure 3.6 Typical ultrasound scan demonstrating normal ovary (**A**) and ovary in the case of polycystic ovary syndrome (**B**).

Table 3.4 Management of amenorrhoea/oligomenorrhoea

Cause	Management
Low BMI	Dietary advice and support
Hypothalamic lesions (e.g. glioma)	Surgery
Hyperprolactinaemia/ prolactinoma	Dopamine agonist (e.g. cabergoline or bromocriptine) or surgery if medication fails
POF	HRT or COCP (see **Chapter 8**)
PCOS	Lifestyle changes, endometrial protection (e.g. COCP, metformin, clomiphene, surgery, IVF)
Asherman syndrome	Adhesiolysis and IUD insertion at time of hysteroscopy (see **Chapter 17**)
Cervical stenosis	Hysteroscopy and cervical dilatation (see **Chapters 16** and **17**)

BMI, body mass index; COCP, combined oral contraceptive pill; HRT, hormone replacement therapy; IUD, intrauterine device; IVF, in vitro fertilization; PCOS, polycystic ovary syndrome; POF, premature ovarian failure.

resonance imaging of the brain should be carried out if symptoms are consistent with a pituitary adenoma. Hysteroscopy is not routine, but is a suitable investigation when Asherman syndrome or cervical stenosis is suspected. Karyotyping is diagnostic of Turner syndrome and other sex chromosome abnormalities.

The management of amenorrhoea/oligomenorrhoea is outlined in **Table 3.4**. More specific descriptions of management are detailed in the chapters indicated in that table.

POLYCYSTIC OVARY SYNDROME

PCOS is the most common endocrinological disorder in women of reproductive age, affecting around 8–15%, with complex reproductive, metabolic and psychological features. PCOS is a syndrome of ovarian dysfunction along with the cardinal features of hyperandrogenism and polycystic ovary morphology (**Figure 3.6**). The prevalence of polycystic ovaries seen on ultrasound is around 25% of all women but is not always associated with the full syndrome. Clinical manifestations include menstrual irregularities, signs of androgen excess (e.g. hirsutism and acne) and obesity. Elevated serum LH levels, biochemical evidence of hyperandrogenism and raised insulin resistance are also common features. The aetiology of PCOS is not completely clear, although the frequent familial trend points to a genetic cause.

CLINICAL FEATURES

- Oligomenorrhoea/amenorrhoea in up to 75% of patients, predominantly related to chronic anovulation
- Hirsutism and male pattern alopecia
- Subfertility
- Obesity in at least 40% of patients
- Acanthosis nigricans (areas of increased velvety skin pigmentation occur in the axillae and other flexures)
- May be asymptomatic

DIAGNOSIS

According to the Rotterdam diagnostic criteria, patients must have two of the following three features:

1. ovulatory dysfunction (amenorrhoea/ oligomenorrhoea)
2. clinical or biochemical hyperandrogenism
3. polycystic ovaries on ultrasound

The ultrasound criteria for the diagnosis of a polycystic ovary are eight or more subcapsular follicular cysts <10 mm in diameter and increased ovarian stroma. While these findings support a diagnosis of PCOS, they are not by themselves sufficient to identify the syndrome. Insulin resistance is a common feature of PCOS, but is not usually clinically assessed. The endocrinological and metabolic features of PCOS are associated with an increased risk of gestational and type 2 diabetes, endometrial cancer, obstructive sleep apnea and cardiovascular events.

MANAGEMENT

The management of PCOS involves the protection of the endometrium from the action of unopposed oestrogen by providing progestogens in anovulatory patients, reducing androgenic and metabolomic symptoms, treating subfertility in those trying to conceive and reducing long-term risk factors associated with endocrine and metabolic abnormalities.

Pharmacological management

Endometrial protection

- Combined oral contraceptive pill (COCP)
- Progesterone-only preparations:
  - cyclical oral progesterone, to regulate withdrawal bleeds
  - levonorgestrel intrauterine system (LNG-IUS), to provide local synthetic progestogens

Treatment of androgenic and metabolic symptoms

- For hirsutism – eflornithine cream (Vaniqua™) applied topically
- Cyproterone acetate (an antiandrogen contained in the Dianette™ contraceptive pill, sometimes used alone)
- Metformin, which is beneficial alone or in combination with other treatments to improve insulin resistance, hyperandrogenaemia, anovulation and acne while aiding weight loss
- Inositol could be considered in women with PCOS, which may improve metabolic abnormalities, but with limited clinical benefits in ovulation, hirsutism or weight reduction

Subfertility

In women with anovulatory PCOS, letrozole is the first-line pharmacological infertility therapy, while clomiphene, metformin and gonadotrophins are also options. Such medications are used either alone or in combination to induce ovulation. If these treatments are unsuccessful in inducing ovulation, laparoscopic ovarian surgery (ovarian drilling) could be a second-line therapy for women with PCOS. In vitro fertilization (IVF) is offered as a third-line treatment when ovulation induction therapies have failed.

Reducing long-term health consequences

Lifestyle advice includes weight management, dietary modification and exercise, which are essential elements for patients with PCOS, as these patients are at an increased risk of developing diabetes and cardiovascular disease later in life. The reduction of other risk factors, such as hyperlipidemia and hypertension, is important, and aerobic and weight-bearing exercise has been shown to reduce weight and improve insulin resistance. Anxiety and depressive symptoms are common and should be screened for and treated to improve emotional well-being and quality of life.

Surgical therapy

- Surgical treatments for hirsutism (e.g. laser or electrolysis)
- Ovarian drilling, that is, a laparoscopic procedure to destroy some of the ovarian stroma that may prompt ovulatory cycles
- Bariatric/metabolic surgery could be considered to improve weight loss

PREMENSTRUAL SYNDROME

Premenstrual syndrome (PMS) is the occurrence of cyclical somatic, psychological and emotional symptoms that occur in the luteal (premenstrual) phase of the menstrual cycle and resolve by the time menstruation ceases. Premenstrual symptoms occur in almost all women of reproductive age. In 3–60% of cases, symptoms are severe, causing disruption to everyday life, in particular interpersonal relationships.

AETIOLOGY

The precise aetiology of PMS is unknown, but cyclical ovarian activity and the effects of oestradiol and progesterone on certain neurotransmitters, including serotonin and gamma-aminobutyric acid, appear to play a role.

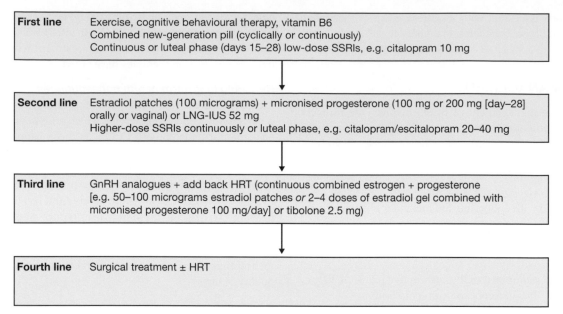

First line	Exercise, cognitive behavioural therapy, vitamin B6 Combined new-generation pill (cyclically or continuously) Continuous or luteal phase (days 15–28) low-dose SSRIs, e.g. citalopram 10 mg
Second line	Estradiol patches (100 micrograms) + micronised progesterone (100 mg or 200 mg [day–28] orally or vaginal) or LNG-IUS 52 mg Higher-dose SSRIs continuously or luteal phase, e.g. citalopram/escitalopram 20–40 mg
Third line	GnRH analogues + add back HRT (continuous combined estrogen + progesterone [e.g. 50–100 micrograms estradiol patches *or* 2–4 doses of estradiol gel combined with micronised progesterone 100 mg/day] or tibolone 2.5 mg)
Fourth line	Surgical treatment ± HRT

Figure 3.7 Algorithm for the treatment of premenstrual syndrome (PMS). (GnRH, gonadotrophin-releasing hormone; HRT, hormone replacement therapy; SSRI, selective serotonin reuptake inhibitor.) (From Royal College of Obstetricians and Gynaecologists (2017). Green-top guideline No 48: Management of premenstrual syndrome. *BJOG: An International Journal of Obstetrics & Gynaecology*, 24(3): e73–e105. With permission from John Wiley & Sons.)

HISTORY AND EXAMINATION

To make a diagnosis, symptoms should be recorded prospectively, over at least two consecutive menstrual cycles, as retrospective recall of symptoms is unreliable. The cyclical nature of symptoms and their impact on daily activities is the cornerstone of the diagnosis. A short course of GnRH analogues is sometimes used if the history is insufficient to make a diagnosis.

BOX 3.3: Symptoms of PMS

- Mood swings
- Feeling depressed, irritable or bad tempered
- Feeling anxious, upset or emotional
- Tiredness or difficulty sleeping
- Headaches
- Changes in appetite and food cravings
- Feeling clumsy
- Fluid retention and feeling bloated
- Changes to skin or hair
- Sore or tender breasts

MANAGEMENT

The management of PMS is depicted in **Figure 3.7**.

Lifestyle changes

Lifestyle changes include stress reduction, alcohol and caffeine limitation, and exercise. Cognitive behavioural therapy (CBT) and other psychological counselling treatments should also be considered as an initial treatment option for severe PMS.

Medical treatments

Hormonal

The hormonal management of PMS works by effectively stopping ovulation and cyclical hormone changes:

- COCP – bicycling or tricycling pill packets (i.e. taking two or three packets in a row without a scheduled break)
- transdermal oestrogen by patch, gel or implant – these contain lower doses of oestrogen than the COCP and can be given with a shortened

7-day course of a progestogen each month for endometrial protection

- GnRH analogues – treatment requires a continuous combined form of HRT or tibilone (selective oestrogen receptor modulator) therapy to be administered concurrently to reduce the risk of osteoporosis, and surveillance with bone mineral density scans for those on long-term GnRH analogues

Non-hormonal

- *Selective serotonin reuptake inhibitors (SSRIs)* – these significantly improve PMS and can be given at low doses initially and titrated to higher doses. SSRIs are particularly effective when used in combination with CBT.
- *Vitamins and other supplements* – vitamin B6 has been shown to be effective in randomized controlled trials and there is also limited evidence for the benefits of using magnesium, calcium and isoflavones.
- *Alternative therapies* – although there is mixed evidence for some benefit from therapies such as St John's wort, ginkgo biloba, saffron, vitex agnus-castus (a herb known as chasteberry), evening primrose oil, reflexology and acupuncture, further robust studies are warranted before recommending them for PMS.

Surgical treatments

Surgery aims to stop the ovarian cycle with bilateral salpingo-oophorectomy and hysterectomy. This should be considered as a last resort, when other treatments have failed. Before surgery, a pre-operative trial of GnRH analogue should be used to 'test' expected symptom relief and confirm tolerance to HRT.

KEY LEARNING POINTS

- The hypothalamus, the pituitary gland, the ovary and the end organ endometrium have an intricate interplay.
- Normal puberty and a regular menstrual cycle require the function of each organ and healthy hormonal interaction.
- DSDs may be diagnosed at birth but some cause delayed puberty or primary amenorrhoea.
- Oligomenorrhoea and amenorrhoea may be primary or secondary and may be caused by hypothalamic, pituitary, ovarian or other hormonal disorders. They can also be caused by endometrial problems.
- PCOS is a common disorder associated with oligomenorrhoea or amenorrhoea.
- PMS is common and can be treated with simple remedies or with those that stop the ovarian hormone cycle.

FURTHER READING

European Society of Human Reproduction and Embryology (2018). International evidence-based guideline for the assessment and management of polycystic ovary syndrome (PCOS). https://www.eshre.eu/Guidelines-and-Legal/Guidelines/Polycystic-Ovary-Syndrome.

Hughes IA, Houk C, Ahmed SF, Lee PA; LWPES Consensus Group; ESPE Consensus Group (2006). Consensus statement on management of intersex disorders. *Archives of Disease in Childhood*, 91(7): 554–563.

Royal College of Obstetricians and Gynaecologists (2017). Green-top guideline No 48: Management of premenstrual syndrome. *BJOG: An International Journal of Obstetrics & Gynaecology*, 24(3): e73–e105.

Tempest N, Hill CJ, Maclean A, Marston K, Powell SG, Al-Lamee H, Hapangama DK (2022). Endometrial glands: Implications in endometrial regeneration and pathologies. *Human Reproduction Update*, 28(2): 153–171.

SELF-ASSESSMENT

For interactive SBAs and EMQs relating to this chapter, visit www.routledge.com/cw/crosbie.

CASE HISTORY 1

A 14-year-old girl attends the gynaecological outpatient department with delayed menarche. She is 145 cm tall and has normal female external genitalia but has no secondary sexual characteristics. Transabdominal ultrasound scan demonstrates a small uterus but neither ovary can be identified.

A What is the most likely diagnosis and what further symptoms she may have?
B What additional investigations would you request?
C How would you manage her?

ANSWERS

A Turner syndrome (lacking X-chromosomal material, e.g. 45,XO) is the likely diagnosis here. She may have other features, such as a short webbed neck, cubitus valgus, shield chest, a history of middle ear infections, epicanthus and micrognathia. Her blood pressure may be high, and there may be signs of congenital cardiac abnormalities (e.g. bicuspid valve or coarctation of the aorta) and endocrine and autoimmune disease (e.g. diabetes, thyroid disease or inflammatory bowel disease).

B Assessing her hormone profile will demonstrate high gonadotrophins, low oestrogen and low AMH. Further tests should include karyotyping and cardiac, renal, bone and endocrinology investigations.

C Treatment is via a specialist multidisciplinary team and involves HRT and appropriate management of comorbid conditions. Puberty induction and maintenance of feminization throughout life is needed, using ovarian hormone replacement (transdermal route preferred) and if possible growth hormone to increase final height during childhood/adolescence. Subfertility is common, but pregnancy can be achieved with assisted reproduction techniques with egg donation or ovarian cryo-preservation, but pregnancy is associated with increased risks due to associated comorbidities (e.g. dissecting aortic aneurysm). Lifelong surveillance with multidisciplinary teams to manage her likely multiple comorbidities is recommended. Psychological support is also important.

CASE HISTORY 2

A 28-year-old woman consults her general practitioner (GP), complaining of having no periods after coming off the COCP 12 months ago. She complains of increasing weight, excessive facial hair and male pattern hair loss.

A What additional features of the history will be helpful?
B If she has been in a relationship, what initial bedside test should her GP consider?
C Outline the investigations and management of this case.

ANSWERS

A This young woman presents with a typical history of PCOS (post-pill amenorrhoea usually only lasts up to 6 months). Her menstrual history before starting the COCP may reveal oligomenorrhoea and she may have symptoms and signs of clinical hyperandrogenism, including acne, alopecia and hirsutism. Her previous obstetric history and future plans for fertility are important in selecting investigative and management plans. Her current sexual history and contraindications to hormonal contraceptives are also important.

B Pregnancy test is indicated to exclude a pregnancy.

C Initial investigations may include transvaginal ultrasound scan (demonstrating typical enlarged ovaries containing >10 small follicles) and increased stromal echogenicity and/or a blood test to confirm biochemical hyperandrogenism with free testosterone (high LH/FSH ratio and normal oestrogen but a lack of progesterone may also indicate PCOS). Positive findings from either investigation in combination with amenorrhoea are sufficient to make a diagnosis of PCOS. Education and support to achieve a normal weight and adapt a healthy lifestyle will promote spontaneous ovulation and reduce the long-term consequences of PCOS. The first-line medical treatment in those who do not wish to get pregnant is the COCP for endometrial protection, but LNG-IUS or cyclical progestins are further options. However, if she wishes to conceive, referral to a specialist clinic for ovulation induction with letrozole, clomid or metformin needs to be arranged.

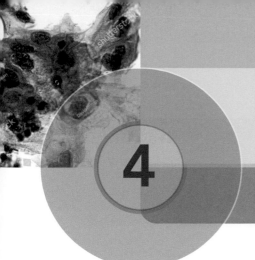

Disorders of menstrual bleeding

4

DHARANI K HAPANGAMA

Learning Objectives
- Understand the symptoms and aetiology of abnormal uterine bleeding.
- Describe the terminology of abnormal uterine bleeding.
- Understand the symptoms, investigations and management of heavy menstrual bleeding.
- Appreciate the impact of heavy menstrual bleeding on quality of life.
- Understand the causes and investigation of painful periods.
- Understand the action of medication used for heavy menstrual bleeding and painful periods.

INTRODUCTION

The impact of disorders of menstrual bleeding, now termed abnormal uterine bleeding (AUB), is considerable, with prevalence ranges from 3% to 30% in the reproductive-age population. AUB is one of the most common reasons for women to attend their general practitioner (GP) and, subsequently, a gynaecologist, and there is an age-related increase in AUB at the start and end of reproductive life (adolescents and perimenopausal age groups). Although rarely life threatening, menstrual disorders can be a major social, psychological and occupational burden. Patients present with symptoms of heavy menstrual bleeding (HMB), intermenstrual bleeding (IMB), post-coital bleeding (PCB) and postmenopausal bleeding (PMB). Initial investigations include pelvic and speculum examinations (if indicated), swabs for

microbiology and cervical screening, transvaginal ultrasound scan (TVUSS), outpatient hysteroscopy and endometrial biopsy as necessary.

There are several classification systems for AUB, some of which link symptoms to pathology. Such systems help clinicians to adopt a similar categorization of the pathology they are seeing, which helps audit and research. One system that is increasingly recognized is the system developed by the International Federation of Gynecology and Obstetrics (FIGO), which is named after the following visually objective structural criteria – polyps, adenomyosis, leiomyoma and malignancy – and the following causes unrelated to structural anomalies – coagulopathy, ovulatory disorders, endometrial, iatrogenic and not classified causes – namely PALM-COEIN (see 'Further reading'). Note that further descriptions in this chapter for causes of AUB do not refer specifically to this system.

10.1201/9781003218036-4

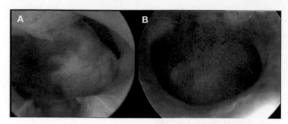

Figure 4.1 Hysteroscopic view of an endometrial polyp (**A**) and a normal uterine cavity (**B**).

Associated with structural abnormalities (PALM)

- Endometrial polyps (**Figure 4.1**)
- Adenomyosis: 70% of cases will have AUB/HMB
- Leiomyomas (fibroids): 30% of HMB is associated with fibroids
- Endometrial hyperplasia or malignancy of endometrium/cervix

Not associated with structural abnormalities (COEIN)

- Coagulation disorders (e.g. von Willebrand disease)
- Ovarian disorders (e.g. polycystic ovary syndrome)
- Endometrial dysfunction
- Diagnosis of exclusion of iatrogenic causes:
  - drug therapy (e.g. warfarin)
  - intrauterine devices
- Not otherwise classified (e.g. uterine aterio-venous malformations, thyroid dysfunction)

Other symptoms may be described in patients with HMB that may indicate underlying pathology, as shown in **Table 4.1**. Despite appropriate investigations, when no pathology can be identified endometrial dysfunction is the diagnosis of exclusion. Disordered endometrial prostaglandin production, abnormalities of endometrial vascular development, endometrial regeneration, hypoxia and immune cell function have all been implicated in the aetiology of endometrial dysfunction.

HEAVY MENSTRUAL BLEEDING

HMB is the most common type of menstrual bleeding disorder. There has previously been some confusion over the various terminologies used for abnormalities of excessive menstrual blood loss. HMB is now the preferred description, as it is simple and easily translatable into other languages. It replaces the older term 'menorrhagia'.

The methods to quantify menstrual blood loss are both inaccurate (poor correlation with haemoglobin level) and impractical. The previous definition of HMB as blood loss of greater than 80 mL per period has now been replaced by the following more clinically relevant and patient-focused definition proposed by the National Institute for Health and Care Excellence (NICE): 'excessive menstrual blood loss that interferes with the physical, social, emotional, and/or material quality of life'.

Each year in the UK, 1 million women between the ages of 30 and 49 years consult their GP with HMB, with the associated estimated loss of 5 million workdays. Indeed, 20–30% of women of reproductive age are reported to suffer from HMB.

The aetiology of HMB includes the following common causes.

HISTORY AND EXAMINATION

The clinical history and examination should be focused on understanding the nature of the bleeding,

Table 4.1 Symptoms that may be associated with heavy menstrual bleeding (HMB) and related pathologies

Symptoms associated with HMB	Related pathologies
Irregular bleeding, IMB, PCB	Endometrial or cervical polyp or other cervical abnormality, anovulatory bleeding, hormonal medications
Excessive bruising/ bleeding from other sites	Coagulation disorder (coagulation disorders will be present in 20% of those presenting with 'unexplained' HMB)
History of post-partum haemorrhage	
Excessive post-operative bleeding	
Excessive bleeding with dental extractions	
Family history of bleeding problems	
Unusual vaginal discharge	Pelvic inflammatory disease, cervical pathologies
Urinary symptoms, abdominal mass or abdominal fullness	Pressure from fibroids
Weight change, acne, hirsutism/alopecia, skin changes, fatigue	Thyroid disease, polycystic ovary syndrome

IMB, intermenstrual bleeding; PCB, post-coital bleeding.

any related symptoms that suggest underlying causes and the impact of the symptoms on quality of life, and should also aim to rule out red-flag signs of malignancy to guide the choice of first-line investigations for patients with HMB.

The relevant questions to determine the heaviness of the period and the extent to which it disrupts the activities of daily living and causes anaemia are covered in **Chapter 2**. In younger women, it is important to question whether HMB started at menarche, as this is much less likely to be associated with pathology. The regularity of the menstrual cycle is also important, as heavy anovulatory bleeds may be associated with early puberty, polycystic ovary syndrome or the perimenopause.

After examining the patient for signs of anaemia, it is important to perform an abdominal and pelvic examination in patients complaining of HMB. This enables any pelvic masses to be palpated, the cervix to be visualized for polyps/carcinoma, swabs to be taken if pelvic infection is suspected and cervical screening to be performed if it is due. The exception to this rule is for young women and girls with HMB and no associated symptoms, in whom it may be appropriate to initiate pharmacological treatment without pelvic examination.

INVESTIGATIONS

The NICE guidelines for HMB indicate that the following investigations may be useful.

- Full blood count (FBC).
- **Pelvic ultrasound scan.** This is used in patients suspected of having large fibroids (pressure symptoms or enlarged uterus palpable), endometrial polyps, pelvic mass or adenomyosis and in those for whom examination is inconclusive or difficult, for example in patients with an elevated body mass index.
- **Endometrial biopsy.** This is recommended in perimenopausal individuals >45 years of age, who are at an increased risk of hyperplasia and malignancy. Endometrial biopsy is also recommended before endometrial ablation, to confirm normal endometrial histology. Hysteroscopy (**Figure 4.2**) is indicated for those suspected of having a submucosal fibroid or endometrial polyp, which is usually done in the outpatient setting. Hysteroscopy allows for concomitant treatment of intrauterine pathologies, such as resection of submucosal fibroids and polyps, as well as initiating treatments, such as with the levonorgestrel intrauterine system (LNG-IUS, Mirena™) (**Figure 4.3**).
- **Coagulation screen.** This should only be considered if there has been HMB since menarche or there is a family history of coagulation defects.
- **Hormone testing.** This is not performed routinely; it is performed only if an

endocrinopathy (e.g. polycystic ovary syndrome or thyroid dysfunction) is suggested by the history.

- **High vaginal and endocervical swabs.** These should be taken if there are signs of pelvic infection, as such swabs are important for identifying sexually transmitted infections.

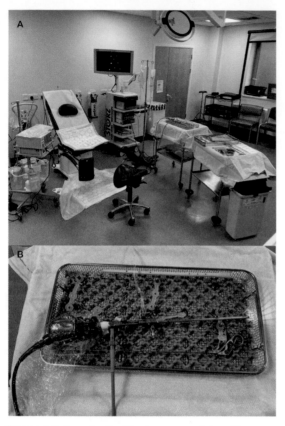

Figure 4.2 An outpatient hysteroscopy clinic setting (**A**) and hysteroscope (**B**).

BOX 4.2: Role of endometrial biopsy in HMB

An endometrial biopsy is indicated prior to ablative techniques or if there is:

- PMB and endometrial thickness >4 mm on TVUSS
- persistent PMB irrespective of endometrial thickness
- HMB in a patient older than 45 years of age
- HMB associated with IMB
- treatment failure

MANAGEMENT

All patients complaining of excessive menstrual blood loss that interferes with their physical, social, emotional and/or material quality of life should be offered treatment. The effectiveness of medical

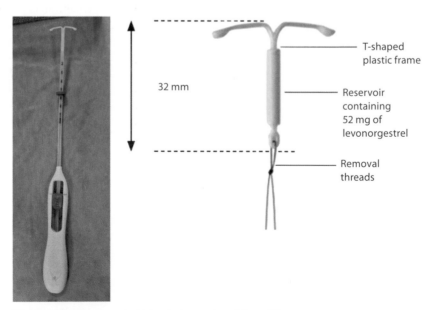

32 mm

T-shaped plastic frame

Reservoir containing 52 mg of levonorgestrel

Removal threads

Figure 4.3 Levonorgestrel intrauterine system (Mirena™).

treatments is often temporary, while surgical treatments are mostly incompatible with desired fertility.

When counselling patients for HMB treatment, the discussion should cover:

- all available treatment options
- the benefits and risks of each option
- the patient's wish for future fertility
- suitable treatments for those trying to conceive
- the presence or absence of structural abnormalities (fibroids, polyps or adenomyosis)
- associated symptoms, such as pain or pressure symptoms
- any contraindications to medical therapies or existing comorbidities
- the patient's suitability for surgery or an anaesthetic
- the patient's previous surgical history on the uterus or abdominal surgery

---

BOX 4.3: Management of HMB

Medical therapy

- Tranexamic acid/non-steroidal anti-inflammatory drugs (NSAIDs: mefenamic acid)
- LNG-IUS
- Combined oral contraceptive pill (COCP)
- Progestogens

Surgery

- Endometrial ablation
- Myomectomy in those who wish to retain fertility with large fibroids
- Hysterectomy

Other treatments

- Umbilical artery embolization (UAE) for fibroids
- High-intensity focused ultrasound (HIFU) therapy
- Transcervical fibroid ablation (e.g. high-resolution ultrasound, Sonata™)

MEDICAL

The initial management of HMB in the absence of structural or histological abnormality is medical treatment. NICE guidelines suggest the following order.

1. LNG-IUS (Mirena™) for long-term symptom control of up to 5 years. The LNG-IUS (as further described in **Chapter 6**) has revolutionized the treatment of HMB by providing a highly effective alternative to surgical treatment with few side effects and less risk (**Figure 4.3**). Reductions in mean blood loss of around 95% are achieved by 1 year after LNG-IUS insertion and around 7 or 8 users out of 10 will have amenorrhoea. NICE guidelines (2018; see 'Further reading') and the Royal College of Obstetricians and Gynaecologists have suggested that the LNG-IUS be considered in the majority of patients as an alternative to surgical treatment.

2. Tranexamic acid, an antifibrinolytic that reduces blood loss by 50% and is taken during menstruation; mefenamic acid, which inhibits prostaglandin synthesis, reduces blood loss by 25% and improves pain; the COCP, which will induce slightly lighter periods and, as successive packets can be taken back to back (tricycling), can reduce bleed frequency; and progestogen-only contraceptives, which may suppress menstruation in some patients.

3. Cyclical oral progestogens such as norethisterone can be taken in a cyclical pattern from day 6 to day 26 of the menstrual cycle.

4. Gonadotrophin-releasing hormone (GnRH) agonists. These drugs are usually taken as slow-releasing depot injections and act on the pituitary to stop the production of gonadotrophins, thus switching off the ovaries and resulting in amenorrhoea. They are usually used in the short term due to the associated hypo-oestrogenic state and consequential osteoporosis. They may be used pre-operatively to shrink fibroids or cause endometrial suppression to enhance visualization at hysteroscopy. In severe HMB, they can allow the patient the opportunity to improve their haemoglobin by providing a respite from bleeding.

5. Alternative new pharmacological treatments for HMB. Ulipristal acetate, a progesterone receptor modulator, was previously licensed for general use in patients with HMB and fibroids. Its use has now been restricted in the UK

and worldwide, due to the rare complication of serious liver injury associated with its use. It can be used for intermittent treatment of moderate to severe symptoms of uterine fibroids before the menopause and only when surgical procedures (including uterine fibroid embolization) are not suitable or have failed. Oral GnRH antagonists have been shown in phase 3 trials to be an effective treatment for fibroid-associated HMB, and three drugs of this class (elagolix, relugolix and linzagolix) are now licensed for use in several countries worldwide. These medications are usually combined with add-back hormone replacement therapy (HRT) to overcome hypo-oestrogenic side effects.

SURGICAL

Details of surgical interventions including pre-operative assessment, consent and complications are covered in **Chapter 17**.

Minimally invasive treatments for heavy menstrual bleeding

Surgical treatment is normally restricted to individuals for whom fertility is no longer desired and medical treatments have failed or when there are associated symptoms such as pressure symptoms from fibroids or prolapse.

Endometrial ablation
All endometrial destructive procedures employ the principle that ablation of the endometrium to sufficient depth to completely remove the stem-cell-rich basalis layer prevents its regeneration. Ablation is suitable for patients with a uterus no bigger than 10 weeks' size and with fibroids less than 3 cm. The risks of a pregnancy after an ablation procedure theoretically include prematurity and placenta accreta spectrum disorder (morbidly adherent placenta); therefore, ablation is only recommended for individuals who have completed their family or those who do not wish to have children.

First-generation techniques, including transcervical resection of the endometrium with electrical diathermy or rollerball ablation, have now been replaced by newer, second-generation, techniques that use hydrothermal (e.g. ThermaChoice®), radiofrequency (e.g. Novosure™), cryoablation (e.g. Her Option™) or microwave (e.g. Microsulis™) energy to destroy the endometrium with a better side-effect profile.

According to the recent Cochrane review (see 'Further reading'), endometrial ablation provides significant reduction in menstrual bleeding, with similar rates of patient satisfaction and quality of life to hysterectomy at 2 years after treatment. Some patients require repeat surgical procedures (including hysterectomy) due to treatment failure (3.3–13% at 1-year post-ablation). Endometrial ablation is often carried out in the outpatient setting and is associated with fewer adverse events, including quicker return to work and resumption of normal daily activities, than following hysterectomy. Although data from long-term follow-up is lacking, younger patients with HMB are more likely to undergo hysterectomy after endometrial ablation than LNG-IUS and, conversely, older patients with HMB are more likely to require a hysterectomy after failed LNG-IUS than endometrial ablation.

Minimally invasive treatments for heavy menstrual bleeding with fibroids
Umbilical artery embolization
UAE is a treatment useful for HMB associated with fibroids, as discussed in **Chapter 12**. UAE significantly reduces fibroid-related bleeding, with symptomatic improvement in over 80% of patients, but its long-term effectiveness and impact on future fertility is uncertain.

Laparoscopic or open myomectomy
This may be another option for patients with HMB secondary to large fibroids with pressure symptoms who wish to conceive in the future (and are at an age when this plan is realistic) (see **Chapter 12**). The procedure carries a small risk of emergency hysterectomy and, if the uterine cavity is opened, future pregnancies are at an increased risk of uterine rupture and placenta accreta spectrum disorders.

Transcervical (hysteroscopic) resection of fibroid
Transcervical resection of a large submucosal fibroid using a variety of energy sources may reduce HMB

and may also increase the chance of conception in patients wishing to conceive.

Non-surgical treatments for fibroids

In patients who wish to retain their uterus, there are many minimally invasive treatment options for fibroids, such as magnetic resonance- or ultrasound-guided HIFU, laparoscopic/hysteroscopic cryomyolysis, microwave ablation and laser ablation, and they are being used clinically for fibroid-associated HMB. However, the effectiveness of and the long-term safety data for these techniques is still lacking.

Hysterectomy

A hysterectomy is the surgical removal of the uterus, as described in **Chapter 17**. It can be avoided by medical and ablation procedures. However, it can be necessary to control HMB in those patients who have not responded. It is a first-line treatment in those individuals who have HMB associated with large fibroids who also have severe pressure symptoms or in those with associated uterine prolapse. The route of hysterectomy for HMB should be determined on an individual basis. Hysterectomy for HMB is now routinely performed via minimal access route, whereby the uterus, cervix and fallopian tubes are resected laparoscopically with conservation of the ovaries if they appear to be normal. However, hysterectomy is associated with premature ovarian failure in around 25% of patients, even when the ovaries are preserved. As most aggressive epithelial ovarian cancers are thought to originate in the fallopian tubes, their removal at hysterectomy for HMB is recommended. Evan large fibroid uteri can be resected laparoscopically after morcellation procedures, but the possibility of occult malignancy (e.g. leiomyosarcoma) should be excluded first. Transabdominal hysterectomy may be necessary for patients with larger fibroids and other comorbidities that are not compatible with laparoscopy. Although vaginal hysterectomy may be considered in patients with significant prolapse, the removal of the fallopian tubes is not always possible via this route. Subtotal hysterectomy, whereby the uterus is removed but the cervix is retained, is an option for some patients, but future removal of the cervical stump can be challenging.

BOX 4.4: Management of acute HMB

1. Admit
2. Intravenous access and resuscitation or transfusion as required
3. Pelvic examination
4. FBC, coagulopathy screen and biochemistry
5. Tranexamic acid, orally or intravenously
6. TVUSS
7. High-dose progestogens to arrest bleeding
8. Consider suppression with GnRH in the medium term
9. Immediate surgical intervention for causes such as prolapsing fibroid polyp
10. Longer-term plan when a diagnosis has been made

ACUTE HEAVY MENSTRUAL BLEEDING

Acute HMB is an episode of heavy bleeding that requires immediate intervention to reduce or arrest further blood loss. Acute HMB may present in patients with chronic HMB or in those without a prior history. Patients are usually admitted to hospital, where they require stabilization, examination to exclude cervical abnormalities and pelvic masses, medication to arrest bleeding (tranexamic acid, high-dose progestogens or GnRH analogues) and correct anaemia (blood or iron infusion), investigation and treatment of the underlying cause and are discharged with a long-term plan to avoid further admissions.

DYSMENORRHOEA

Dysmenorrhoea is defined as painful menstruation. It is experienced by 45–95% of women of reproductive age. Primary dysmenorrhoea is cyclical period pain without any obvious identifiable pathology. It is usually present from menarche. Patients complain of abdominal and pelvic pain, often with associated headaches, flushing, nausea, sweating and cramps, with the latter probably related to prostaglandin and associated inflammatory mediators. Treatment can be initiated with NSAIDs and/or hormonal contraceptives in women with a typical history and this can be done without further investigations. In the case of treatment failure, investigations can be started for causes of secondary dysmenorrhoea.

Secondary dysmenorrhoea develops over time and may be associated with underlying pathology, specifically endometriosis, adenomyosis, pelvic inflammatory disease (PID), cervical stenosis and haematometra. It may be associated with other chronic pain symptoms such as non-cyclical pelvic pain, dyspareunia, pain with urination or defecation, and rectal bleeding.

HISTORY AND EXAMINATION

What constitutes a painful period is patient dependent and therefore the available treatments are neither universally effective nor acceptable. To ascertain the how the period pain affects the patient's quality of life and disrupts their daily activities, the following questions may be useful:

- Do you need to take painkillers for this pain? Which tablets help?
- Have you needed to take any time off work/ school due to the pain?

When evaluating dysmenorrhoea, abdominal and pelvic examinations should be performed, except in adolescents, for whom empirical treatment for primary dysmenorrhoea is standard. Certain signs associated with endometriosis include a tender pelvic mass (an endometrioma), a fixed uterus (due to associated adhesions) and induration/tethering or endometriotic nodules typically palpable in the posterior vaginal fornix. An enlarged, tender uterus may be found with adenomyosis. Abnormal discharge and tenderness with more acute symptoms may be seen with PID, which can be associated with a tubo-ovarian abscess.

INVESTIGATIONS

The following investigations are appropriate in women with secondary dysmenorrhoea.

- High vaginal and endocervical swabs are recommended when PID and an infective cause is suspected.

- TVUSS may be useful to detect endometriomas, adenomyosis (enlarged uterus with heterogeneous texture), tubo-ovarian abscess or fibroids.
- If initial assessment suggests severe endometriosis involving the bowel, magnetic resonance imaging is indicated, as it provides useful information regarding the presence and the extent of deep infiltrating endometriosis, allowing patients to be referred to a specialized centre managing severe endometriosis that can plan surgery and counsel patients appropriately.
- Diagnostic laparoscopy may be performed to investigate secondary dysmenorrhoea when the history is suggestive of endometriosis and when empirical treatment with medical therapy has failed or is inappropriate. Discussion about invasive investigations, particularly laparoscopy, should include its surgical and anaesthetic risks, as well as the possibility that it will find no obvious cause for their symptoms. Laparoscopy is not usually indicated as the initial investigation for primary dysmenorrhoea, unless medical treatment fails.
- Cervical stenosis is an infrequent cause of dysmenorrhoea, and if the history or TVUSS suggest cervical stenosis, hysteroscopy (with or without ultrasound guidance) can be used to confirm the diagnosis.

MANAGEMENT

- Simple analgesia with NSAIDs is effective for many affected individuals. Examples are naproxen, ibuprofen and mefenamic acid.
- Hormonal contraceptives such as the COCP are widely used, but a Cochrane review of randomized controlled trials (see 'Further reading') provides little evidence supporting the COCP as an effective treatment for primary dysmenorrhoea or endometriosis-associated pain. Progestogens – given orally (desogestrol), parenterally as a depot injection (medroxyprogesterone) or as a subdermal implant (etonogestrel) – may be useful to

achieve amenorrhoea and thus provide effective relief in primary and secondary dysmenorrhoea.

- There is evidence that LNG-IUS is beneficial for dysmenorrhoea and indeed can be an effective treatment for underlying causes, such as endometriosis and adenomyosis. It is often used before or after surgical treatment, fitted at the time of laparoscopy.
- GnRH analogues are not a first-line treatment or an option for prolonged management of primary dysmenorrhoea due to their hypo-oestrogenic side effects, but there is strong evidence that GnRH analogues provide an effective means of reducing pain in patients with endometriosis. GnRH analogues are often used with add-back HRT to reduce hypo-oestrogenic side effects. These can be used to manage symptoms if awaiting hysterectomy or as a form of assessment of the benefits of hysterectomy. If the pain does not settle with the GnRH analogue, it is less likely to be resolved by hysterectomy. The new orally active GnRH antagonists are also shown to be effective for endometriosis-associated pain, and are licensed to be used for this indication in some countries.
- Uterus-sparing new non-pharmacological treatments for adenomyosis-associated dysmenorrhea are being evaluated. They include surgical resection and ablation, including UAE, radiofrequency ablation and HIFU, but evidence from randomized controlled trials supporting their effectiveness and safety is lacking.
- With regard to surgery, signs or symptoms of pathology such as endometriosis may warrant surgical laparoscopy to perform adhesiolysis, excise endometriosis and remove endometriomas. If severe endometriosis is diagnosed, surgical treatment should be offered via specialist centres with a multidisciplinary team including specialist gynaecologists and colorectal and urological surgeons, with input from fertility specialists, pain specialists, radiologists, psychologists, etc., for the best outcomes.

- There is some evidence to suggest that a low-fat, vegetarian diet, exercise and physiotherapy may improve dysmenorrhoea. Applying heat and using transcutaneous electrical nerve stimulation (TENS) may also reduce pain, but robust data are lacking for their impact on improving quality of life.

KEY LEARNING POINTS

- HMB is one of the most frequent reasons for consultation in primary care and referral to secondary care.
- HMB may be associated with symptoms that indicate pathology, such as fibroids or adenomyosis.
- First-line treatment of HMB is usually medical: LNG-IUS, NSAIDs or other reversible hormonal treatments.
- Second-generation endometrial ablation techniques should be offered before hysterectomy for HMB.
- Women with other associated pathology, for example pressure symptoms with fibroids or uterovaginal prolapse, may opt for hysterectomy.
- Primary dysmenorrhoea is rarely pathological.
- Secondary dysmenorrhoea may be associated with pathology, such as endometriosis, adenomyosis or chronic PID.
- First-line treatment of dysmenorrhoea is medical: NSAIDs, the COCP or progestogens.
- Women with secondary dysmenorrhoea and signs or symptoms of other pathology, or who are not responding to medical treatment, may be investigated with laparoscopy.

FURTHER READING

Becker CM, Bokor A, Heikinheimo O, Horne A, Jansen F, Kiesel L, King K, Kvaskoff M, Nap A, Petersen K, Saridogan E, Tomassetti C, van Hanegem N, Vulliemoz N, Vermeulen N; ESHRE Endometriosis Guideline Group (2022). ESHRE guideline: endometriosis. *Human Reproduction Open*, 2022(2): hoac009.

Bofill Rodriguez M, Dias S, Jordan V, Lethaby A, Lensen SF, Wise MR, Wilkinson J, Brown J, Farquhar C (2022). Interventions for heavy menstrual bleeding; overview of Cochrane reviews and network meta-analysis. *Cochrane Database of Systemic Reviews*, 5(5): CD013180.

Brown J, Crawford TJ, Datta S, Prentice A (2018). Oral contraceptives for pain associated with endometriosis. *Cochrane Database of Systemic Reviews*, 5(5): CD001019.

Munro MG, Critchley HOD, Fraser IS; FIGO Menstrual Disorders Committee (2018). The two FIGO systems for normal and abnormal uterine bleeding symptoms and classification of causes of abnormal uterine bleeding in the reproductive years: 2018 revisions. *International Journal of Gynecology & Obstetrics*, 143(3): 393–408. https://doi.org/10.1002/ijgo.12666.

NICE (2018). *Heavy Menstrual Bleeding: Assessment and Management*. NICE guideline [NG88]. Last updated: 24 May 2021. https://www.nice.org.uk/guidance/ng88.

SELF-ASSESSMENT

For interactive SBAs and EMQs relating to this chapter, visit www.routledge.com/cw/crosbie.

CASE HISTORY 1

A 28-year-old woman has presented to her GP with HMB of 2 years' duration. She also complains of dysmenorrhoea that is getting worse. On examination, there is tethering and tenderness in the posterior fornix.

A What additional features of the history are important?
B What are the initial investigations?
C What is your management plan?

ANSWERS

A When taking the history, it is important to determine how much the patient's periods are interfering with their daily life and sexual relations. The timing of the pain in the menstrual cycle is important. Their plans for pregnancy will influence the choice of treatment, as will any previous treatments and drug allergies or contraindications.

The patient tells you that they need analgesia and frequent sanitary changes. The patient works as a nurse and is finding some shifts difficult and so has taken some sick days. The pain is worse before the period rather than with the menstrual bleed. Additionally, they have been trying to conceive for the last year and have experienced painful sexual intercourse.

B Appropriate investigations include FBC, TVUSS, high vaginal swab and endocervical swab to exclude an infective cause for pain; however, the history is typical of HMB and dysmenorrhoea associated with endometriosis.

C Treatment options are limited by the desire to conceive. It is appropriate to offer simple analgesia and laparoscopy to diagnose/treat endometriosis. It may be appropriate to perform tubal insufflation at the same time, as there has been a slight delay in conception.

CASE HISTORY 2

A 48-year-old woman presents to the gynaecology emergency room complaining of an excessively heavy period, which makes her dizzy. She gives a history of having progressively heavy, irregular bleeding for at least a year, which is interfering with her daily life. She's up to date with cervical screening. On examination, you identify a large, smooth but hard mass prolapsing through the cervix.

A What is your diagnosis?
B What initial investigations will you do?
C Outline the management.

ANSWERS

A Prolapsing pedunculated submucosal fibroid polyp is the diagnosis.
B The following investigations should be undertaken: FBC to assess the severity of anaemia and coagulation screen, TVUSS to confirm pelvic anatomy and urgent hysteroscopy and endometrial biopsy to exclude underlying malignancy.
C Initial management will include stabilizing the patient, intravenous cannulation and blood cross-matching and starting intravenous or oral tranexamic acid and oral norethisterone 5 mg three times per day to arrest bleeding, and GnRH analogues can be considered for continuous relief of bleeding until definitive management is organised. The patient may need blood or an iron transfusion and, at the time of the diagnostic hysteroscopy, transcervical resection of the fibroid could be done either by securing the pedicle and resecting or with the available devices, such as MyoSure™. Offering her an LNG-IUS to be fitted after resection of the fibroid will ensure long-term reduction of bleeding.

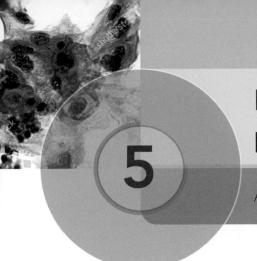

Implantation and early pregnancy

ANDREW HORNE

> **Learning Objectives**
> - Understand the social and emotional context of early pregnancy loss.
> - Understand why a high suspicion of ectopic pregnancy is needed in all women of reproductive age with symptoms.
> - Obtain a detailed knowledge of the clinical presentation and management of miscarriage and ectopic pregnancy.
> - Obtain an awareness of less common early pregnancy conditions, including recurrent miscarriage, gestational trophoblastic disease and hyperemesis gravidarum.

IMPLANTATION AND THE ESTABLISHMENT OF PREGNANCY

After ovulation, the cells of the dominant follicle form the corpus luteum (CL), and the CL produces large amounts of progesterone. Progesterone prepares the endometrium (decidualization) to support a pregnancy. Successful implantation occurs when the oocyte is fertilized in the fallopian tube and implants in the endometrium, around 7 days after ovulation (**Figure 5.1**). The implanted blastocyst secretes human chorionic gonadotrophin (hCG). Exponentially increasing hCG acts on the CL to rescue it from luteolysis to maintain progesterone secretion, prevent menstruation and support the early conceptus. The CL supports the pregnancy for approximately 8 weeks, after which the early placental tissue becomes the main source of progesterone support (luteo–placental shift).

hCG can be detected in the urine in sensitive pregnancy tests 1 or 2 days before the expected date of menstruation. Most women delay taking a pregnancy test until after a missed period. However, it is relatively common for positive pregnancy tests to occur just prior to the time of the expected period, and for menstruation to occur as expected or 1 or 2 days later with a negative pregnancy test thereafter. This transiently positive hCG is a result of pregnancy failure during the early stages of implantation and is known as a 'biochemical pregnancy'.

A transvaginal ultrasound scan (TVUSS) can detect an early intrauterine gestational sac, the first sign of a normal pregnancy, at around 5 weeks' gestation. A few days later, a circular yolk sac can be seen within the gestational sac, and the embryonic fetus can usually be identified after 5.5 weeks' gestation (**Figure 5.2**). The fetal heartbeat may be visible as early as 6 weeks' gestation.

10.1201/9781003218036-5

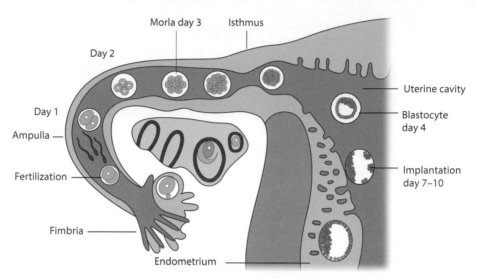

Figure 5.1 Pre-implantation development and intrauterine implantation.

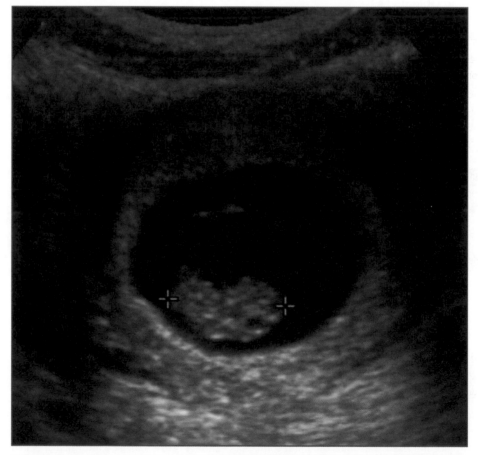

Figure 5.2 Image of an early intrauterine pregnancy with yolk sac and pole (~5–6 weeks).

- The gestational age is calculated from the last menstrual period rather than the time of conception. When someone is 6 weeks' pregnant, this means that they have conceived 4 weeks previously (assuming they have regular menstrual cycles). This is important, as it sometimes causes the patient some confusion.
- In the early stages of a normally developing intrauterine pregnancy, serum concentrations of hCG double every 48 hours, although variations exist.
- A normal pregnancy with serum hCG concentrations of >1,500 IU/L can be confirmed as intrauterine on a TVUSS.

MISCARRIAGE

Miscarriage is a pregnancy that ends spontaneously before 24 weeks' gestation.

CLINICAL PRESENTATION

The most common sign of miscarriage is vaginal bleeding.

INCIDENCE AND AETIOLOGY

Miscarriage is common, occurring in 10–20% of clinical pregnancies, with the risk increasing with maternal age. Clinically, miscarriages can be classified into different types based on the clinical presentation and investigation findings. **Table 5.1** illustrates

Table 5.1 Types of miscarriages with the relevant ultrasound findings and clinical presentation

Type of miscarriage	Ultrasound scan findings	Clinical presentation	Management
Threatened miscarriage	Intrauterine pregnancy (appropriately developed ±FH)	Vaginal bleeding and abdominal pain Speculum: cervical os closed	Supportive
Inevitable miscarriage	Intrauterine pregnancy (no FH)	Vaginal bleeding and abdominal pain Speculum: cervical os closed or open, blood seen	Expectant, medical or surgical approach
Incomplete miscarriage	Retained products of conception	Vaginal bleeding and abdominal pain Speculum: cervical os open, products of conception located in cervical os	Remove pregnancy tissue at time of speculum, if possible Expectant, medical or surgical approach
Complete miscarriage	Empty uterus (need serum hCG to exclude ectopic pregnancy if there is no previous ultrasound scan identifying intrauterine pregnancy)	Pain and bleeding has resolved Speculum: cervical os closed	Supportive
Missed miscarriage (silent/delayed miscarriage)	Intrauterine pregnancy (no FH)	Asymptomatic Often diagnosed at booking ultrasound scan Speculum: cervical os closed	Expectant, medical or surgical approach

Note that a pelvic examination is not usually required if the patient has had an ultrasound scan (so arrange an ultrasound scan first if you possibly can). FH, fetal heartbeat; hCG, human chorionic gonadotrophin.

the clinical presentation, examination findings and management of the different types of miscarriages.

AETIOLOGICAL FACTORS

- Chromosomal abnormalities (estimated at 50–70%)
- Other developmental abnormalities
- Medical/endocrine disorders
- Uterine abnormalities
- Infections
- Drugs/chemicals

INVESTIGATIONS

It is fundamentally important to assess the patient who is miscarrying clinically ('ABCDE'*, abdomino-pelvic examination) in conjunction with the results of the following investigations. The patient may be emotionally distraught and distressed by their physical symptoms, and a sensitive, yet clinically robust, approach is necessary.

- Transabdominal examination/TVUSS: a single ultrasound scan can diagnose a miscarriage if there is a pregnancy within the uterine cavity and certain criteria are met, that is, one of the following:
  - if the crown–rump length is 7.0 mm or more with a transvaginal ultrasound scan and there is no visible heartbeat
  - if the mean gestational sac diameter is greater than 25.0 mm with a transvaginal ultrasound scan and there is no visible fetal pole
- In both scenarios, a second opinion should be sought and/or another scan performed a minimum of 7 days later before diagnosing miscarriage.
- Haemoglobin and 'group and save' (or cross-match if patient is severely compromised): this assesses the degree of vaginal loss and rhesus status.

---

* ABCDE refers to airway, breathing, circulation, disability and exposure. The ABCDE approach is applicable in all clinical emergencies for immediate assessment and treatment. The approach is widely accepted by experts in emergency medicine and likely improves outcomes by helping healthcare professionals to focus on the most life-threatening clinical problems.

MANAGEMENT

A miscarriage can be managed using an expectant (natural), medical or surgical approach, depending on clinical presentation and patient choice.

EXPECTANT MANAGEMENT

Expectant management allows for the avoidance of surgery and is usually offered as the first-line option (7–14 days) following a confirmed diagnosis of miscarriage. After a spontaneous miscarriage in which pain and bleeding resolve, a repeat ultrasound scan is not required to confirm completion. Patients may be advised to take a urinary pregnancy test after 3 weeks and attend if it is still positive. Those undergoing expectant management may require unplanned surgery if they start to bleed heavily. Women with a threatened miscarriage should be asked to seek medical attention if their bleeding gets heavier (with or without the passage of tissue) or persists beyond 14 days.

Expectant management may not be suitable in patients with evidence of current infection, those at significant risk of haemorrhage (previous severe haemorrhage associated with a miscarriage, bleeding disorders or late first trimester), those who decline blood transfusion and those with previous traumatic experiences associated with pregnancy events; an individualized plan by a senior clinician should be reached with the patient in these circumstances.

MEDICAL MANAGEMENT

Medical treatment is increasingly used in an outpatient setting to allow pregnant women to miscarry at home. It involves the single or repeated administration, vaginally or orally (patient preference), of the prostaglandin E analogue misoprostol. There may be a role for pretreatment with the progesterone antagonist mifepristone in some cases, and practice varies. The side effects include pain, vomiting and diarrhoea, and patients are routinely provided with pain relief and antiemetics. As with expectant management, there is no need for routine scan follow-up, although a post-treatment pregnancy test is recommended. Patients undergoing medical management of miscarriage should be informed that they may need surgical treatment if medical treatment fails (10% failure rate) or if they bleed heavily.

SURGICAL MANAGEMENT

Surgical management of miscarriage is preferred if there is persistent excessive bleeding or haemodynamic instability, or if patients favour this option. It can be done by manual vacuum aspiration under local anaesthetic in an outpatient setting if the patient is not compromised. More commonly, it is done as a day case in theatre under general anaesthesia. Vaginal or oral misoprostol is frequently used to ripen the cervix to facilitate cervical dilatation for suction curette insertion and may reduce the risk of cervical trauma and haemorrhage. Synthetic osmotic dilators (e.g. Dilapan-S®) also have been shown to be effective for this purpose. However, surgical evacuation has its drawbacks, including risks of uterine perforation, visceral injury (bowel or bladder), infection, cervical trauma, bleeding and blood transfusion, retained pregnancy tissue, intrauterine adhesions (Asherman syndrome) and, rarely, laparoscopy or laparotomy in the event of uterine perforation causing visceral injury and/or haemorrhage.

COUNSELLING

Miscarriage can be a very distressing experience and the psychological impact, sense of bereavement and feelings of depression and anxiety should not be underestimated. Patients who have suffered miscarriages are counselled to ensure that they understand that most miscarriages are non-recurrent and that they are not to blame for their loss. Patients and their partners may be signposted to appropriate bereavement support services and organizations, including the Miscarriage Association (https://www.miscarriageassociation.org.uk).

RECURRENT MISCARRIAGE

Recurrent miscarriage is defined as the loss of three or more consecutive pregnancies and it affects 1% of couples. Risk factors for recurrent miscarriage include advancing maternal and paternal age, obesity, balanced chromosomal translocations, uterine structural anomalies and antiphospholipid syndrome (APS). The investigation of recurrent miscarriage includes testing for antiphospholipid antibodies and imaging of the uterus. Products of conception in subsequent miscarriages are sent for cytogenetic analysis and, if an unbalanced structural chromosomal abnormality is identified, parental peripheral blood karyotyping is performed. Aspirin and low-dose heparin reduces the miscarriage rate in women with APS by 50%. Balanced translocations may be overcome by pre-implantation genetic diagnosis or gamete donation. Congenital uterine abnormalities, including uterine septum and cervical incompetence, may be amenable to surgery. Although treatment with progesterone, corticosteroids or metformin has been advocated, there is insufficient evidence to recommend their routine use at present. However, there may be a role for progesterone supplementation for women with a history of recurrent miscarriage and a current threatened miscarriage. Most couples have normal investigations, and psychological support and serial ultrasound scans during pregnancy are beneficial.

ECTOPIC PREGNANCY

DEFINITION

An ectopic pregnancy (EP) is defined as the implantation of a pregnancy outside the uterine cavity. Over 98% of EPs implant in the fallopian tube (**Figure 5.3**). Rarely, EPs can implant in the interstitium of the tube, the ovary, the cervix, the abdominal cavity or

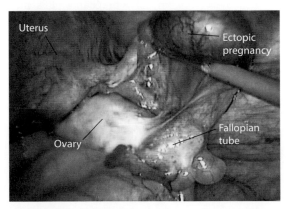

Figure 5.3 Image of tubal ectopic pregnancy taken at laparoscopy.

caesarean section scars. A heterotopic pregnancy is the simultaneous development of two pregnancies: one within and one outside the uterine cavity.

INCIDENCE AND AETIOLOGY

EPs account for 1 in 80 pregnancies and for 9–13% of maternal deaths in the Western world and 10–30% of maternal deaths in low-resource countries. The incidence of a heterotopic pregnancy in the general population is low (1 in 25,000–30,000), but is significantly higher after in vitro fertilization (IVF) treatment (1%) after the transfer of two blastocysts.

> **BOX 5.2: Aetiological factors for EP**
>
> - Fallopian tube damage due to pelvic infection (e.g. *Chlamydia/Gonorrhoea*), previous EP and previous tubal surgery
> - Functional alterations in the fallopian tube due to smoking and increased maternal age
> - Additional risk factors, including previous abdominal surgery (e.g. appendicectomy or caesarean section), subfertility, IVF, the use of intrauterine contraceptive devices, endometriosis and conception on oral contraceptive/morning after pill

CLINICAL PRESENTATION

The majority of patients with an EP present with a subacute clinical picture of abdominal pain and/or vaginal bleeding in early pregnancy. EPs may also present with non-specific urinary or gastrointestinal symptoms and rectal pressure or pain during defecation. Rarely, patients present very acutely with rupture of the EP and massive intraperitoneal bleeding. The free blood in the peritoneal cavity can cause diaphragmatic irritation and shoulder tip pain. The diagnosis of ruptured EP is usually clear, as these cases present with signs of an acute abdomen and hypovolaemic shock with a positive pregnancy test. A high suspicion of EP is needed in all women of reproductive age with symptoms. It is, however, important to know that women commonly experience bleeding or abdominal pain with a viable intrauterine pregnancy.

INVESTIGATIONS

The following are useful investigations for the diagnosis of EP. It is fundamentally important to assess the patient clinically ('ABC', abdominopelvic examination) in conjunction with the results of investigations to optimally manage the patient.

- *TVUSS.* The identification of an intrauterine pregnancy (intrauterine gestation sac, yolk sac ± fetal pole) on TVUSS effectively excludes the possibility of an EP in most patients, except in those patients with rare heterotopic pregnancy. A TVUSS showing an empty uterus with an adnexal mass has a sensitivity of 87.0–99.0% and a specificity of 94.0–99.9% in the diagnosis of EP. The presence of moderate to significant free fluid in the peritoneal cavity or pouch of Douglas during TVUSS is suggestive of a ruptured EP.
- *Serum hCG.* hCG increases by more than 63% every 48 hours in a normally developing intrauterine pregnancy. In patients with EP, the rise of hCG is often suboptimal. However, hCG levels can vary widely in individuals and during various stages of early pregnancy; thus, consecutive measurements 48 hours apart are often required for comparison purposes.

> **BOX 5.3: Pregnancy of unknown location**
>
> - In up to 40% of women with an EP, the diagnosis is not made on first attendance and they are labelled as having a pregnancy of unknown location (PUL).
> - A PUL is defined as an empty uterus with no evidence of an adnexal mass on TVUSS (in a patient with a positive pregnancy test). It is a 'working' diagnosis rather than a diagnosis, and an EP has not yet been excluded.
> - The mainstay of investigation of a PUL is consecutive measurement of serum hCG. An endometrial biopsy (to determine the presence or absence of chorionic villi) can occasionally be helpful when hCG levels are static. All PULs must be investigated to determine the location of the pregnancy and followed up to ensure hCG levels become negative.

- Haemoglobin and 'group and save' (or cross-match if patient is severely compromised). This is used to assess the degree of intra-abdominal bleeding and rhesus status. Most hospitals have a major haemorrhage protocol for exsanguinating patients that makes blood and blood products readily available for patients in extremis.

MANAGEMENT

An EP can be managed using an expectant, a medical or a surgical approach, depending on clinical presentation and patient choice.

EXPECTANT MANAGEMENT

Expectant management is based on the assumption that a significant proportion of all EPs will resolve without any treatment. This option is suitable for patients who are haemodynamically stable and asymptomatic (and remain so). The EP mass should measure less that 35 mm on TVUSS with no visible heartbeat. Serum hCG levels should be less than 1,000 IU/L (although consideration could be given for expectant management with levels up to 1,500 IU/L with senior medical input). The patient should be willing to return for follow-up care, as serial hCG measurements will be required until levels are undetectable (less than 20 IU/L).

MEDICAL MANAGEMENT

Intramuscular methotrexate can be offered to patients with minimal symptoms (pain), an adnexal mass <35 mm in diameter with no fetal heartbeat and a current serum hCG concentration less than 5,000 IU/L. The higher the initial hCG, the more likely medical treatment will fail. Methotrexate blocks the action of folic acid within cells inhibiting deoxyribonucleic acid (DNA) synthesis, particularly within trophoblastic cells. The dose of methotrexate is calculated based on the patient's body surface area at 50 mg/m^2. After methotrexate, serum hCG is measured on days 4 and 7 and then weekly thereafter until undetectable (levels must fall by >15% between days 4 and 7 and continue to fall with treatment). Medical treatment should therefore be offered only

if facilities exist for regular follow-up visits. The few contraindications to medical treatment include (1) chronic liver, renal or haematological disorder; (2) active infection; (3) immunodeficiency; and (4) breastfeeding. There are side effects, including stomatitis, conjunctivitis, gastrointestinal upset and photosensitive skin reaction, and about two-thirds of patients will suffer from non-specific abdominal pain. It is important to advise patients to avoid sexual intercourse during treatment and to avoid conceiving for 3 months after methotrexate because of the risk of teratogenicity. It is also important to advise them to avoid alcohol and prolonged exposure to sunlight during treatment. Around 15% of patients treated with methotrexate require a second dose because of an inadequate hCG fall, and a similar number require surgical management after methotrexate treatment.

SURGICAL MANAGEMENT

The standard surgical treatment approach is laparoscopy (see **Figure 5.3**). Laparotomy is reserved for severely compromised patients or when there are no endoscopic facilities or expertise. The operation of choice is removal of the fallopian tube and the EP within (salpingectomy). Tubal conservative procedures include a salpingotomy (a small incision can be made over the site of the EP (antimesentric border of the fallopian tube) and the EP extracted via this opening, followed by primary closure of the incision) or a salpingostomy (a small incision can be made over the site of the EP and the EP extracted via this opening, followed by healing of the incision by secondary intention). Conservative tubal surgery is recommended only if the contralateral tube is absent or damaged, as it is associated with a higher rate of subsequent EP. Pregnancy rates are high if the contralateral tube is normal because the oocyte can be picked up by the ipsilateral or contralateral tube. After an EP, the risk of recurrence is between 8% and 18%.

COUNSELLING

Similar to miscarriage, an EP can be a very distressing experience and the psychological impact, sense of bereavement and feelings of depression and

Table 5.2 Summary of other early pregnancy disorders

Disorder	Definition	Risk factors	Clinical presentation	Management
GTD (abnormal trophoblast proliferation)	Spectrum of conditions that includes complete and partial hyatidiform mole, invasive mole and choriocarcinoma	Previous molar pregnancy High or low maternal age Asian origin	Ultrasound features of intrauterine vesicles ('cluster of grapes') Persistently raised hCG levels after miscarriage	Registration Uterine evacuation by suction curettage (without misoprostol) Serial hCG measurements Avoid oestrogens
Hyperemesis gravidarum		Multiple pregnancies with GTD	Excessive nausea and vomiting, often accompanied by dehydration	Antiemetics Fluid and electrolyte replacement Multivitamins Thromboprophylaxis

GTD, gestational trophoblastic disease; hCG, human chorionic gonadotrophin.

BOX 5.4: Anti-D administration (see Chapter 6 in *Obstetrics by Ten Teachers*)

- Rhesus isoimmunization can occur after early pregnancy problems, and there are some circumstances in which patients who are rhesus negative require anti-D prophylaxis.
- All rhesus-negative patients who have a surgical procedure to manage an EP or miscarriage should be offered anti-D immunoglobulin at a dose of 50 μg (250 IU) as soon as possible and within 72 hours of the surgery.
- A Kleihauer test is not needed to quantify fetomaternal haemorrhage in the first trimester of pregnancy.
- Anti-D is not required for threatened, incomplete or complete natural miscarriage (local guidelines may differ).
- Anti-D may not be required after the medical management of miscarriage or EP but guidelines differ, and prophylaxis is often given.

anxiety can be considerable. Patients and their partners may be signposted to appropriate bereavement support services, such as the Ectopic Pregnancy Trust (https://ectopic.org.uk).

OTHER EARLY PREGNANCY PROBLEMS

Table 5.2 summarizes other, less common, early pregnancy disorders. It is important to remember that non-gynaecological conditions, including urinary tract infection and medical/surgical problems (e.g. appendicitis), can present in early pregnancy.

FURTHER READING

National Institute for Health and Care Excellence (2019). *Ectopic Pregnancy and Miscarriage: Diagnosis and Initial Management.* NICE guideline [NG126].

Royal College of Obstetricians and Gynaecologists (2020). *Green-top Guideline No. 38: Gestational Trophoblastic Disease.*

Royal College of Obstetricians and Gynaecologists (2016). *Green-top Guideline No. 69: The Management of Nausea and Vomiting of Pregnancy and Hyperemesis Gravidarum.*

Royal College of Obstetricians and Gynaecologists (2011). *Green-top Guideline No. 17: Recurrent Miscarriage, Investigation and Treatment of Couples.*

SELF-ASSESSMENT

For interactive SBAs and EMQs relating to this chapter, visit www.routledge.com/cw/crosbie.

CASE HISTORY 1

Miss Y is a 22-year-old who presents at 9 weeks' gestation with abdominal pain and vaginal bleeding. She had an ultrasound scan at 7 weeks' gestation, which confirmed an intrauterine pregnancy. Her observations on admission are blood pressure 135/80 mmHg, pulse 84/minute and temperature 37.6°C.

A   What is your differential diagnosis?
B   What are the key points in her history, examination and investigation?
C   Discuss her management.

ANSWERS

A   Threatened miscarriage. An EP has been excluded by her previous ultrasound.
B   With a known intrauterine pregnancy, the typical features of threatened miscarriage are vaginal bleeding with or without abdominal pain. Importantly, the patient is haemodynamically stable.
C   The patient should be offered another pelvic ultrasound scan. If a miscarriage is confirmed on imaging, the patient can be managed using an expectant, a medical or a surgical approach (depending on patient choice). The patient should also be offered counselling. If the pregnancy is viable on ultrasound, the patient should be reassured and discharged.

CASE HISTORY 2

Mrs M is a 32-year-old woman who presents after 6 weeks of amenorrhoea with abdominal pain and dizziness. Her observations on admission are blood pressure 90/50 mmHg, pulse 115/minute and temperature 36.9°C. She has a positive urinary pregnancy test.

A   What is your differential diagnosis?
B   What are the key points in her history, examination and investigation?
C   Discuss her management.

ANSWERS

A   EP. The findings of cardiovascular instability, in the presence of pregnancy, are an EP until proven otherwise.
B   An EP should be suspected in any woman of reproductive age who presents with symptoms. This patient has classical symptoms of EP: pain and dizziness. She also has signs of hypovolaemic shock. She has a positive urinary pregnancy test.
C   'ABC'. The patient should have a large bore cannula inserted and should be given intravenous fluids. Bloods should be taken for full blood count and 'group and save'. She should remain nil by mouth. She requires an abdominopelvic examination. A senior colleague should be informed about her admission and the possibility of her requiring an urgent laparoscopy.

The patient had a laparoscopy and was discovered to have a large right ruptured EP in her fallopian tube with 1.5 L of blood in her pelvis. She had a salpingectomy and subsequently recovered well.

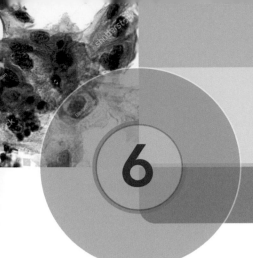

Contraception and abortion

6

SHARON CAMERON

Learning Objectives
- Understand the mechanism of action of contraceptive methods.
- Describe factors that affect contraceptive effectiveness.
- Understand the non-contraceptive benefits of different methods.
- Understand the use of medical eligibility criteria for contraception.
- Understand the mechanism of action of medical abortion.
- List what to cover during a consultation about a request for an abortion.
- Understand when to start contraception post-pregnancy.

INTRODUCTION

Correct and consistent use of effective methods of contraception can prevent most unintended pregnancies. Abortion is a common outcome of unintended pregnancy, and in settings that restrict abortion, abortions are often conducted under unsafe conditions and result in women dying or suffering serious injuries. Unintended pregnancies can also lead to delayed or no antenatal care, which can pose health risks to mothers and babies. It is estimated that, worldwide each year, there are 25 million unsafe abortions, approximately 31,000 deaths from unsafe abortion and seven million women who suffer injury/disability from unsafe abortion. These are preventable through contraception and, as a backup, access to safe abortion.

BOX 6.1: Global unmet need for contraception

- Over 200 million women worldwide would like to avoid a pregnancy, but are not using an effective method of contraception. This is due to a lack of supplies, cultural and political barriers, and a poor quality of services.
- An estimated 25 million unsafe abortions take place each year.
- There are approximately 31,000 deaths from unsafe abortion each year.
- Seven million women suffer injury/disability from unsafe abortion each year.

10.1201/9781003218036-6

CONTRACEPTIVE TARGETS IN THE FEMALE REPRODUCTIVE TRACT

Contraceptive methods prevent pregnancy by targeting one or more key reproductive processes or sites in the male or female reproductive tract. None of the existing methods of contraception is 100% effective at preventing pregnancy. The effectiveness of a method depends on both its mechanism of action and correct and consistent use. Compliance depends on the acceptability of the method to the user and tolerability with any untoward effects that they experience related to use of the method. Even in settings in which contraception is readily available and free (such as the UK), unintended pregnancy rates remain high. Many women who present with an unintended pregnancy have used a contraceptive method, but it is usually a method of low effectiveness (e.g. condom) or a method that has been used incorrectly or inconsistently (e.g. missed oral contraceptive pills). The uptake of existing methods is limited by their acceptability and, for many methods, discontinuation rates are high.

An individual's choice of contraception is just as likely to be based upon information from the media, friends and family as from a healthcare professional. The most effective methods of contraception are long-acting reversible contraception (LARC) methods, such as the copper intrauterine device (Cu-IUD), levonorgestrel intrauterine device (LNG-IUD) and progestogen-only implant. Unfortunately, myths and misconceptions among both the general population and healthcare professionals surrounding the use of LARC are major factors that limit their uptake. Education, dispelling myths and promoting the significant non-contraceptive benefits of LARC methods could improve uptake and continuation and could have the potential to prevent many more unintended pregnancies for more women.

MECHANISM OF ACTION

The current available methods of contraception work in the following ways:

- preventing ovulation – this is the mechanism of action of the following methods: combined hormonal contraception (CHC: pill, patch and vaginal ring), the progestogen-only injectable, the progestogen-only implant, oral emergency contraception (EC) and lactational amenorrhoea
- preventing sperm from reaching the oocyte, that is, female sterilization and male sterilization (vasectomy)
- preventing an embryo from implanting in the uterus – this is a mechanism of action of the Cu-IUD and LNG-IUD
- allowing sperm into the vagina but poisoning them – this is the mechanism of action of spermicides
- allowing sperm into the vagina but blocking further passage – this is the mechanism of action of the diaphragm and cap, and is also one of the mechanisms of action of progestogens through their effect on the cervical mucus
- preventing sperm from entering the vagina – this is the mechanism of action of:
  - male and female condoms
  - avoiding sex during the fertile time of the cycle
  - fertility awareness-based methods

EFFICACY AND EFFECTIVENESS

The efficacy of a method depends on its mechanism of action. However, effectiveness depends on compliance and continuation with the method. Compliance is influenced by the route of administration (**Table 6.1**). Continuation with a method depends on the acceptability to the user. The most effective method for any woman, therefore, is a method that will be used correctly and consistently. The length of action of currently available contraceptives has an influence on the acceptability and efficacy and is shown in **Table 6.1**.

Failure rates during perfect use, defined as following the directions for use, show how effective methods can be. Failure rates during typical use show how effective the different methods are during actual use (including inconsistent or incorrect use).

Table 6.2 shows estimates of the probabilities of pregnancy during the first year of typical use of each method (based upon data from the USA). For some

Table 6.1 Route of administration of currently available contraceptives and their duration

Route of administration	Duration
COCP and POP	24 hours
Combined hormonal contraceptive patch	7 days
Combined hormonal contraceptive vaginal ring	21 days or 3 months
Progestogen-only injectable	14 weeks
Progestogen-only implant	3 years
Cu-IUD	3 years, 5 years, 10 years or more
LNG-IUD	3 years, 5 years or 6 years

COCP, combined oral contraceptive pill; Cu-IUD, copper intrauterine device; LNG-IUD, levonorgestrel intrauterine device; POP, progestogen-only pill.

Table 6.2 Percentage of women experiencing an unintended pregnancy within the first year of use with typical use and perfect use

Method	Unintended pregnancies (%)	
	Typical use	Perfect use
None	85	85
Fertility awareness-based methods	15	
Male condom	13	2
Female diaphragm	17	16
Combined contraceptive pill, patch or vaginal ring or progestogen-only pill	7	0.3
Progestogen-only injectable	4	0.2
Cu-IUD	0.8	0.6
52 mg LNG-IUD	0.1	0.1
Progestogen-only implant	0.1	0.1
Female sterilization	0.5	0.5

Modified from WHO (2015).
Note: Highlighted boxes show the forms of LARC.
Cu-IUD, copper intrauterine device; LARC, long-acting reversible contraception; LNG-IUD, levonorgestrel intrauterine device.

methods, such as implants and intrauterine contraceptives, the efficacy is high and proper and consistent use is nearly guaranteed once inserted, with extremely low pregnancy rates found in all studies. For other methods, such as the oral contraceptive pill and progestogen-only injectable, efficacy is high, but they can potentially be misused (e.g. forgetting to take pills or failure to get repeat injections). Characteristics of the user that determine the risk of pregnancy include compliance, age (reducing fertility in the late 30s) and frequency of intercourse.

LARC methods have been defined in the UK as methods that require administration less than once per month (i.e. implant, intrauterine devices (IUDs) and injectables), although, in most other countries, the injectable is considered not a LARC but a 'medium-acting' method. LARC methods are the most effective contraceptive, as once inserted they do not require any action by the user until they need to be renewed (3 years for the etonorgestrel implant and 5–10 years or longer for IUDs). In contrast, the shorter-acting methods do require compliance by the user (e.g. to take a daily pill, change a weekly patch or use a condom for every act of sex). Discontinuation rates of short-acting methods (the pill, patch and ring) and even the progestogen-only injectable are all high, with approximately half of users stopping this method by 1 year. In contrast, discontinuation rates of LARC methods are lower, with studies reporting that 80% or more of users still use the implant or IUD at 1 year.

LARC methods have 'typical use' failure rates within the first 12 months of use that are similar to 'perfect use' failure rates. In contrast, for short-acting methods, typical failure rates are much higher than perfect failure rates. Typical use failure rates should be used when providing information to women about the effectiveness of a method. The use of simple diagrams can help put the effectiveness of a method into context. Without contraception, approximately 85% of couples conceive within 12 months.

SAFETY

Most women who use contraception are fit and healthy. However, some health conditions may be associated with real or theoretical risks if a particular contraceptive method affects the health condition.

In an attempt to produce a set of international norms for providing contraception to individuals with a range of medical conditions that may contra-indicate a contraceptive method, the World Health Organization (WHO) developed medical eligibility criteria for contraceptive use. The WHO *Medical Eligibility Criteria for Contraceptive Use* (MEC, 2015) is a guidance document that contains recommendations for whether or not women with given medical conditions or characteristics are eligible to use a particular contraceptive method, based on evidence and also expert consensus opinion. The MEC categories have four levels, as shown in **Table 6.3**. Category 1 includes conditions for which there is no restriction for the use of the method, while category 4 includes conditions that represent an unacceptable health risk if the contraceptive method is used (absolutely contraindicated). Some MEC 4 conditions that restrict the use of CHC are shown in the box 'Examples of World Health Organization medical eligibility criteria category 4 conditions'. For some conditions, the MEC category may differ depending on whether the condition was pre-existing when the contraceptive was initiated or developed during use of the method. If a woman develops a condition while using a method of contraception, then it is possible that the method contributed to the onset of the condition and they may need to stop using it.

Table 6.3 Medical eligibility criteria for contraceptive eligibility

Category	Description
1	A condition for which there is no restriction for the use of the contraceptive method
2	A condition for which the advantages of using the method generally outweigh theoretical or proven risks
3	A condition for which the theoretical or proven risk usually outweighs the advantages of using the method
4	A condition that represents an unacceptable health risk if the contraceptive method is used

Modified from WHO (2015).

BOX 6.2: Examples of World Health Organization medical eligibility criteria category 4 conditions

- Age >35 and smoking
- Blood pressure >160/100 mmHg
- Hypertension with vascular disease
- Deep vein thrombosis, current or past
- Myocardial infarction, current or past
- Cerebrovascular accident, current or past
- Multiple serious risk factors for cardiovascular disease
- Known thrombogenic mutations
- Current breast cancer

However, if a woman with a particular condition (often one that makes pregnancy less safe) wishes to start a method of contraception, there may be less of an issue with safety.

INTERACTION WITH OTHER MEDICINES

There are a number of medicines (some anticonvulsants, antifungals, antiretrovirals and antibiotics) that induce cytochrome P450 enzymes in the liver and will reduce the efficacy of hormonal contraception such as the CHC pill, patch and ring, the progestogen-only implant and the progestogen-only pill (POP) (**Table 6.4**). If a woman using enzyme-inducing medication wishes to use one of these hormonal methods, then the consistent use of condoms is also advised. Alternatively, they could consider the progestogen-only injectable, Cu-IUD or LNG-IUD, as the efficacy of these methods is not affected by drugs that are enzyme inducers. The effectiveness of the combined oral contraceptive pill (COCP) (and all other methods) is not affected by the administration of most broad-spectrum antibiotics.

SIDE EFFECTS

The common side effects that women report with all hormonal methods are unexpected bleeding, weight gain, headaches, mood swings and loss of libido. Concern about weight gain attributed to hormonal

Table 6.4 Drugs known to decrease the efficacy of hormonal contraception through the induction of liver enzymes (oral contraceptive pills, patch, ring and implant)

Type of drug	Liver enzyme induction
Anticonvulsant	Carbamazepine
	Eslicarbazepine
	Oxcarbazepine
	Phenobarbital
	Phenytoin
	Primidone
	Topiramate
Antibiotic	Rifampicin
	Rifabutin
Antifungal	Griseofulvin
Antiretroviral	**Protease inhibitors**
	Amprenavir
	Atazanavir
	Nelfinavir
	Lopinavir
	Saquinavir
	Ritonavir
	Non-nucleoside reverse transcriptase inhibitors
	Efavirenz
	Nevirapine

contraception has been shown to be one of the greatest perceived disadvantages of hormonal contraception. With the exception of the progestogen-only injectable in adolescents, there is no good evidence that hormonal methods cause weight gain. There is also no evidence that intrauterine methods (Cu-IUD or LNG-IUD) cause weight gain. Furthermore, there is no good evidence that hormonal contraception has adverse effects on either mood or libido.

Unexpected bleeding is common (15%) when women start a COCP and may settle with time. If not, then changing to another contraceptive pill with a different dose of hormones may help. If bleeding problems persist for more than 3 months, then current UK guidelines advise that investigations be undertaken to exclude other causes (e.g. cervical conditions such as polyps, chlamydial infection or intrauterine cavity lesions such as submucous fibroids or polyps).

NON-CONTRACEPTIVE HEALTH BENEFITS

Hormonal contraceptives may be used for their beneficial side effects, in which case the risk–benefit ratio changes and MEC categories may no longer apply (**Table 6.5**). Barrier methods, particularly condoms, protect against sexually transmitted infections (STIs).

ACCEPTABILITY

Acceptability determines whether women choose to start a method and whether they continue to use that method. The box 'Determinants of contraceptive method acceptability' lists such factors, including personal characteristics (e.g. age), fertility intentions (e.g. if planning a baby sooner, later or not at all), the experience of others (e.g. friends and family), the method's ease of use, the ease of access to the

Table 6.5 Non-contraceptive health benefits of hormonal contraception

Method	Conditions for which there are benefits	Additional benefits
LNG-IUD (52 mg)	Heavy menstrual bleeding Endometriosis Adenomyosis Dysmenorrhoea Endometrial hyperplasia	Endometrial protection
CHC	Heavy menstrual bleeding Irregular menses Hirsutism Acne Premenstrual syndrome	Reduces risk of ovarian cancer Reduces risk of endometrial cancer
Progestogen-only injectable	Heavy menstrual bleeding Endometriosis Dysmenorrhoea	

CHC, combined hormonal contraception; LNG-IUD, levonorgestrel intrauterine device.

method (including whether or not a health professional needs to be seen to obtain the method), the method's perceived intrusiveness and the non-contraceptive benefits of the method (e.g. reduction in menstrual flow or pain).

> **BOX 6.3: Determinants of contraceptive method acceptability**
>
> - Personal characteristics (e.g. age)
> - Fertility intentions
> - Perceptions of effectiveness
> - Perceptions of safety
> - Fear of side effects
> - Familiarity
> - Experience of others
> - Ease of use and of access
> - Need to see a health professional
> - Intrusiveness
> - Non-contraceptive benefits

PRACTICAL PRESCRIBING

Women considering using a particular method of contraception require clear, accurate information in a format that is easily understandable to them. The information provided should cover the following aspects:

- how to use the method (pill, patch or ring) and what to do when misused (e.g. missed pill)
- typical failure rates
- common side effects
- health benefits
- fertility return on stopping
- when a review is required or when the implant or IUD needs to be replaced

METHODS OF CONTRACEPTION

COMBINED HORMONAL CONTRACEPTION

CHC methods contain two hormones: an oestrogen and a progestogen. They are available as an oral pill, a transdermal patch or a vaginal ring. They are similar in terms of effectiveness, safety and side effects.

These methods all work by inhibition of ovulation via negative feedback of oestrogen and progestogen on the pituitary, with suppression of follicle-stimulating hormone (FSH) and luteinizing hormone (LH).

PILL

Most of the commonly used COCPs are 'low dose' and contain ethinyl oestradiol in a dose of 15–35 µg (**Figure 6.1**). Some newer pills contain oestradiol valerate or 17-beta oestradiol, which is more similar in structure to the 'naturally occurring' oestradiol, but confer no other proven benefits.

Most 'traditional' preparations contain 21 pills followed by a 7-day pill-free interval (or seven placebo tablets in place of a 7-day pill-free interval). Some preparations contain 24 days of pills with a shorter pill-free interval. Preparations are commonly monophasic (i.e. the same dose of hormones throughout), but some are phasic (the dose varies). There is no advantage of phasic preparations. Although traditional 21-day pills usually result in a withdrawal bleed during the pill-free interval, there is no reason why the pill cannot be taken continuously. Women with dysmenorrhoea or headaches during the pill-free interval are often advised to take the pill continuously to avoid recurrence of symptoms during the hormone-free interval or to tricycle the pill (taking three packets without any break) to have a bleed every three months. Tailored pill use is also recommended. Tailored pill taking is where women continue to take the pill until they want to start a bleeding episode. Then they have the pill-free interval at this time.

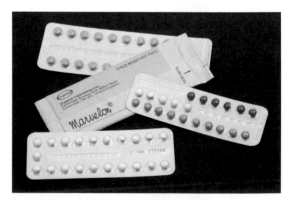

Figure 6.1 The oral contraceptive pill.

The progestogens that are used in currently available pills are sometimes referred to as second-generation (levonorgestrel and norethisterone), third-generation (gestodene desogestrel) and fourth-generation progestogens (drospirenone and dienogest). Preparations containing third- and fourth-generation progestogens were developed to have the advantages of progestogens with less androgenic activity, but they seem to be associated with a higher risk of venous thrombosis than pills containing second-generation progestogens. In view of this, COCPs containing second-generation progestogens are generally recommended as the first choice.

PATCH AND RING

The combined hormonal contraceptive patch releases 33.9 µg ethinyl oestradiol/day and 203 µg norelgestromin/day. It is applied to the skin of the lower abdomen, buttock or arm for 7 days, although it can be applied to any skin-covered area except the breast (**Figure 6.2A**). The regimen usually involves the application of patches for a total of 21 days followed by a 7-day hormone-free interval. Continued use (or tricycling or tailored use) is also possible. Some women may experience problems with patch adherence or skin sensitivity to the patch.

The combined hormonal contraceptive ring is a flexible ring of 54 mm in diameter that releases 15 µg ethinyl oestradiol and 120 µg etonorgestrel daily and, as such, is the lowest dose CHC method (**Figure 6.2B**). The ring is self-inserted and worn in the vagina. There are rings that are worn for 21 days and others that are worn for 3 months, followed by a 7-day hormone-free interval, during which a withdrawal bleed occurs. Continuous use of the ring (or tricycling or tailored use), like for the pill and patch, is also possible. There should be no discomfort from the ring and it can be removed for a short time (less than 3 hours) and can be cleaned and replaced.

MISSED PILLS, PATCHES AND RINGS

Missing a single COCP is insufficient to reverse ovarian suppression; however, missing several pills or extending the hormone-free interval by missing pills at the end of a packet or forgetting to restart the new packet on time could theoretically increase the risk of ovulation. Additional contraceptive cover (condoms or abstinence) is required for most monophasic pills containing ethinyl oestradiol during the next 7 days of pill taking (**Figure 6.3**). Additional precautions are also required if a patch is not applied for 48 hours or a ring is removed for more than 48 hours. If unprotected sexual intercourse has occurred during this time, then there is a risk of pregnancy and so EC (see **Box 6.8** 'Emergency contraception') is recommended.

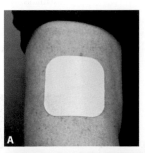

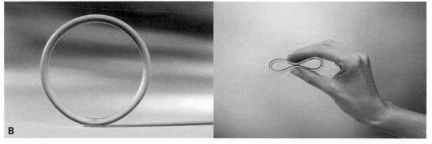

Figure 6.2 (**A**) Combined hormonal patch. (**B**) Combined hormonal vaginal contraceptive ring.

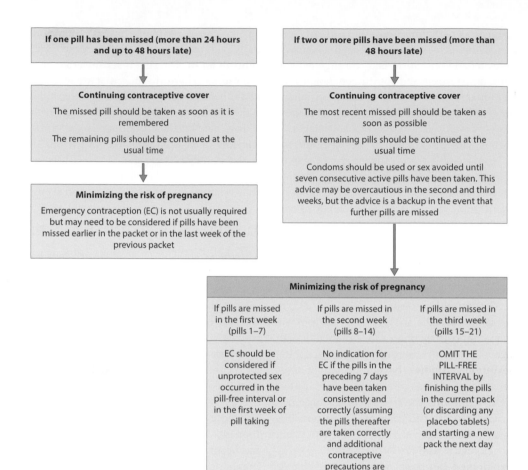

Figure 6.3 Missed pill guidelines. (Adapted from Faculty of Sexual and Reproductive Healthcare, 2020.)

SAFETY

Cancer

Large observational studies have shown that women who are current or ever users of COCPs have a 12% reduction in their risk of death from any cancer. Ever use of oral contraception has been associated with a 46% reduced risk of ovarian cancer compared with never use, and with 10 years of use of a COCP there is a halving of the risk of ovarian cancer. This protection is also evident for women with a family history of breast cancer (who may be particularly at risk of ovarian cancer). In the same studies, the risk of endometrial cancer was almost halved among women who had ever used the contraceptive pill compared with never users. A reduction in the risk of colon cancer was also observed. The reason for this reduction in the risk of cancers with contraceptive pill use is not known. Protection against ovarian cancer could be due to the suppression of follicular rupture from the surface of the ovary each month. Protection against endometrial cancer could be due

---

BOX 6.4: Cancer risks among users of COCPs

- A 12% reduction in the risk of any cancer.
- Reduced risk of colorectal cancer.
- Reduced risk of endometrial cancer.
- Reduced risk of ovarian cancer.
- Increased risk of breast cancer during use (decreases on stopping, with the risk being similar to if never used by 10 years after stopping).

to the progestogen content of the pill, which opposes the mitogenic effects of oestrogen on the endometrium. This protection against ovarian and endometrial cancer seems to persist for more than 15 years after stopping the pill.

Most (but not all) observational studies have reported an increase in the risk of breast cancer among current users of COCPs. A meta-analysis of observational studies of breast cancer and hormonal contraception suggests that current users of COCPs have an increased risk of breast cancer while taking the pill, but that, soon after discontinuing, this risk diminishes, so that their risk 10 years after stopping is the same as an individual who never used the pill. It has been suggested that starting to use the pill may accelerate the appearance of breast cancer in susceptible women. Alternatively, women using the pill might have their tumours diagnosed earlier, although it is difficult to explain why a tendency to earlier diagnosis would persist for years after stopping.

Observational studies have also reported an increase in the risk of cervical cancer among users of COCPs. While this may be due to confounding factors such as users being less likely to use condoms (that protect against human papillomavirus (HPV)), a biological association cannot be excluded. However, women can be reassured that participating in a cervical screening programme can detect oncogenic HPV subtypes and precancerous cells that can be effectively treated. Having HPV vaccination (against oncogenic HPV subtypes 16 and 18) before sexual activity commences, using condoms and not smoking also significantly reduces the risk of cervical cancer.

Venous thromboembolism and arterial disease

CHC (pill, patch and ring) increases the tendency to thrombosis in both venous and arterial circulation. The adverse effect on venous thrombosis is related to the dose of oestrogen and appears less with combined pills containing second-generation progestogens than with those containing third- or fourth-generation progestogens. However, whichever progestogen is used, the absolute risk of venous thromboembolism (VTE) is very small and much less

BOX 6.5: Risk of VTE in users and non-users of CHC

- 5 per 10,000 in non-pregnant non-users
- 10 per 10,000 in COCP users
- 29–400 per 10,000 during pregnancy/ post-partum

than that associated with pregnancy (see **Box 6.5** 'Risk of VTE in users and non-users of CHC').

The risk of VTE is greatest during the first year of CHC use, possibly due to the unmasking of inherited thrombophilias. Screening for known thrombophilias is not cost-effective, but women should be asked about a personal and family history of VTE if considering using this method, as these are contraindications to using a CHC method. Women who are using CHC and undertaking long-distance travel should take appropriate exercise on the journey and consider wearing graduated compression socks.

Arterial disease is much less common than VTE but is more serious. It is related to age, and the risk is strongly influenced by smoking. Individuals over 35 years old who smoke are not eligible to use a CHC method. The combined pill is also contraindicated in patients who experience migraine with aura (homonymous hemianopia, unilateral paraesthesia, weakness, aphasia or unclassifiable speech disorder occurring before the headache), as this condition is related to cerebral vasospasm and these individuals may therefore be at higher risk of stroke if they use CHC.

PROGESTOGEN-ONLY CONTRACEPTIVE METHODS

Progestogen-only methods are available as an oral method, an injectable, an implant or an IUD. The mechanism of action of this method and the bleeding pattern appear to depend on the dose of progestogen and also the route of administration.

The injectable, the implant and some POPs (containing the progestogen desogestrel or drospirenone) inhibit ovulation. Other POP formulations only inhibit ovulation inconsistently. All progestogen-only contraceptive methods, regardless of the route of administration, thicken the cervical mucus, so reducing sperm penetrability and transport. The LNG-IUD has little effect on ovarian activity but causes marked endometrial atrophy, which prevents implantation if ovulation and fertilization occur.

PROGESTOGEN-ONLY PILL

Almost all types of POP need to be taken every day. The exception is a new POP containing drospirenone, which is designed to be taken for 24 days followed by a 4-day pill-free interval. Both the desogestrel-containing POP and the drospirenone-containing POP inhibit ovulation in 99% of cycles. Other POPs inhibit ovulation in less than half of cycles, relying on the cervical mucus effect for contraception. Side effects of all POPs include irregular bleeding, persistent ovarian follicles (simple cysts) and acne.

If a POP is missed, then the woman should continue taking the POP and use extra precautions (e.g. condoms) for the next 48 hours until the progestogen effect on the mucus is built up. If unprotected sex occurs during this time, then EC is required.

IMPLANT

A single rod implant containing the progestogen etonorgestrel is the currently available method in the UK and Europe. Nexplanon® contains 68 mg of 3-keto-desogestrel (a metabolite of desogestrel) providing contraception for 3 years. Implants that are in use in other parts of the world include Uniplant® (single rod, nomegestrol, lasts 1 year) and Jadelle® (two rods, levonorgestrel, lasts 5 years).

Nexplanon® is a flexible rod, similar in size to a match stick (40 mm × 2 mm) and is inserted subdermally 8 cm above the medical epicondyle, usually of the non-dominant arm (**Figure 6.4**). Insertion is conducted under local anaesthesia using a specially designed insertion device. Nevertheless, poor insertion technique can still result in deep insertion with consequent difficult removal, so insertion should be conducted only by clinicians who have undertaken appropriate training. The implant is not usually visible but should be easily palpable. It contains a small quantity of barium, which permits it to be visualized by X-ray. It can also be localized using low-frequency ultrasound probes, which can help aid the removal of implants that are not easily palpable.

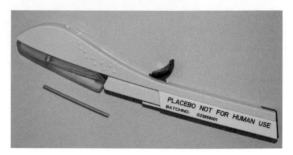

Figure 6.4 Nexplanon®.

Once inserted, there is no need for any routine follow-up until the device is due for replacement or the user wishes it to be removed. After removal, serum levels of etonorgestrel are undetectable within 1 week, and fertility is restored immediately after removal.

PROGESTOGEN-ONLY INJECTABLE

The most commonly used injectable worldwide is a depot injection of medroxyprogesterone acetate, which can be administered intramuscularly (buttock, upper arm or lower abdomen) as the formulation Depoprovera® (150 mg) or subcutaneously as the micronized lower-dose formulation of Sayana® Press (104 mg). Intramuscular and subcutaneous preparations have similar features: the same mode of action (inhibition of ovulation), the same efficacy, similar injection intervals (every 13 weeks) and similar bleeding patterns (over 50% amenorrhoea rates at 1 year). As subcutaneous injections are easier to give, this preparation offers the possibility of training users to self-administer. This can increase access to this method and may increase its acceptability (**Figure 6.5**).

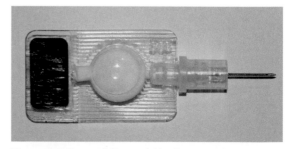

Figure 6.5 Sayana® Press single-dose container.

The progestogen-only injectable is the only hormonal method that may delay the return of fertility after discontinuation. In some cases, it may take up to 1 year after the last injection for ovulation to return. There is no permanent impairment of fertility, but this delay makes the injectable an inappropriate method for individuals wanting short-term contraception.

Both the intramuscular and subcutaneous preparations may cause weight gain in a minority of women and a loss of bone mineral density (BMD) (5% loss of BMD at lumbar spine) in the first few years of use. However, patients should be advised that BMD loss seems to plateau, has not been associated with osteoporotic fractures and appears to be reversible on stopping.

There is robust evidence from countries with a high prevalence of human immunodeficiency virus (HIV) (sub-Saharan Africa) that users of the progestogen-only injectable are not at any increased risk of acquisition of HIV than users of the implant or IUD. However, condom use in addition to the injectable should also be encouraged to protect against the transmission or acquisition of HIV.

PROGESTOGEN-RELEASING INTRAUTERINE DEVICE

The currently available hormonal IUDs release the progestogen levonorgestrel into the uterus. There are three doses of LNG-IUD that are available in Europe. The 52 mg LNG-IUD (Mirena®, Levosert®) (see **Chapter 4**: **Figure 4.3**) is licensed for 6 years for contraceptive use (Levosert® is licensed for 6 years), but, if it is inserted in individuals 45 years or older, UK guidelines advise that this device may be left in situ for contraception until the menopause or age 55. There is also a 19.5 mg LNG-IUD (Kyleena®), which is licensed for 5 years' use, and a 13.5 mg LNG-IUD (Jaydess®), which is licensed for 3 years for contraceptive use. Both the 19.5 mg and 13.5 mg LNG-IUDs have a slightly narrower insertion device and a shorter frame than the 52 mg device, which may make insertion easier in young people or those who are nulliparous. The 19.5 mg and 13.5 mg LNG-IUDs also have a silver band at the proximal end, which helps distinguish it from the 52 mg LNG-IUD on ultrasound.

The LNG-IUD works by exerting a potent hormonal effect on the endometrium, which prevents endometrial proliferation and implantation. Its progestogenic effect on thickening the cervical mucus also impedes the entry of sperm.

The LNG-IUD does not prevent ovulation. In the first few months of use, many patients experience unpredictable bleeding; they should be advised that this usually improves with time and many will eventually have lighter or absent periods. The provision of quality information about side effects in advance of fitting a LNG-IUD is important to reduce unnecessary discontinuation rates. Reported side effects of the LNG-IUD include acne, breast tenderness, mood disturbance and headaches.

The most notable non-contraceptive benefit of the 52 mg LNG-IUD is reducing heavy menstrual bleeding (reduced by 90% at 12 months). It is more effective than oral treatments (e.g. norethisterone, the COCP and tranexamic acid) at reducing menstrual blood flow (see **Chapter 4**). It is also effective for treating dysmenorrhoea and pain associated with endometriosis and adenomyosis, and protecting the endometrium against hyperplasia.

> **BOX 6.6: Intrauterine contraceptives (Cu-IUD, LNG-IUD)**
>
> - Last 3–10 years (or more) depending on type and the age of the individual at insertion
> - Failure rate less than 1 in 100
> - Prevent fertilization
> - Thicken cervical mucus
> - Inhibit implantation

While the 19.5 mg and 13.5 mg LNG-IUD are not licensed for use as a treatment for heavy menstrual bleeding, they do reduce blood loss but are less likely to give amenorrhoea than the 52 mg LNG-IUD.

INTRAUTERINE CONTRACEPTION

Intrauterine methods of contraception include the Cu-IUD and the LNG-IUD (see previous section). The duration of use of the Cu-IUD is between 3 and 10 years, depending on the device used and the age of the individual at insertion. If a woman has a Cu-IUD inserted at 40 years of age or older, it can be left in situ until the menopause. For women who have a 52 mg LNG-IUD inserted at 45 years or over, the device can be left for contraceptive purposes until the menopause (or age 55 years).

There are a number of Cu-IUDs available and they vary in size, shape, copper content and duration of use. Most consist of a plastic frame with copper wire wound around the stem and some may have copper on the arms of the device. The LNG-IUD consists of an elastomere frame with a reservoir on the stem containing levonorgestrel. With both the Cu-IUD and the LNG-IUD, threads protrude through the cervical canal into the upper vagina to permit easy removal. Once inserted, the effectiveness of IUDs does not rely on the user and so typical failure rates are much lower than the shorter-acting methods of contraception. In addition to routine contraception, the Cu-IUD can also be used for EC.

Research shows that both the general population and healthcare professionals often lack accurate knowledge and often hold negative misconceptions about IUDs. Evidence suggests that the Cu-IUD and the LNG-IUD do not cause a delay in return to fertility or increase the risk of infertility, and patients should be advised of this.

MODE OF ACTION

IUDs stimulate an inflammatory reaction in the uterus. The concentration of macrophages and leucocytes, prostaglandins and various enzymes in both uterine and tubal fluid change significantly. It is thought that these effects are toxic to both sperm and egg and interfere with sperm transport. If a fertilized egg reaches the uterine cavity, implantation is inhibited.

BLEEDING PATTERN WITH INTRAUTERINE DEVICE

Although women with the LNG-IUD tend to experience lighter, less painful menses after insertion; those using the Cu-IUD may experience more painful or heavier menses. The use of a non-steroidal anti-inflammatory drug at menses may help lessen the pain and blood loss. Tranexamic acid during

menses may also reduce blood loss with a Cu-IUD. Alternatively, they could switch to the LNG-IUD.

Patients using an IUD should be informed that their overall risk of ectopic pregnancy is much reduced compared with those who are using no contraception. However, if a pregnancy does occur with an IUD in situ then the 'relative' risk of that pregnancy being ectopic is higher. Some studies have reported that 50% of the rare pregnancies that do occur are ectopic. If anyone does become pregnant with an IUD in situ, an ultrasound scan should be conducted to exclude ectopic pregnancy. It is generally advisable that, where possible, IUDs should be removed in view of the greater risk of miscarriage, preterm delivery, septic abortion and chorioamnionitis if the device is left in situ. Although there is a theoretical concern about teratogenicity if a pregnancy is exposed to the LNG-IUD, to date no birth defects have been reported in the small number of cases exposed.

INSERTION OF INTRAUTERINE DEVICE

An IUD can be fitted at any point in the cycle provided there is no risk of pregnancy. Insertion is associated with the following risks.

Perforation

Uterine perforation with insertion of an IUD is rare: approximately 1 in 1,000. Factors associated with an increased risk of perforation include relative inexperience of the clinician, breastfeeding and being less than 6 months post-partum. Usually, the woman presents with 'missing' threads and a history of severe pain following insertion. An ultrasound of the uterus confirms no IUD is seen in the uterus, and an abdominal X-ray shows an IUD. Laparoscopic retrieval of the device from the pelvis (often attached to omentum) is possible in most cases, but laparotomy may rarely be required to remove the IUD.

Expulsion

One in 20 IUD devices will be expelled in the first 3 months after insertion. After this, the risk of expulsion diminishes. Given that some expulsions are not always obvious, IUD users should be advised to perform self-checks for the presence of threads in the upper vagina to ensure the device is still present.

Infection

The overall risk of pelvic infection in the first 3 weeks following insertion of an IUD is low (1 in 100). Thereafter, the risk of infection is the same as women not using contraception. In most cases of infection, the IUD can be left in situ and antibiotic therapy commenced. If the IUD is removed, then the clinician should provide oral EC if required (i.e. due to recent unprotected sex). In addition, women with symptoms of pelvic infection with an IUD should be tested for STIs. To minimize the risk of pelvic infection, screening women at risk of STIs before insertion is advised. Prophylactic antibiotics (at least to cover chlamydia) can be given to women at high risk of an STI if insertion needs to be done before the results of tests are known (e.g. Cu-IUD insertion for EC).

'Missing' threads

'Missing' threads may indicate pregnancy, expulsion or perforation. However, it is often the case that the threads are merely sitting in the cervical canal or uterus. A pregnancy test should be performed and EC/alternative contraception provided until the IUD can be confirmed to be in situ, either by visualization of the threads on speculum examination or an ultrasound confirming the presence of the IUD within the uterus.

BARRIER CONTRACEPTION

CONDOMS

Male condoms are cheap and widely available. They protect against STIs including HIV. They are currently the only available reversible male method. Typical failure rates are in the region of 24%, as they rely on users putting them on correctly before penetration and before every act of sex. The female condom is a lubricated polyurethane condom that is inserted into the vagina. It also protects against STIs (**Figure 6.6**).

DIAPHRAGM AND CAP

These are latex or non-latex devices that are inserted into the vagina to prevent the passage of sperm to the cervix (**Figure 6.7**). They can be inserted in

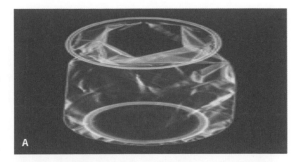

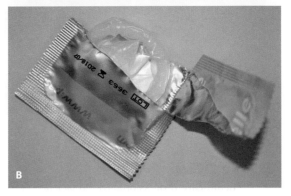

Figure 6.6 (A) Female condom. **(B)** Male condom.

advance of sex. Caps fit over the cervix, whereas diaphragms form a hammock between the postfornix and the symphysis pubis. Caps and diaphragms are often used in conjunction with a spermicide. Disadvantages of these devices are that women need to be able to insert and remove them, and typical failure rates in the region of 18% are reported. In some individuals, their use may be associated with increased vaginal discharge and urinary tract infections.

SPERMICIDES

Spermicide alone is not recommended for the prevention of pregnancy, as it is of low effectiveness. Nonoxynol-9 is a spermicidal product sold as a gel, cream, foam, sponge or pessary for use with diaphragms or caps. Some data have suggested that frequent use of Nonoxynol-9 might increase the risk of HIV transmission. It is therefore no longer recommended for women who are at high risk of HIV infection.

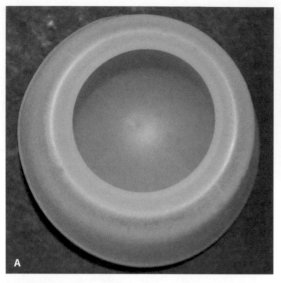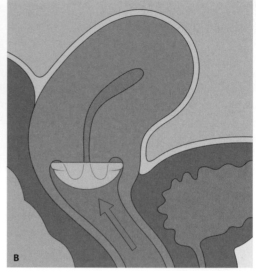

Figure 6.7 (**A**) A cap. (**B**) Correct position of a cap.

FEMALE STERILIZATION

This is a permanent method of contraception that prevents sperm reaching the oocyte in the fallopian tube. It can be performed by laparoscopy or laparotomy (e.g. at caesarean section).

LAPAROSCOPIC STERILIZATION

Laparoscopic sterilization most commonly occludes the fallopian tube with filshie clips (**Figure 6.8**). Effective contraception should be used until the next menses after the procedure due to the risk of

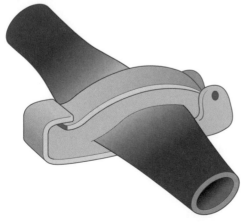

Figure 6.8 Filshie clip.

pregnancy from implantation of an early fertilized egg in the same cycle as sterilization.

Careful assessment of surgical risk at laparoscopic sterilization is required for women who pose a higher surgical risk due to significant obesity or previous abdominal surgery.

Women who are requesting sterilization at the same time as having a caesarean section must be counselled and must give consent for this well in advance of the procedure.

As sterilization results in permanent loss of fertility and involves a surgical procedure, it is important that valid consent is obtained. Individuals would be deemed unable to consent if it is clear that, having been provided with appropriate support and information, they cannot comprehend, retain, assess or use the information provided to them to make a decision. In such cases, legal advice should be sought.

VASECTOMY

This is the technique of interrupting the vas deferens to provide permanent occlusion. The so-called no-scalpel vasectomy involves a puncture wound in the skin of the scrotum under local anaesthesia to access and then divide and occlude the vas using cautery (**Figure 6.9**).

BOX 6.7: Advice to be given to women considering sterilization

- The method is considered irreversible.
- The failure rate is 1:200 (comparable to long-acting reversible methods).
- There are risks and complications (1:1,000 risk of trauma to the bowel, bladder or blood vessels).
- Vasectomy is safer and quicker, has less morbidity and can usually be performed under local anaesthesia.
- A significant proportion of women regret sterilization. Risk factors for regret are being under 30 years, nulliparity, recent pregnancy (birth, abortion or miscarriage) and relationship issues.
- Sterilization does not protect against STIs.
- Effective contraception is required until the menstrual period following the procedure.
- Pregnancy following sterilization is rare but, if it does occur, there is an increased relative risk of the pregnancy being ectopic.

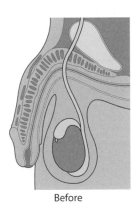 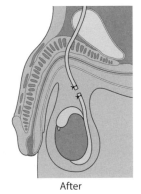

Before   After

Figure 6.9 Vasectomy.

There is a small risk of a scrotal haematoma and infection with the procedure. Post-vasectomy semen analysis should be conducted at 12 weeks to confirm the absence of spermatozoa in the ejaculate. Alternative contraception should be used until azoospermia is confirmed. The failure rate of vasectomy is significantly less than that of female sterilization at approximately 1 in 2,000. In addition, vasectomy has the advantage that it can usually be performed under local anaesthesia.

FERTILITY AWARENESS-BASED METHODS

Fertility awareness-based methods rely on the signs and symptoms that reflect the physiological changes that occur during the menstrual cycle that define the fertile period, with avoidance of intercourse at that time. The use of fertility awareness-based methods requires motivation and a regular menstrual cycle, and so cannot be used for women at the extremes of reproductive age or with irregular periods. Typical failure rates are high.

The method depends on the use of one or more of the following indicators to enable the avoidance of intercourse during the fertile days.

CALENDAR OR RHYTHM METHOD

Fertile days are calculated based upon the cycle length recorded over at least six cycles. The first fertile day is calculated as the shortest cycle minus 20. The last fertile day is calculated as the longest cycle minus 10. For individuals with a 28-day cycle, this equates to abstinence for 10 days in each cycle (i.e. days 8–18).

TEMPERATURE METHOD

This relies on the increase in basal body temperature (0.5°C) produced by the rise in progesterone following ovulation. Daily temperatures must be measured using the same route. Infection, exercise and some medications can affect body temperature and interfere with this method.

CERVICAL MUCUS METHOD

Mucus on toilet tissue after wiping the vulva can be examined for consistency. Mid-cycle 'fertile' mucus due to rising oestradiol levels is clear, watery and slippery, rather like raw egg white. Following ovulation, progesterone renders it thick and opaque. Semen in the vagina makes it difficult to recognise the mucus.

CERVICAL PALPATION

At mid-cycle, the cervix rises 1–2 cm and feels softer and moist.

PERSONAL FERTILITY MONITOR

This hand-held monitor analyses diposable urine dipsticks that record the presence of metabolites of oestrogen (estrone glucuronide) and LH in the urine. It recognises urinary oestrogen concentrations corresponding to the midfollicular phase of the cycle and the preovulatory LH peak, so that the beginning and end of the fertile phase can be identified. A red light indicates the fertile phase (risk of conception) and a green indicates the infertile phase. Users need to perform urine dipstick tests on early morning urine. A red light is usually shown for 6–10 days in the cycle.

DIGITAL FERTILITY AWARENESS-BASED METHODS

The use of mobile phone fertility apps for contraception has been growing among those keen to use a non-hormonal method of contraception. The apps facilitate input, storage and analysis of cycle characteristics together with some physiological data (e.g. basal body temperature) or hormonal tests such as urinary LH. The app then analyses the data and advises the woman on 'fertile days' and the need to abstain from sex or use barrier contraception.

LACTATIONAL AMENORRHOEA

If a mother is within 6 months post-partum, is amenorrhoeic and is fully or nearly fully breast-feeding, then their risk of pregnancy is about 2%. After 6 months, or if menses occur or breastfeeding is reduced, then another method of contraception must be used.

EMERGENCY CONTRACEPTION

The Cu-IUD is the most effective method of EC available (failure rate 1 in 1,000) and should ideally be offered as the first choice to women. When used for EC, its effect on the endometrium may prevent implantation if fertilization has occurred. The Cu-IUD can be removed once pregnancy has been excluded or can be left in place for ongoing contraception. There is some recent evidence that the LNG-IUD may also be effective for EC but, given the limited evidence, UK guidelines do not currently endorse its use for this purpose.

The two oral methods of EC that are licensed for use are levonorgestrel (LNG 1.5 mg) and the progesterone receptor modulator ulipristal acetate (UPA 30 mg). UPA is more effective than LNG for EC, and UPA can be used up to 120 hours after sex, whereas LNG is licensed for use up to 72 hours. Both methods work by delaying ovulation, so that any sperm present in the reproductive tract will have lost the ability to fertilize the oocyte once it is eventually released. Oral EC is estimated to prevent only two-thirds of pregnancies that might have occurred in the absence of EC. Oral EC is much less effective than regular contraception. Women should be encouraged to start an effective method of contraception immediately after EC, to protect against pregnancy from further acts of intercourse.

BOX 6.8: Emergency contraception

- The most effective method of EC is a Cu-IUD (effective).
- A Cu-IUD can be inserted up to 5 days after ovulation for EC.
- UPA and LNG are available as oral methods of EC.
- UPA is more effective than LNG and can be given within 120 hours of intercourse.
- Effective ongoing contraception should be started after EC.

OPPORTUNITIES TO PROVIDE CONTRACEPTION

There are important opportunities to discuss and provide effective contraception when patients present to gynaecology clinics (**Table 6.6**). These include presentation to a general gynaecology clinic, presentations for EC, presentation to request an abortion and also antenatally or after childbirth or following a miscarriage or an ectopic pregnancy. The antenatal/post-partum period is a particularly important opportunity, as studies consistently show that 95% of post-partum women want to avoid pregnancy in the next 12 months and, in women who are not fully breastfeeding, fertility may return as soon as just 1 month post-partum. In addition,

Table 6.6 Opportunities to provide contraception

Opportunity	Rationale
Gynaecology clinic	Gynaecological benefits of many hormonal methods of contraception
EC	Two- to threefold higher risk of unintended pregnancy if women have further unprotected sex in the same cycle after EC Cu-IUD can be used for EC and to provide ongoing contraception
Request for abortion	Most women ovulate in the month following an abortion Women who choose to start a LARC method at the time of abortion have a significantly reduced risk of a further abortion in the next few years
Antenatal/ post-partum period	50% of women resume sex by 6 weeks after childbirth Non-breastfeeding women may ovulate at day 21
Early pregnancy unit	Effective contraception is required following ectopic pregnancy treated with methotrexate teratogenic Not all pregnancies ending in miscarriage have been intended and so effective contraception may be required

Cu-IUD, copper intrauterine device; EC, emergency contraception; LARC, long-acting reversible contraception.

closely spaced pregnancies increase the risks of preterm delivery, low birth weight and small-for-gestational-age babies. The risk of child mortality is highest for very short birth to pregnancy intervals (<12 months). It is estimated that 30% of maternal and 10% of child deaths worldwide could be prevented if couples spaced pregnancies more than 2 years apart.

THE FUTURE

Given the wide range of existing contraceptive methods and delivery systems (pill, patch, ring, injectable and intrauterine) and hormonal methods with established safety, the question is often posed: Do we need new methods of contraception?

We should remember that, even in high-income countries, unintended pregnancy rates remain high. The uptake of existing methods is limited by their acceptability to women, and for many methods discontinuation rates are high. As science advances our understanding of reproductive physiology, women should be able to benefit from more sophisticated methods of contraception that may be devoid of side effects and offer more health benefits (such as protection against STIs or breast cancer). It is also important that male methods are developed, as they are currently limited to condoms or vasectomy.

KEY LEARNING POINTS

- In sexually active women, contraception is required until the menopause (or the age of 55 years).
- LARC methods are currently the most effective contraceptive methods, with typical failure rates close to perfect failure rates.
- The uptake of contraception and its continuation is limited by its acceptability to the user.
- If no contraceptive method is used, or a method fails, then women need easy access to EC.

ABORTION

No method of contraception is perfect and so there will always be the need for safe abortion. Safe abortion saves lives and prevents the severe morbidity associated with unsafe abortion. Modern methods of inducing an abortion are safer than all common gynaecological operations, such as sterilization and hysterectomy, and there is a lower risk of dying than during childbirth. Evidence shows that the liberalization of abortion laws does NOT lead to more abortions. Restricting access to abortion simply leads to unsafe abortion, with a consequent increase in the risk of death or severe morbidity for pregnant women.

LAWS AND REGULATION OF ABORTION

In most countries, abortion is subject to laws and regulations. In countries with the most restrictive laws (including abortion being illegal), the rates of death and severe morbidity as a result of unsafe abortion are highest. The WHO's Global Abortion Policies Database is a website that provides up-to-date information for each country.

In Great Britain (England, Scotland and Wales), abortion is subject to the 1967 Abortion Act, which states that abortion can be performed if two registered medical practitioners acting in good faith agree that the pregnancy should be terminated on one of the recognized legal grounds (**Table 6.7**). There is actually no medical need for two doctors

to be involved, and the British Medical Association Ethics Committee has long argued that the law should be changed and that abortion should be 'decriminalized altogether'. This means it would be regulated in the same way as other medical treatments. Criminalizing anyone for having an abortion is incompatible with human rights, as is requiring doctors and health workers to report women who have had abortions.

In the UK, any medical practitioner who has an objection to abortion is not required to participate in abortion services, unless the treatment is necessary to save the life of the pregnant woman. However, a medical practitioner who conscientiously objects to abortion should still provide advice and refer the patient promptly to another doctor who does not hold such views.

The 1967 Abortion Act does not apply to Northern Ireland where, until 2019, abortion was only legal in exceptional circumstances to save the life of the mother. In 2019, abortion became decriminalized in Northern Ireland, paving the way for the provision of services. However, the provision of services remains poor, meaning that many pregnant women in Northern Ireland who seek an abortion may still to travel to other parts of the UK for abortion or continue an unintended pregnancy.

Table 6.7 Great Britain legal grounds for termination of pregnancy

Ground	Description
A	Continuance of the pregnancy would involve risk to the life of the pregnant woman greater than if the pregnancy were terminated
B	Termination is necessary to prevent grave permanent injury to the physical or mental health of the pregnant woman
C	Pregnancy has not exceeded its 24th week and continuance of the pregnancy would involve risk, greater than if the pregnancy were terminated, of injury to the physical or mental health of the pregnant woman
D	Pregnancy has not exceeded its 24th week and continuance of the pregnancy would involve risk, greater than if the pregnancy were terminated, of injury to the physical or mental health of any existing child(ren) of the family of the pregnant woman
E	There is a substantial risk that if the child were born, it would suffer from such physical or mental abnormalities as to be seriously handicapped
F	To save the life of the pregnant woman
G	To prevent grave permanent injury to the physical or mental health of the pregnant woman

The vast majority (>95%) of all abortions in Great Britain are carried out under Ground C of the 1967 Abortion Act (**Table 6.7**), with approximately 1% carried out for serious fetal abnormality (Ground E). With the exception of emergency abortion to save the life of the mother or severe fetal abnormality, the upper legal limit for abortion is 24 weeks (23 completed weeks), which reflects fetal viability as a result of improvement in neonatal care.

The UK National Institute for Health and Care Excellence (NICE) guideline on the care of women requesting an abortion recommends that women should be able to access abortion services without delay. At early gestation, medical abortion has the greatest efficacy and there is less pain and bleeding and the lowest risk of complications. In addition, (depending on legislation in the country), women can choose to self-administer the medications for medical abortion at home. Studies show that most women requesting an abortion are certain of their decision and so routine counselling for decision making is not required. However, anyone who is uncertain should be offered sympathetic non-directional support in decision-making. No woman seeking an abortion should be subjected to compulsory counselling or a mandatory period of reflection.

METHODS OF ABORTION

The methods of abortion are medical abortion – that is, the use of medications to end a pregnancy – and surgical abortion, namely transcervical procedures to end a pregnancy, including manual vacuum aspiration, electrical vacuum aspiration, and dilatation and evacuation.

Neither medical nor surgical abortion is a complex procedure and both have a very low rate of complications. Indeed, the WHO advise that, in the first trimester, it can be safely performed by a range of healthcare providers including an appropriately trained nurse or midwife (if country legislation permits this). Both medical and surgical methods can be used to induce abortion throughout pregnancy. Ideally, patients should be given a choice of method, although the method used may also depend on factors such as the gestational stage, pre-existing medical conditions and local availability of surgery.

PRE-ABORTION ASSESSMENT

During the consultation around a request for abortion, healthcare providers should refrain from imposing personal values or beliefs on a patient and should instead focus on their needs and show empathy and respect for their decision to end a pregnancy. It is also important to appreciate that the patient may be anxious and sensitive to perceived negative attitudes or of feeling judged given the stigma that surrounds abortion in society. If the consultation is being conducted by telephone, on a video call or online, the healthcare professional should be confident that the patient is able to speak privately without risk of being overheard. It is necessary to determine that the patient seeking an abortion is sure of their decision and is not being coerced into terminating the pregnancy.

Clinical history taking should identify any medical conditions that might affect suitability for a particular method of abortion and any extra considerations that might determine the setting for the abortion, including those with serious medical conditions who may require input from another speciality. It is also important to ask every patient about sexual and domestic violence and abuse (physical and emotional) and, where necessary, to refer them to appropriate support services.

The gestation of pregnancy should be determined. This can be assessed from the first day of the last menstrual period. Routine pre-abortion ultrasound scanning is not necessary but, if available, should be used if there is clinically relevant uncertainty about the pregnancy duration or if there is reason to suspect an ectopic pregnancy, such a pain, bleeding or significant risk factors (e.g. previous ectopic pregnancy, sterilization procedure or tubal disease).

It is also good practice to undertake an STI risk assessment on everyone and then to screen, where appropriate (e.g. for chlamydia and gonorrhoea), which might be implicated in postabortion infection.

Pre-abortion assessment does not require routine blood tests. A determination of rhesus status may be considered if the duration of the pregnancy is over 12 weeks and anti-D is available. Measurement of haemoglobin or other blood tests are not required unless there are good clinical indications for doing so, such as for those with symptomatic anaemia.

Women seeking abortion should be offered information about all of their contraceptive options, but they should not be pressured to choose or start a method.

MEDICAL ABORTION

The majority of women undergoing abortion in countries where medical abortion is available choose to have abortion performed medically. This involves the combination of mifepristone (a progesterone receptor modulator) followed by a prostaglandin analogue, misoprostol.

Progesterone is necessary to maintain uterine quiescence, so the administration of mifepristone (oral) brings about an increase in uterine contractility, as well as some softening and dilation of the cervix. Mifepristone also sensitizes the uterus to exogenous prostaglandins so that these have a synergistic effect. This permits lower doses of misoprostol to be used to bring about expulsion. The effect of mifepristone is maximal at 48 hours; therefore, if misoprostol is administered at an interval of 24–48 hours later, there is an increase in cramping pain, bleeding and expulsion of the fetus through the slightly dilated cervix. Evidence-based guidelines from the WHO recommend that patients can safely self-administer these medications at home (if the country legislation permits) and expel the pregnancy at home up to 12 weeks' gestation. Simple oral analgesia (e.g. ibuprofen, dihydrocodeine) is usually provided for pain relief. Pain and bleeding tend to increase with gestation. Patients can be advised that at 9 weeks' gestation they will bleed for, on average, 2 weeks following the medical abortion. **Table 6.8** sets out advice for women on what to expect with medical abortion.

After 12 weeks' gestation, the same combination of mifepristone and misoprostol is used, except that the regimen requires repeated doses of misoprostol to be administered every 3 hours until expulsion occurs. After 12 weeks' gestation, the discomfort experienced, increased bleeding and passage of a larger fetus mean that these cases are managed in a clinical facility, although there is no evidence that home management is unsafe. In the second trimester, the average induction to abortion time (from first dose of misoprostol to expulsion) is 7 hours.

Table 6.8 What to expect with medical abortion

Possibility/event	Frequency/further information
Incomplete abortion requiring surgical evacuation	Less than 5%
Ongoing pregnancy	1–2%
Severe infection	Less than 1%
Haemorrhage (>1,000 mL)	0.1%
Median duration bleeding (at 8 weeks' gestation)	12 days
Median blood loss (at 8 weeks' gestation)	72.5 mL
Factors associated with greater pain	Advanced gestation, nulliparity, dysmenorrhoea
Location of expulsion	Home (depending on legislation and stage of pregnancy) or clinical facility

After 21 completed weeks (i.e. 21 weeks and 6 days), the Royal College of Obstetricians and Gynaecologists recommends that for women undergoing medical abortion, feticide should be used to eliminate the possibility of the aborted fetus displaying any signs of life. This is usually conducted by intracardiac injection of potassium chloride or an intrafetal or intramniotic injection of digoxin. The neural pathways necessary to experience pain are not fully developed in the fetus until after 24 weeks.

SURGICAL METHODS

VACUUM ASPIRATION

Vacuum aspiration is the method that should be used to conduct a surgical termination of pregnancy up to 14 weeks. The procedure involves gently dilating the cervix with graduated dilators (usually to the size in mm that the uterus is in weeks' gestation) and then evacuating the cavity with gentle suction. This usually takes less than 10 minutes to perform. Sharp curettage should never be performed (there is an increased risk of perforation and intrauterine adhesions). Vacuum aspiration can be performed using either a manual handheld aspirator (manual vacuum aspiration) or electrical vacuum aspiration. There is little to choose between manual and electrical vacuum aspiration. Manual vacuum aspiration may be more practical and portable for use in the outpatient setting. Electrical vacuum aspiration gives a more constant suction.

Surgical termination can be performed under either local or general anaesthesia. Local anaesthesia in the first trimester is preferred, as it minimizes any small risk of anaesthetic drugs. It is important to provide pretreatment of the cervix for all patients undergoing surgical abortion to bring about cervical dilation, which makes instrumentation of the cervical canal easier and minimizes the risk of incomplete abortion. The optimal regimen for cervical pretreatment is 400 µg misoprostol given sublingually 1 hour prior to the surgical procedure. Alternatively, 200 mg mifepristone can be given orally 24 hours before surgery.

It is recommended that prophylactic antibiotics should be given (periabortal) with surgical abortion, as this has been shown to significantly reduce the risk of postabortal infection following this procedure. The optimal antibiotic regimen is not known, but doxycycline, penicillins and nitroimidazoles have all been shown to be effective. Prophylactic antibiotics are not considered necessary following medical abortion, as the overall incidence of postabortal infection is lower after medical than after surgical abortion.

DILATION AND EVACUATION

After 14 weeks, the surgical technique of choice is dilatation and evacuation (often known as D&E). In skilled hands, this procedure has a low complication rate and is highly acceptable to women. It is widely used in North America, but is less common in Europe. It is necessary to achieve good cervical dilation before the procedure (up to 20 mm) in order to remove larger fetal parts. This is achieved using one or a combination of the following: osmotic dilators (hygroscopic sticks placed in the cervix several hours before the procedure that absorb fluid from surrounding tissues, causing them to swell and bring about cervical dilation), misoprostol (vaginal or sublingual) and/or mifepristone (oral). At surgery, the cervix is then further dilated using graduated dilators and the contents of the uterus removed by a combination of aspiration and extraction of fetal tissue using appropriate instruments; ultrasound is performed to confirm complete evacuation.

SEQUELAE OF ABORTION

Both medical and surgical abortion are safe and have a high success rate. Adverse outcomes, when they do occur, include failure to end the pregnancy (ongoing pregnancy) and incomplete abortion requiring evacuation. Both abortion methods are also associated with a low incidence of complications. Complications include infection and haemorrhage. In the absence of a serious complication (such as operative complication or severe infection), there is no impact on future fertility. While several studies have suggested an increased risk of preterm delivery following abortion, findings of recent studies have suggested that modern medical and surgical methods of inducing abortion are not associated with this risk.

There is no association with breast cancer. There is no adverse effect on mental health, although women with an existing mental health issue or a history of poor mental health are at an increased risk of an exacerbation postabortion, as they are post-partum. Women for whom the pregnancy was originally intended, women who are unsupported, and women who are ambivalent about the decision to terminate or who belong to a group that feels that abortion is morally wrong are at a higher risk of ongoing distress or regret following the procedure. Women should be given information on how to seek help under such circumstances.

FOLLOW-UP AFTER ABORTION

There is no medical need for a follow-up after an uncomplicated medical or surgical abortion. Rather, good verbal and written advice about signs and symptoms that might indicate the need to seek medical attention should be provided, together with access to 24-hour emergency care. Women should also be provided with their chosen method of ongoing contraception at the time of the abortion procedure. For anyone who had a medical abortion at home, there should be an effective method of confirming the success of the abortion. This is commonly a self-performed urine pregnancy test at home: either a low-sensitivity urine pregnancy test (detection limit 1,000 IU human chorionic gonadotrophin [hCG]) from 2 weeks after treatment or a high-sensitivity test (detection 50 IU hCG or less) from 4 weeks after treatment.

POSTABORTAL CONTRACEPTION

Most women ovulate in the first month after abortion, and more than half of women will have resumed sex by 2 weeks postabortion. Guidelines therefore advise that effective contraception should be commenced immediately to avoid another unintended pregnancy. However, women should never be pressured into choosing contraception or into choosing a particular method. All methods of contraception can be started at the time of surgical abortion, including an IUD, which can be inserted following evacuation. All methods of hormonal contraception can be started with medical abortion at the time of mifepristone, and an IUD can be inserted as soon as expulsion of the pregnancy takes place.

There is evidence that women who choose to use the most effective LARC methods postabortion (and start these immediately after the abortion) have a significantly reduced risk of having a subsequent unintended pregnancy, compared with women choosing other methods. There has been much effort in recent years to ensure that abortion services provide high-quality information about contraception and are able to provide all methods at the time of discharge following the procedure (including the provision of LARC). All hormonal methods can be safely commenced at the time of abortion. Intrauterine methods can be inserted at the time of surgical abortion and following expulsion of the pregnancy at medical abortion.

FURTHER READING

Faculty of Sexual and Reproductive Healthcare (2020). *Clinical Effectiveness Unit Guidance: Recommended Actions after Incorrect Use of Combined Hormonal Contraception*. https://www.fsrh.org/documents/fsrh-ceu-guidance-recommended-actions-after-incorrect-use-of/.

Faculty of Sexual and Reproductive Healthcare (n.d.). Standards & Guidance. https://www.fsrh.org/standards-and-guidance/.

Global Library of Women's Medicine (n.d.). Fertility regulation. https://www.glowm.com/volume-content/item/6/recordset=64585&value=501#sub-501.

NICE (2019). *Abortion Care*. NICE guideline [NG140]. https://www.nice.org.uk/guidance/NG140.

RCOG (n.d.). Making abortion safe. https://elearning.rcog.org.uk/catalog?pagename=Making-Abortion-Safe.

WHO (2015). *Medical Eligibility Criteria for Contraceptive Use*, 5th edn. Geneva: WHO. https://www.who.int/publications/i/item/9789241549158.

WHO (2022). *Abortion Care Guideline*. Geneva: WHO. https://www.who.int/publications/i/item/9789240039483.

WHO (n.d.). Global Abortion Policies Database. https://abortion-policies.srhr.org/countries/.

SELF-ASSESSMENT

For interactive SBAs and EMQs relating to this chapter, visit www.routledge.com/cw/crosbie.

CASE HISTORY

A 44-year-old woman requests sterilization, as she does not want any more children. She has three children. Her partner will not consider a vasectomy. She has regular but heavy menses. She is currently using no method of contraception. She smokes and suffers from migraine.

A   What are the key points to cover in the counselling on sterilization?
B   What alternative methods of contraception might be appropriate for this woman?
C   What methods of contraception is she not medically eligible for?

ANSWERS

A   Important points to cover are that sterilization should be considered irreversible, that it has a failure rate of approximatly 1:200 and that it is a surgical procedure with associated risks and complications. It is no more effective than long-acting reversible methods and sometimes these methods are used to manage menstrual bleeding problems that increase with age. In addition, pregnancy following female sterilization is rare but, if it does occur, there is an increased risk of ectopic pregnancy. Moreover, the reversal of sterilization is a highly skilled procedure of obtaining tubal reanastomosis and is not commonly performed or available, so in vitro fertilization (IVF) would be required if a pregnancy was later desired.

B   The LNG-IUD provides comparable contraceptive effectiveness and also has the non-contraceptive benefit of reduced menstrual blood loss. Other progestogen-only methods such as the POP or progestogen-only implant may also be appropriate, but irregular bleeding is common and POP has higher typical failure rates. The injectable could also be considered.

C   CHC is contraindicated, as the woman is a smoker who is over 35 years and also has migraine. The Cu-IUD is not ideal, as this may exacerbate the existing heavy menses.

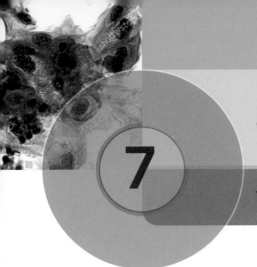

Subfertility

7

YING CHEONG

Learning Objectives
- Understand the definition and causes of subfertility.
- Describe the concept of ovarian reserve.
- Understand the history, examination and investigations relevant to subfertility.
- Understand the provision and regulation of fertility treatment.
- Explain the processes and procedures involved in assisted reproductive treatment.
- Understand the outcomes and success rates of assisted reproductive treatment.

INTRODUCTION

A delay in conception is one of the most common reasons that a woman will consult their doctor. The most common accepted definition for subfertility is failure to conceive after 12 months of regular unprotected intercourse. The incidence of subfertility is thought to be one in seven heterosexual couples. There has been an increase in the number of couples accessing treatment services over the last 10 years in the UK. This may be related to social demographic changes, with more couples delaying childbirth, and an increased acceptance of fertility treatments. The diagnosis of subfertility may be primary in couples that have never conceived together or secondary in couples that have previously conceived together (although either partner may have conceived in a different relationship, which requires further elucidation). The approach to fertility investigation and management should always be couple-centred. Specialist teams should be available to offer evidence-based advice and treatment to couples, supported by counselling services and accurate information.

NATURAL CONCEPTION

A healthy couple having regular intercourse have a 15–20% chance of conceiving in a single menstrual cycle. As a species this makes our reproduction relatively inefficient. There is of course a cumulative increase in pregnancy rates over time as couples try to conceive. Within 6 months, 70% of couples will

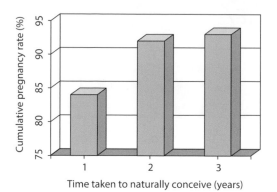

Figure 7.1 The natural conception rate over a 3-year period.

have conceived; after 12 months, 80% of couples will have conceived; and, by 24 months, 90% of couples will achieve a pregnancy (**Figure 7.1**). The most important factor affecting fertility is female age, which is related to a decline in the quality and quantity of eggs. Female fertility falls sharply after 35 years of age, with a further dip after 40. However, there is considerable variation, and biological age (or ovarian reserve) does not always correlate with chronological age. Male age is also important; semen quality falls in men over the age of 50.

Both frequency and timing of sexual intercourse have a strong impact on conception rates. Couples having intercourse three times a week are three times more likely to conceive than those having intercourse once a week. Maximum 'efficiency' is probably intercourse at least two to three times per week outside menstruation. There should, however, be awareness among physicians and patients of the added stress and anxiety that 'over-medicalizing' this advice can bring to couples. Increased frequency of intercourse should be encouraged in the peri-ovulatory period. Eggs are thought to be fertilizable for about 12–24 hours post-ovulation, while sperm can survive in the female reproductive tract for up to 72 hours. Ovulation usually occurs about 14 days prior to menstruation, with the luteal phase being relatively stable in length. The 'fertile window' for women will therefore be different depending on the average length of their menstrual cycle (e.g. for a 28-day menstrual cycle, the optimal fertile window is days 12 to 15).

External factors influence the chance of conception. Smoking can decrease the quality and quantity of eggs and sperm. The role of alcohol and caffeine remains controversial, with no compelling evidence to totally abstain while trying to conceive, but moderation is probably sensible. Body mass index (BMI) exerts a strong influence on fertility, with male and female BMI at either extreme associated with a reduced chance of conceiving. However, there is little evidence for so-called fertility diets to improve natural fertility. Stress can have a direct influence on the hypothalamic–pituitary–ovarian (HPO) axis, interfering with regular ovulation, and may indirectly reduce conception by reducing libido and frequency of intercourse.

All women trying to conceive should take folic acid 400 µg daily to reduce fetal neural tube defects until 12 weeks' gestation and should take vitamin D 10 µg daily throughout pregnancy. Women at higher risk of neural tube defects, including those with a family history of neural tube defects and those taking anti-epileptic drugs, should take folic acid 5 mg daily.

CAUSES OF SUBFERTILITY

The main cause of subfertility varies across the world. In the UK, around 30% of subfertility is caused by a male factor, 30% is caused by a female factor, 25% is unexplained and 15% has both male and female or other causes. This can be further broken down into specific causes (some of which are male and some of which are female), as shown in **Figure 7.2**.

FEMALE SUBFERTILITY

Ovulatory disorders, tubal damage and uterine disorders (e.g. fibroids) are most common, with endometrial pathology, specific gamete defects and endometriosis contributory. Cigarette smoking reduces fertility. General medical conditions including diabetes, epilepsy, thyroid disorders and bowel disease can reduce the chance of conception. Decreased ovarian reserve associated with advanced female age is increasingly important, as

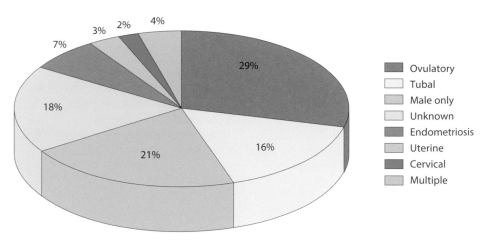

Figure 7.2 Causes of subfertility.

couples are more commonly delaying pregnancy until their 30s and 40s.

OVULATORY DISORDERS

The most common cause of ovulation disturbance is polycystic ovary syndrome (PCOS; see **Chapter 3**). Women with PCOS who suffer from oligomenorrhoea due to anovulation may require treatment; however, the hormonal treatments taken to regulate periods or improve hirsutism are contraindicated in women trying to conceive (e.g. the combined oral contraceptive pill).

Hypothalamic disorders (including hypothalamic hypogonadism), pituitary disease (hyperprolactinaemia) and endocrine abnormalities (thyroid disease) are less common causes of anovulation.

TUBAL PROBLEMS

Tubal disease is usually associated with pelvic inflammatory disease or endometriosis. Chlamydial infection is a leading cause of hydrosalpinx: a blocked fallopian tube, often with a thickened wall, flattened epithelial mucosa and peri-tubal adhesions.

Previous pelvic or abdominal surgery can result in post-operative scar tissue or adhesions that can also compromise tubal patency and function. The fallopian tube is not a passive conduit. Tubal function requires both patency and normal physiology for gamete and embryo transport.

UTERINE PROBLEMS

Uterine factors such as fibroids can interfere with fertility, but their impact depends on their size and location. Submucosal fibroids reduce fertility, but there is insufficient evidence to implicate intramural and subserosal fibroids in reducing fertility. Endometrial polyps sometimes reduce the chance of implantation. Endometrial scarring (Asherman syndrome) from surgery or infection can be associated with lighter or no periods and a significantly reduced chance of conception.

MALE FACTOR

Compromised sperm number or quality is an important contributor to subfertility. There is some evidence that sperm counts are falling, which may be the result of environmental or dietary issues. Spermatogonial cells that produce sperm can be damaged by inflammation (orchitis), and the epididymis that stores mature sperm can also be damaged. Certain iatrogenic influences, including pelvic radiotherapy and surgery for undescended or torted testes, reduce sperm production and damage or block the male reproductive tract. Medical conditions such as diabetes and certain occupations involving contact with chemicals or radiation are associated with male factor subfertility. Occasionally, sperm production may be normal but there are erectile difficulties or problems with ejaculation.

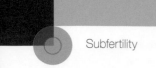

Table 7.1 Key points to cover in the history taking and examination of patients presenting with subfertility

Female	Male
History	
Age	Age
Length of time spent trying for pregnancy	Length of time spent trying for pregnancy
Any previous pregnancies?	Fathered any previous pregnancies?
Coital frequency	History of mumps or measles
Occupation	History of testicular trauma or surgery to testis
General gynaecological history	Occupation
Previous history of pelvic inflammatory disease	Medical and surgical history
Medical and surgical history	
Previous fertility treatment	
Cervical smear history	
General health – screen for history of thyroid disorders	
Examination	
Pelvic examination – any uterine pathology such as fibroids and adnexal masses or tenderness	Testicular examination – testicular volume, consistency, masses, absence of vas deferens, varicocele, evidence of surgical scars
General blood pressure, pulse, height and weight	

Genetic causes of male factor infertility include aneuploidy of sex chromosomes (Klinefelter [XXY] syndrome, most commonly) and structural abnormalities of the autosomes, such as inversions, deletions or balanced translocations. Microdeletions of the azoospermia factor (AZF) regions of the Y chromosome are associated with low sperm counts and motility.

HISTORY AND EXAMINATION

A thorough and detailed history is taken from patients presenting with subfertility. As this is a couple-centred issue, it is advisable for both partners to be present at the consultation. Key features of history taking and examination are presented in **Table 7.1**. In many clinics, a template is employed to ensure that all of these features are covered.

INVESTIGATIONS

Diagnosing a cause of subfertility enables treatment to be targeted to a specific pathology. However, even with a detailed series of investigations, a specific cause may not be found for many couples. There is some debate as to when investigations should start. Most

authorities suggest that a couple who have not conceived after 1 year of regular unprotected intercourse should be investigated; however, age and level of anxiety should be taken into account. Investigations may start earlier if the couple have known predisposing factors, including amenorrhoea, oligomenorrhoea, pelvic inflammatory disease, women with low ovarian reserve or male-factor subfertility.

FEMALE INVESTIGATIONS

A blood hormone profile test should be undertaken. In a woman with a regular menstrual cycle, this should include early follicular phase follicular-stimulating hormone (FSH), oestradiol and luteinizing hormone (LH). Anti-Müllerian hormone (AMH) (see **Box 7.1** 'Measurement of ovarian reserve') is proving particularly helpful in the assessment of ovarian reserve and is independent of the menstrual cycle, which is practical. A mid-luteal progesterone measurement should be taken to confirm ovulation. In women with an irregular menstrual cycle, thyroid function, prolactin and testosterone can also prove useful.

Chlamydia testing should be offered prior to any uterine instrumentation. If assisted reproductive technology (ART) is to be offered, viral screening for human immunodeficiency virus (HIV) and hepatitis B and C is important.

A transvaginal ultrasound scan (TVUSS) should be performed, where possible. This provides an accurate assessment of pelvic anatomy, including uterine size and shape, the presence of any fibroids, and ovarian size, position and morphology, with antral follicle count (AFC) an important parameter of ovarian reserve. Pathology, such as hydrosalpinges and endometriotic cysts, can be detected, and access to the ovaries for ART can be assessed. Tubal patency testing may be necessary, as described in the following section, 'Tubal assessment'.

BOX 7.1: Measurement of ovarian reserve

- Female reproductive potential is directly proportional to the number of oocytes in the ovaries, which is called ovarian reserve.
- Ovarian reserve declines after the age of 35 years in an average, healthy individual, or at an earlier age due to genetic predisposition, surgery or following exposure to toxins, such as chemotherapy.
- Ovarian reserve can help to predict response to ovarian stimulation in ART.
- AFC seen on TVUSS is a good indicator of ovarian reserve (AFC <4 predicting low ovarian response, >16 predicting high response).
- AMH is produced in the granulosa cells of ovarian follicles and does not change in response to gonadotrophins during the menstrual cycle. As a result, it can be measured and compared at any point in the cycle and, at present, is the most successful biochemical marker.
- Neither AMH nor AFC is a perfect indicator, and most clinics utilize both to assess ovarian reserve.

TUBAL ASSESSMENT

Tubal patency and an assessment of the uterine cavity are traditionally investigated by hysterosalpingography (HSG) using X-ray, hysterocontrast synography (HyCoSy) using ultrasound or, more recently, 3D HyCoSy (**Figure 7.3**). HSG and HyCoSy are comparable in terms of their effectiveness as screening tests for tubal patency. Both require instrumentation of the uterine cavity and instillation of radio-opaque dye

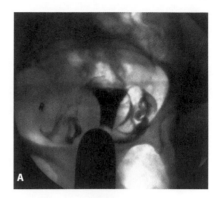

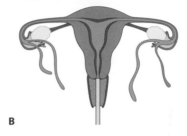

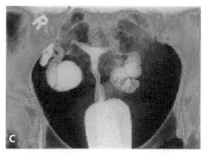

Figure 7.3 (**A**) Hysterosalpingogram showing normal patency of the fallopian tubes. (**B**) Pictorial illustration of a normal hysterosalpingogram. (**C**) Abnormal hysterosalpingogram with pocketed areas suggesting blocked tubes.

(HSG) or sono-opaque contrast medium (HyCoSy) via a very fine catheter. During HSG, the time lapse of the flow of dye is captured by X-rays, while, in HyCoSy, it is visualized via an ultrasound scan. If there is a blockage of the fallopian tube, dye will be seen to accumulate in a pocket representing the blocked end of the fallopian tube. There is some evidence that patients deemed at high risk of pelvic pathology could benefit from a more invasive laparoscopy and hysteroscopy as a dual diagnostic and potentially therapeutic procedure. It is crucial to remember that tubal patency is not equivalent to tubal function. Currently, there is no effective test to check for tubal function.

Table 7.2 World Health Organization parameters for semen analysis – Fifth centile

Parameter	Lower and reference limits
Semen volume (mL)	1.5 (1.4–1.7)
Sperm concentration (million/mL)	15 (12–16)
Total sperm number (million per ejaculate)	39 (33–46)
Progressive motility (%)	32 (31–34)
Morphology normal forms (%)	4 (3–4)
Vitality – live sperm (%)	58 (55–63)
pH	>7.2

MALE INVESTIGATIONS

The only routine investigation for males is a semen fluid analysis (SFA). Most centres recommend a 2- to 4-day abstinence from ejaculation before providing the semen sample. The new World Health Organization criteria (2021) for semen analysis are presented in **Table 7.2**. These are not average or median measurements, but represent lower reference limits (fifth centile). If the initial SFA is abnormal, it should be repeated 3 months later to allow adequate time for spermatogenesis, because occasionally an abnormal SFA will result from acute insults such as viral infections.

Some clinics will also assess total motile count, the presence of round cells or leucocytes to assess for inflammation, and the presence of sperm antibodies. For men with a very low sperm count or azoospermia, a hormone profile including FSH, LH and testosterone should be performed. This may have later importance in male health, as testicular failure may be associated with symptomatic low testosterone. A karyotype and a cystic fibrosis screen are also recommended.

Microdeletions of the AZFa and AZFb regions of the Y chromosome are not tested for routinely because they are not amenable to treatment. However, they carry a poor prognosis for surgical sperm retrieval procedures and may be tested for in this context in the presence of azoospermia.

Less evidence-based tests include measuring deoxyribonucleic acid (DNA) fragmentation levels in the sperm.

MANAGEMENT

The management of the couple's subfertility should be evidence-based. It relies on an accurate diagnostic evaluation, considering the couple's history, clinical examination and investigations. Management may be expectant, medical, surgical or a combination of these. Medical and surgical management are complementary to each other and fertility treatment must be individualized to optimize outcomes (**Table 7.3**).

OVULATION INDUCTION

For patients with ovulatory problems, ovulation induction is usually the first line of management, so long as there is tubal patency and normal semen analysis. The most common ovulation induction agent used is the anti-oestrogen clomiphene citrate. Clomiphene citrate induces gonadotrophin release by occupying the oestrogen receptors in the hypothalamus, thereby interfering with normal feedback mechanisms, boosting the release of FSH and so stimulating the ovary to produce more follicles. Approximately 70% of women on clomiphene citrate will ovulate, with a pregnancy rate of 15–20% per month. There is a risk of multiple pregnancies (12%), and women on clomiphene are monitored by ultrasound to track follicle growth, to time ovulation and to reduce the risk of multiple pregnancies. In clomiphene-resistant women, alternative strategies include augmentation with metformin, the use of aromatase inhibitors (although they are not licensed for this indication in some countries) and the use of injectable gonadotrophins. Ovulation can also be induced by laparoscopic ovarian drilling in PCOS. For unknown reasons, passing electrical energy through polycystic ovaries can induce ovulation. However, as laparoscopic ovarian drilling is a surgical procedure with associated risks, it is only appropriate to offer such treatment to women who are resistant to clomiphene treatment.

In women with anovulation of hypothalamic origin, ovulation induction using injectable gonadotrophins is more effective.

Table 7.3 Summary of the medical and surgical management of subfertility

Treatment	Treatment criteria
Medical	
Ovulation induction – clomiphene or FSH	Anovulation – PCOS, idiopathic
Intrauterine insemination – with or without stimulation with FSH	Unexplained subfertility
	Anovulation unresponsive to ovulation induction
	Mild male factor
	Minimal to mild endometriosis
Donor insemination – with or without stimulation with FSH	Presence of azoospermia
	Single women
	Same-sex couples
IVF	Patients with tubal pathology
	Patients who underwent the treatments listed previously with no success in pregnancy
Donor egg with IVF	Women whose egg quality is poor (e.g. older individuals, premature ovarian failure)
	Previous surgery/chemo-radiotherapy in which ovarian function was adversely affected
Surgical	
Operative laparoscopy to treat disease and restore anatomy	Adhesions
	Endometriosis
	Ovarian cyst
Myomectomy – hysteroscopy, laparoscopy, laparotomy, fibroid embolization	Fibroid uterus
Tubal surgery	Blocked fallopian tubes amenable to repair
Laparoscopic ovarian drilling	PCOS unresponsive to medical treatment

FSH, follicle-stimulating hormone; IVF, in vitro fertilization; PCOS, polycystic ovary syndrome.

SURGERY

Investigation of subfertility and tubal patency testing by minimal access surgery is undertaken if the patient is symptomatic or if specific therapeutic treatment is planned. There is good evidence that laparoscopic ablation of endometriosis can help improve natural conception rates. Often, surgery may be used as an adjunct to ART. For example, the surgical disconnection from the uterus or removal of hydrosalpinges is associated with a significant improvement in in vitro fertilization (IVF) success rates (**Figure 7.4**). Some practitioners still recommend a more traditional open laparotomy approach for myomectomy

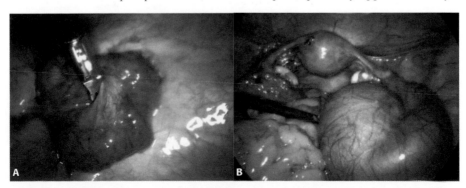

Figure 7.4 (**A**) Photograph of the normal fimbrial end of fallopian tube. (**B**) Photograph of right hydrosalpinx.

for very large uterine fibroids or tubal microsurgery to reverse sterilization or for proximal or distal tubal microsurgery. Submucosal fibroids, endometrial polyps, Asherman syndrome and some congenital uterine anomalies, such as a septum, are usually managed hysteroscopically.

INTRAUTERINE INSEMINATION

Intrauterine insemination (IUI) is performed by introducing a small sample of prepared sperm into the uterine cavity with a fine uterine catheter. IUI may be helpful in cases of mild endometriosis or mild male factor subfertility, in couples who do not have intercourse or in single women or same-sex couples using donor sperm. The success rate of this procedure ranges between 10% and 20% per treatment cycle. This process may be preceded by several days of mild stimulation with subcutaneous injections daily of exogenous FSH, with the aim of stimulating the ovaries to produce two or three mature follicles (this is termed stimulated IUI). Follicular tracking with ultrasound is essential to avoid over- or under-stimulation. Triggering of ovulation (and therefore the timing of the insemination) is achieved

with a subcutaneous injection of human chorionic gonadotrophin (hCG). This mimics the endogenous LH surge, due to crossover of the alpha-subunits of the two hormones.

IN VITRO FERTILIZATION

IVF was originally designed for couples with tubal factor subfertility. Steptoe and Edwards performed the first successful case in 1978. There are now over five million babies worldwide created through IVF. IVF is used for almost all cases of subfertility, including tubal disease, endometriosis, failed ovulation induction, failed IUI or when donor eggs are needed.

Originally, IVF was performed in the natural menstrual cycle, but the use of gonadotrophin-controlled ovarian stimulation made IVF a more efficient process. ART in the UK is regulated by the Human Fertilisation and Embryo Authority (HFEA), which provides guidelines and statistics for patients and clinicians and inspects clinics to ensure adherence to mutually agreed quality standards. IVF can be performed with many different protocols and medications, but the principal steps of IVF are shown in **Figure 7.5** and are as follows.

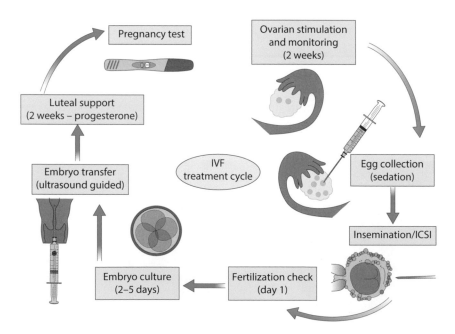

Figure 7.5 Pictorial in vitro fertilization cycle. (ICSI, intracytoplasmic sperm injection.)

PITUITARY DOWNREGULATION

In the most commonly used IVF cycle, the pituitary gland is downregulated to prevent endogenous LH surges and premature ovulation. A gonadotrophin-releasing hormone (GnRH) agonist is used to block the FSH and LH release from the pituitary. Newer approaches involving the use of GnRH antagonists can shorten treatment time and reduce the incidence of ovarian hyperstimulation syndrome.

CONTROLLED OVARIAN STIMULATION

This is achieved using daily subcutaneous doses of gonadotrophin medications, which cause multiple follicle recruitment. Close monitoring with TVUSS predicts the number of follicles and the timing of the egg collection. Ideally, around 15 follicles are recruited. Blood levels may be taken to measure oestradiol levels, and are used by some to measure ovarian response to stimulation. Ultrasound measurement of endometrial thickness is also performed.

INHIBITION OF PREMATURE OVULATION

Feedback from rising oestradiol associated with follicular development should lead to an LH surge from the pituitary, resulting in final oocyte maturation and ovulation. In IVF, this is blocked to allow scheduling of egg collection. This is traditionally done by the administration of GnRH agonists or with a newer, shorter GnRH antagonist protocol.

HUMAN CHORIONIC GONADOTROPHIN TRIGGER

hCG is used as a surrogate for the endogenous LH surge. It causes final maturation of the egg and allows scheduling of the egg collection procedure.

EGG COLLECTION

This procedure is usually performed about 37 hours post-hCG trigger. Under anaesthesia, a needle is inserted into the ovaries under TVUSS control and

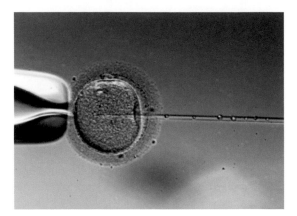

Figure 7.6 Intracytoplasmic sperm injection.

follicular fluid is aspirated from each follicle that contains an oocyte, which is collected by the embryologist into the laboratory.

FERTILIZATION

Fertilization is performed using prepared sperm. Conventional IVF involves the insemination of around 100,000 sperm in a Petri dish with an egg. In cases of poor sperm parameters or in cases of previous poor fertilization, individual sperm can be isolated and directly injected into the cytoplasm of the oocyte (intracytoplasmic sperm injection (ICSI); **Figure 7.6**). Fertilization is checked the next morning and is usually in the region of 60% for IVF and 70% for ICSI.

EMBRYO CULTURE

Embryos are incubated under strict conditions of temperature, pH, humidity and oxygen concentration. A very common type of incubator now used has time-lapse technology, which allows clinicians to review the development of the embryos in real time. The embryo(s) may be transferred back into the uterus after 2, 3 or 5 days of development. Embryos reaching the blastocyst stage on day 5 of development usually exhibit the best chance of implantation. A variety of different protocols are available for embryo selection, including a morphological and a morpho-kinetic assessment.

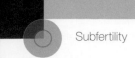

EMBRYO TRANSFER

Embryos are transferred into the uterus using a soft plastic catheter. The choice of how many embryos to transfer is the couple's decision following expert medical and embryological advice; this may be constrained by local regulatory or funding parameters. Embryo transfer is usually performed under trans-abdominal ultrasound control to ensure correct placement of the embryos. In the UK and Europe, there are recommendations regarding the transfer of single embryos to reduce the incidence of multiple pregnancies and their associated risks.

EMBRYO CRYOPRESERVATION

Spare embryos of good quality may be cryopreserved for future use. Vitrification techniques now allow for success rates from frozen embryos to approximate success rates in fresh treatment cycles. This makes the transfer of fresh single embryos with the vitrification of spare embryos more appealing to couples.

LUTEAL PHASE SUPPORT

The use of gonadotrophin agonists or antagonists to prevent a premature LH surge will lead to a reduction in the ability of the corpus luteum to produce progesterone. Patients are therefore supplemented with progesterone following the egg collection. There is no consensus on the ideal dose, route or duration of progesterone supplementation. A pregnancy test is performed around 14 days after embryo transfer.

ASSISTED REPRODUCTIVE TECHNOLOGY SUCCESS RATES

IVF success rates are exquisitely sensitive to female age. In patients under the age of 35, success rates can be as high as 40–45% from a single cycle, while in individuals over the age of 40 they fall below 15%. Undergoing IVF does not preclude the patient from the normal complications of pregnancy, such as miscarriage or ectopic pregnancies. The most significant risk of IVF treatment is ovarian hyperstimulation syndrome, occurring in 1–3% of cases. Patients with severe ovarian hyperstimulation syndrome present with ascites, enlarged multifollicular

ovaries, pulmonary oedema and coagulopathy. These patients need to be admitted to hospital and managed under strict protocols under the care of specialist teams. The use of low-dose stimulation, ultrasound monitoring, GnRH antagonist protocols, GnRH agonist triggers and a more liberal freezing policy have significantly reduced the incidence of this very serious condition.

DONOR GAMETES

Donor sperm can be used to treat patients when the male partner is azoospermic or in the case of single women or female same-sex couples. Both IUI and IVF treatments are possible. Donor eggs may be used if the woman has undergone early menopause or if IVF treatments have been unsuccessful and associated with a reduced ovarian reserve and low egg number and quality. Gamete donation requires careful and thorough counselling, and most countries have legislation to regulate its use.

SURGICAL SPERM RETRIEVAL

When the sperm quality or quantity is low, but sperm are present, ICSI is required to help achieve a pregnancy. However, in the absence of naturally ejaculated sperm (termed azoospermia – which may relate to blockage of the vas deferens or testicular problems), patients may undergo surgical sperm retrieval. This can be performed under sedation or general anaesthesia. A fine needle is inserted into the epididymis or the testicular tissue to obtain sperm or testicular tissue with sperm, respectively. The retrieved sperm can then be cryopreserved or injected into the oocyte as part of a fresh IVF/ICSI cycle.

OOCYTE, SPERM AND EMBRYO DONATION

Donated gametes may be required if one partner cannot produce their own. Sometimes, the couple chooses donated gametes if one has an underlying genetic condition. In the UK, individuals who donate their gametes to help others conceive do not have the right to remain anonymous. Their biological child has the right to know who their biological parents are when the child reaches 18 years old. Under European Union rules, an individual cannot be paid but they can be compensated for donating their gametes. Compensation is higher for those donating their oocytes who undergo invasive and potentially hazardous procedures. In the United States, oocyte donation is encouraged by offering huge financial incentives to donors.

SURROGACY

Surrogacy may be used if a woman has had a hysterectomy, has an underlying medical condition that prohibits pregnancy or has a poor obstetric history. The surrogate is the legal mother who cannot hand over parental responsibility until the child is 6 weeks of age. The oocytes may come from the commissioning couple, the surrogate or a donor.

INVOLUNTARY CHILDLESSNESS

Some couples remain involuntarily childless and the realization that they will never have a biological child of their own can be very traumatic. Couples need support and advice to come to terms with their predicament, which they may not have disclosed to friends and family. Adoption may be a solution for some couples when fertility treatment is not acceptable to them or if it fails.

PRE-IMPLANTATION GENETIC TESTING

Couples who carry a genetic disease (but who are fertile) may choose to use IVF and pre-implantation genetic testing (PGT) to avoid an affected pregnancy. These patients may previously have had affected children or terminations for an affected fetus. IVF will create multiple embryos. These embryos can then be genetically tested for the relevant disease by the removal of several cells at the blastocyst stage that are tested and taken to reflect the genotype of the remaining embryo. Only embryos free of the disease are transferred into the uterus. PGT has now been used worldwide for most monogenic diseases, as well as for translocations. The use of PGT for social sex selection is illegal in the UK, but is available controversially in many other countries.

There is a large attrition rate in PGT from the number of eggs to embryos to unaffected embryos available for transfer. In some cycles, none of the embryos will be unaffected and no embryo transfer will result. Success rates therefore reflect this and vary according to the inheritance pattern of the disorder.

Similar genetic analysis of embryos has been used to detect chromosomal aneuploidy in embryos in patients having IVF treatment, in an attempt to select the embryos with the greatest implantation potential and reduce the time to a pregnancy. This remains controversial and subject to research trials.

FERTILITY PRESERVATION

Patients may face treatments such as chemotherapy, radiotherapy or surgery that could significantly damage their gonads and reduce their reproductive potential. For many years, men have been able to 'bank' sperm ahead of these treatments. Couples can now undergo rapid IVF procedures and cryopreserve embryos for use later on when health is regained.

Recent advances in vitrification have now also allowed young, healthy, single women to go through IVF and freeze their oocytes.

There is very promising evidence, and some successful reports of live births, on the role of laparoscopic ovarian cortex collection and cryopreservation. Tissue could be auto-transplanted back into the patient's pelvis once health is regained. Similar advances have also been made in preserving testicular tissue, although ovarian and testicular tissue cryopreservation are still classed as experimental techniques.

KEY LEARNING POINTS

- A history, an appropriate clinical examination, targeted investigations and advice on evidence-based treatments underpin successful fertility treatment. The approach should always be patient-/couple-centred with counselling when necessary.
- The couple should be given information on the chances of conceiving naturally and how to optimize this. This should include the impact of advancing age and advice on lifestyle issues relating to diet, smoking, BMI and alcohol consumption.

(Contd.)

(Contd.)

- Ovarian reserve decreases significantly with age, with the gradient increasing over the age of 35 onwards.
- Fertility treatment is a combination of expectant, surgical and medical treatments that are complementary to each other.
- Treatments should be tailored to an individual's or the couple's needs, and can include ovulation induction, surgery, IUI and IVF.
- Fertility preservation and PGT are new and effective treatment options for selected patient groups.

FURTHER READING

HFEA. www.hfea.gov.uk.

National Institute for Clinical Excellence (NICE) (2013). *Fertility Assessment and Treatment for People with Fertility Problems*. Clinical guideline [CG11]. Last updated: 6 September 2017. https://www.nice.org.uk/guidance/cg156.

Van Voorlis BJ (2007). Clinical practice. In vitro fertilisation. *New England Journal of Medicine*, 356: 379–386.

World Health Organization (2021). *WHO Laboratory Manual for the Examination and Processing of Human Semen*, 6th edn. https://www.who.int/publications/i/item/9789240030787.

SELF-ASSESSMENT

For interactive SBAs and EMQs relating to this chapter, visit www.routledge.com/cw/crosbie.

CASE HISTORY

A 39-year-old woman, Jane, and her 41-year-old partner, Robert, have come to the fertility clinic after trying for a baby for 1.5 years. The referral letter notes that Jane has irregular periods and Robert had a hernia repair as a child. Neither have any children.

A What important parts of the history must you ask?
B What investigations will you request?
C What treatment will they need?

ANSWERS

A In the fertility clinic, a general gynaecological history must first be obtained and then more specific questions will follow. You must determine how long exactly they have been having unprotected intercourse and what 'irregular periods' means by enquiring about frequency of bleeds, length of bleeds and any other abnormal uterine bleeding. Irregular periods must prompt questions about hirsutism, weight and acne, as these will support the diagnosis of PCOS, a common cause of anovulation. You must ask for how long the irregular bleeds have happened, as you may be mindful of a diagnosis of decreasing ovarian reserve, a cause that may be associated with hot sweats. Do not forget to ask about

smear tests and sexually transmitted infections. Confirm that Jane has never been pregnant before, including miscarriages and ectopic pregnancies. Also check that none of Robert's previous partners has become pregnant.

Ask about frequency of intercourse and any problems with intercourse, because fertility problems are strongly associated with psychosexual problems, both female and male. You need to ask Robert more about the hernia repair: Was it one side or both and at what age?

You find that Jane has always had irregular periods, except when she was on the oral contraceptive pill. She usually has a period every 2–3 months and they vary from very heavy to normal. She has struggled with androgenic symptoms, except when on the oral contraceptive pill. She manages to keep her weight down with difficulty, and keeps her BMI below 30 with a combination of diet and exercise.

Robert had a unilateral uncomplicated hernia repair aged 4 years. He had his sperm count measured about 1 year ago by his general practitioner, which was 'borderline', so they felt it was worth continuing to try naturally for a while. Intercourse is every few days; they no longer try to work out when ovulation has occurred.

B The investigations required are a hormone profile for Jane, a TVUSS to look for PCOS and other abnormalities, and SFA for Robert. Tubal testing at this point is not indicated.

On review, Jane has a hormone profile indicating PCOS, with LH slightly higher than FSH and high AMH. Her TVUSS confirms PCOS, with a corpus luteum suggesting recent ovulation. Robert's SFA shows a sperm count of 10 million/mL with reduced total motility and morphology.

C On review, you should explain that there are two problems: infrequent ovulation and abnormal sperm count. Together with the length of infertility, these problems mean that IVF and ICSI are indicated. There is no need to check for tubal patency as it is irrelevant. Treatment of ovulation induction or IUI will not give good pregnancy rates because the sperm count is low.

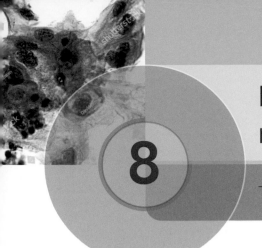

Menopause and post-reproductive health

8

TIMOTHY HILLARD

Learning Objectives

- Know the definition of menopause.
- Understand the physiology of menopause and the causes of premature menopause.
- Understand the effects of menopause and its potential impact on individual women and wider society.
- Be aware of the various issues that should be raised during a menopause consultation.
- Understand the modifiable and non-modifiable aspects of menopausal health.
- Explain the main forms of management of the menopause.
- Know the different types of hormone replacement therapy and their side effects and contraindications.
- Understand the benefits and risks of hormone replacement therapy and the need to individualize treatment.

DEFINITIONS

The menopause is literally defined as a woman's or person's final menstrual period and so the accepted confirmation of this can only be made retrospectively after 1 year of amenorrhoea. The cause of the menopause is cessation of regular ovarian function with the corresponding decline in oestrogen levels. This is usually a gradual process over several years and there is great heterogeneity in the experiences of women as they go through the menopausal transition. Several different descriptive phrases exist (see **Box 8.1** 'Descriptive terms for the menopause')

BOX 8.1: Descriptive terms for the menopause

- Menopause: the last menstrual period.
- Perimenopause: from the onset of ovarian dysfunction until 1 year after the last period and the diagnosis of menopause is made. It is usually characterised by irregular menstruation and the onset of menopausal symptoms. Typically starts after the age of 45 but can occur earlier.
- Climacteric: another term for the perimenopause.
- Postmenopause: all women who have had 1 year or more since their last period are deemed postmenopausal.

(Contd.)

10.1201/9781003218036-8

(Contd.)

- The 'change': a colloquial description of the perimenopause and postmenopause.
- Premature menopause: a menopause that occurs before the age of 40. The correct term is premature ovarian insufficiency (POI).
- Early menopause: a menopause that occurs after the age of 40 but before the age of 45.

PHYSIOLOGY

The average age of the menopause worldwide has not changed for decades (**Figure 8.1**), remaining at a median age of between 51 and 52 years, with 95% of women attaining menopause between the ages of 45 and 55 years. Menopause occurring outside these ages is relatively uncommon. Premature menopause (POI) is discussed later.

ENDOCRINE CHANGES

The current understanding is that the menopause occurs at the time of the depletion of oocytes from the ovary and is irreversible. Unsurprisingly, the endocrinology is not as simple as the ovaries just running out of eggs and losing the capacity to

produce hormones at a particular age. As discussed in **Chapter 3**, reproductive function is maintained by a subtle interplay between the hypothalamic production of gonadotrophin-releasing hormone (GnRH), the anterior pituitary hormones luteinizing hormone (LH) and follicle-stimulating hormone (FSH), the ovarian peptide hormone inhibin B and the steroid hormones oestrogen and progesterone. These hormones change not only during the menstrual cycle but also throughout an individual's reproductive life, with their production changing at differing times and rates according to the age of the woman (**Table 8.1**).

Inhibin B is produced by follicles within the ovary, so, as the number of follicles declines, the production of inhibin decreases. In the perimenopausal years, small declines in inhibin drive an overall increase in the pulsatility of GnRH secretion and overall serum FSH and LH levels, which results in an increased drive to the remaining follicles in an attempt to maintain follicle production and oestrogen levels.

Androgenic hormone production comes from the ovaries, peripheral adipose tissue and the adrenal glands, with the ovaries producing approximately 30–50% of total circulating levels. Although these hormones play no role in the control of ovulation, a decline in ovarian testosterone and other

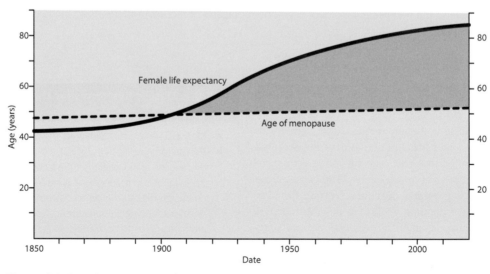

Figure 8.1 Age of menopause and mean life expectancy in the UK since 1850.

Table 8.1 Female hormone production and changes around the menopausal years

Hormones	Perimenopause	Early postmenopause	Late postmenopause and later years
GnRH	Increased pulsatility	Progressive decrease in pulsatility	Reduction in overall levels
LH and FSH	Increased	Increased	Progressive decline
Oestrogen	Slight decline	Rapid decline	Sustained very low levels
Progesterone	Moderate fall	Unpredictable	Undetectable
Inhibin	Slight decline	Significant decline	Undetectable
Testosterone	Progressive decline	Progressive decline	Sustained low levels but may increase after 70 years of age

FSH, follicle-stimulating hormone; GnRH, gonadotrophin-releasing hormone; LH, luteinizing hormone.

androgens accompanies the process of ageing in women. This is shown by the fact that overall androgen concentrations in a woman in their 20s are approximately double those of a woman of 40 years, and then slowly decline throughout life thereafter. Recent research has suggested that levels may start to rise again after 70 years of age, but the significance of this is not yet clear.

DIAGNOSIS

The diagnosis of menopause is largely a clinical diagnosis based on menstrual irregularities and amenorrhoea together with oestrogen deficiency symptoms, such as vasomotor symptoms. The use of serum endocrine tests such as hormone levels are of little value in the perimenopausal years, as they are unpredictable due to the hormonal variations that frequently occur in association with episodic and irregular ovulatory cycles at this time of life. An elevated serum FSH in association with a low serum oestradiol may be suggestive of the menopause, but as this combination of levels can occur during a normal menstrual cycle, this test can be misleading. Two raised FSH levels (>30 IU) at least 6 weeks apart are required to make a diagnosis.

In all women in whom a diagnosis of menopause is being considered, the possibility of pregnancy should also be considered. The diagnosis of menopause in a hysterectomized individual can be more difficult due to the lack of signalling from the bleeding that accompanies the menstrual cycle. However, in these circumstances, the use of other symptoms

of the menopause as biological indicators is usually enough to make a confident diagnosis.

PREMATURE OVARIAN INSUFFICIENCY

A menopause that occurs before the age of 40 years is defined as POI, also sometimes called premature ovarian failure or premature menopause. It occurs in approximately 1% of women under 40 years and in 0.1% of those under 30 years. It can be a very distressing diagnosis to receive, especially if it occurs prior to the completion of any planned family. For young individuals who wish to conceive, gamete donation is the only option.

POI is usually diagnosed following either primary or secondary amenorrhoea. Patients who have a diagnosis of POI can experience unpredictable spontaneous ovarian activity, resulting in irregular vaginal bleeding and a small risk of pregnancy.

While no cause is found in most cases of primary POI, a suspected case should be fully investigated, where possible, for causes that are associated with issues that require separate treatment, as detailed in **Table 8.2**.

POI has significant long-term health implications and all women with POI should be offered supportive care and counselling delivered by a specialist unit to ensure that they fully understand their condition and the specifics of their reproductive needs and that they receive an individualized package of care with close attention to both short-term and long-term management of their health.

Table 8.2 Principal causes of premature ovarian insufficiency

Type	Causes
Primary	Chromosome anomalies (e.g. Turner syndrome, fragile X)
	Autoimmune disease (e.g. hypothyroidism, Addison disease, myasthenia gravis)
	Enzyme deficiencies (e.g. galactosaemia, 17a-hydroxylase deficiency)
Secondary	Infections (e.g. tuberculosis, mumps, malaria, varicella, HIV)
	Surgical menopause after removal of both ovaries
	Chemotherapy or radiotherapy

HIV, human immunodeficiency virus.

IATROGENIC MENOPAUSE

Sometimes, women may be rendered menopausal by a specific treatment that compromises ovarian function. The most obvious example is a surgical menopause when both ovaries are removed. This may be done for benign gynaecological conditions, such as fibroids or endometriosis, or when there is concern about possible ovarian cancer. In addition, bilateral salpingo-oophorectomy may also be performed prophylactically for individuals at high risk of inherited breast and ovarian cancer, such as those with *BRCA1* and *2* pathogenic variants.

Chemo- or radiotherapy for gynaecological or other cancers (e.g. lymphoma) can result in a temporary or permanent loss of ovarian function, and patients should be counselled about this before treatment. In some situations, it may be appropriate to offer oocyte collection and freezing before treatment commences. With survival from childhood cancers now improving, there is an increasing number of young women living longer lives but with a permanent menopause, often from an early age. Such women, especially those under the age of 40 years, must be carefully counselled on what to expect prior to definitive irreversible treatment and then managed as someone with POI thereafter. Special consideration should be given to women whose lifelong treatment demands a hormone-free environment, as these individuals will need to manage on regimes that avoid hormone replacement.

GnRH given in a constant high dose desensitizes the GnRH receptor and reduces LH and FSH release. Therapeutically, GnRH agonists can be used to treat endometriosis and some other gynaecological problems. When administered continuously, they downregulate the pituitary and consequently decrease LH and FSH secretion. This will induce temporary menopause, causing unwanted menopausal symptoms and bone loss. These can be managed with hormone replacement therapy (HRT), known as add-back therapy.

POSTMENOPAUSAL REPRODUCTIVE HEALTH

The UK population is projected to expand by 3.2% from mid-2020 to mid-2030 (Office for National Statistics). The proportion of females of pensionable age in the population will continue to increase and, correspondingly, the number of women experiencing problems during their post-reproductive years will expand by up to one-third over the next 25 years. The menopause has an impact on society in two ways. First, the impact of menopausal symptoms (see the section 'Menopausal symptoms' later in this chapter) can affect a woman's ability to function normally both in terms of their personal life and in their work environment. For example, 19% of the entire NHS workforce of 1.3 million are aged between 45 and 54 years and it is estimated that one in four has considered giving up their job as a result of the menopause and 1 in 10 has actually handed in their notice. Second, the increased risk of longer-term health problems associated with the menopause has an impact on quality of life and longevity, which in turn places a significant strain on the health and social care system. Thus, it is important that strategies are put in place that maintain the health of menopausal women and prevent future disease where possible. A good example would be the management of obesity in the postmenopausal population. While it is well understood that obesity increases the risk of cardiovascular disease and type 2 diabetes, it is less well known that obesity in postmenopausal women increases the risk of hot flushes, breast cancer and endometrial cancer. In addition, as a postmenopausal woman gets older, obesity increases the risk of falls, fractures and stroke, all of which attract a high mortality rate.

Bringing all of these factors together to make a health improvement plan in the early menopause could significantly improve health on an individual level and on a population basis, which could mean significant reductions in healthcare resource use.

HOW WOMEN ARE AFFECTED BY THE MENOPAUSE

The hormonal changes that occur during and immediately after the menopause can lead to profound changes in a variety of different systems. Not only does the timing of when each system is affected vary dramatically between individuals, but also the degree of how the changes influence each individual is remarkably unpredictable. The reasons for these variations are not clearly understood, but there is some evidence that genetic influences play a part.

While most effects of the menopause have long-term implications, the effects of menopause are commonly categorized as having an early onset or an onset in the medium to long term (**Table 8.3**).

Table 8.3 Effects of the menopause by time of onset

Time of onset	Symptoms
Immediate (0–5 years)	Vasomotor symptoms (e.g. hot flushes, night sweats)
	Psychological symptoms (e.g. labile mood, anxiety, tearfulness)
	Loss of concentration, poor memory, brain fog
	Joint aches and pains
	Dry and itchy skin
	Hair changes
	Decreased sexual desire
Intermediate (3–10 years)	Vaginal dryness, soreness
	Dyspareunia
	Urgency of urine
	Recurrent urinary tract infections
	Urogenital prolapse
Long term (>10 years)	Osteoporosis and sarcopenia
	Cardiovascular disease
	Dementia

MENOPAUSAL SYMPTOMS

VASOMOTOR SYMPTOMS

Some of the earliest changes during the menopause are the onset of vasomotor symptoms that typically appear during the perimenopausal years. The colloquial term applied to vasomotor symptoms is a 'hot flush' and these usually coexist with night sweats, that is, when hot flushes occur during sleep.

The exact aetiology of vasomotor symptoms is unknown, but they may be due to loss of the modulating effect of oestrogen on serotonergic receptors within the thermoregulatory centre in the brain, resulting in exaggerated peripheral vasodilatory responses to minor atmospheric changes in temperature.

Hot flushes occur in up to 80% of women and may continue for up to 7 years, sometimes longer. Many women manage these symptoms without the need for specific treatment but, for some, these flushes can be extremely debilitating. Night sweats lead to sleep disturbance, which causes tiredness, exhaustion, poor performance during the day and impaired quality of life. There is also the suggestion that severe vasomotor symptoms are a marker for cardiovascular disease.

While hot flushes tend to appear unpredictably, triggers include alcohol, spicy foods, caffeine and smoking. Individuals with a high body mass index (BMI) tend to get worse vasomotor symptoms.

PSYCHOLOGICAL SYMPTOMS

While there is little evidence to support a direct effect of the menopause as a cause for depression, menopause is associated with low mood, irritability, lack of energy, tiredness and impaired quality of life. Alongside vasomotor symptoms, these symptoms can be very debilitating for some women. While these symptoms may be attributed to hormonal changes, it is important to consider other influences on mood such as relationship and family changes, financial issues, previous history of depression and anxiety, and the woman's or person's attitude to ageing.

COGNITIVE FUNCTION

Many women complain of change in memory, concentration and global cognitive function around the time of the menopause, which is often described as 'brain fog'. Some of these changes can be explained by the impact of vasomotor symptoms and other symptoms on patterns of sleep, but a direct effect of oestrogen deprivation on brain function cannot be excluded.

ENDOMETRIAL EFFECTS

Changes in menstrual bleeding herald the onset of the menopause and occur early during the menopausal transition. The initial scanty vaginal bleeding is due to the reduction in oestrogenic endometrial stimulation with failing ovarian function, ultimately resulting in periods completely stopping when the endometrium is no longer stimulated. Episodic and infrequent ovulation leads to unpredictable progestogen levels, which causes inadequate endometrial shedding with irregular, prolonged and sometimes heavy bleeding.

UROGENITAL TRACT AND VULVOVAGINAL ATROPHY

Once oestrogen levels start to fall in the perimenopausal years, many women, particularly those who are sexually active, become aware of vaginal dryness, irritation, burning, soreness and dyspareunia. Loss of oestrogenic support to the vaginal epithelium leads to reduced cellular turnover and glandular activity, creating a vaginal epithelium that is less elastic and more easily traumatized (**Figure 8.2**).

Embryologically, the urethra and trigone of the bladder are both derived from the lower two-thirds of the vagina, and their associated atrophic changes give rise to irritative bladder symptoms and prolapse, which are covered in **Chapter 10**.

The inherent resistance of the urogenital system to infection is impaired due to an increase in pH of the normally mildly acidic environment within the vagina. The incidence of urinary tract infections is increased, as are episodes of minor cystitis that can accompany sexual activity.

Examination of patients with postmenopausal urogenital atrophy normally demonstrates dryness affecting most of the surfaces of the vagina along with pallor and, in extreme cases, small petechial haemorrhages. Older women may have shrinkage and fusion of the labia with narrowing of the vaginal introitus.

All women experience these changes in the lower genital tract to some degree. It is an intimate area that many patients may have difficulty raising in conversation, even though they may be experiencing severe symptoms, so it is therefore essential that healthcare professionals looking after these individuals proactively ask about these issues, which can easily be corrected.

SEXUAL FUNCTION

Many women complain of loss of sexual desire around the menopause, which can be associated with significant personal and relationship distress. Although sexual desire naturally decreases with age, hormonal changes and, in particular, loss of oestrogen may have a direct effect on sexual desire

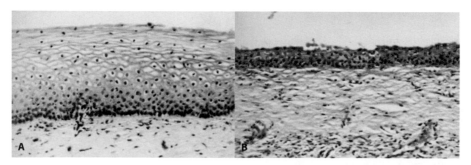

Figure 8.2 Vaginal epithelium in (**A**) a premenopausal woman and (**B**) a postmenopausal woman showing atrophic changes. Note the loss of epithelial structure and architecture. (Reproduced with permission from Whitehead MI, Whitcroft SIJ, Hillard TC (1993). *An Atlas of the Menopause*. Parthenon.)

and function. In addition, menopausal symptoms and vaginal atrophy may lead to tiredness and discomfort, there may be reduced response to sexual stimuli and women may experience more difficulty reaching orgasm. Male partners may also have reduced interest and may have difficulty getting or maintaining an erection. The underlying reasons behind sexual dysfunction are often complex and multifactorial, but is a subject that does require some understanding.

BONE HEALTH AND OSTEOPOROSIS

One of the best understood areas of long-term post-reproductive health is the changes to bone that occur on loss of oestrogenic support of skeletal metabolism. The skeleton is maintained by a constant process of remodelling, with bone being laid down by osteoblasts and resorbed by osteoclasts (**Figure 8.3**). The balance of the rates of resorption versus deposition is affected by many different factors, one of

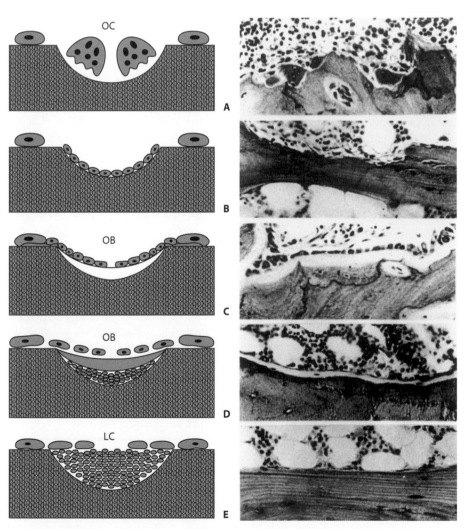

Figure 8.3 The principal stages of the bone remodelling cycle represented diagrammatically (left) with corresponding light micrographs of iliac crest biopsies (right). (**A**) Resorption by osteoclasts (OCs). (**B**) Reversal with disappearance of OCs. (**C**) OC formation with the deposition of osteoid by osteoblasts (OBs). (**D**) Mineralization of the osteoid. (**E**) Completion of the cycle with bone lining cells (LCs) on the surface. (Light micrographs reproduced with permission from Dempster DW (1992). *Disorders of the Bone and Mineral Metabolism*. Raven Press.)

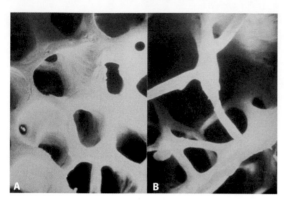

Figure 8.4 Electron micrograph of trabecular bone showing (**A**) normal structure and (**B**) osteoporotic bone. Note the loss of architecture and density in (**B**) making the bone weaker and more prone to fracture. (Reproduced with permission from Whitehead Malcolm I, Whitcroft SIJ, Hillard TC (1993). *An Atlas of the Menopause*. Parthenon.)

BOX 8.2: Risk factors for osteoporosis

- Family history of osteoporosis or hip fracture
- Smoking
- Excess alcohol
- Long-term steroid use
- POI and hypogonadism
- Medical treatment of gynaecological conditions with induced menopause
- Disorders of thyroid and parathyroid metabolism
- Immobility
- Disorders of gut absorption, malnutrition or liver disease

which is oestrogen. An important consideration is the attainment of peak bone mass. Bone density naturally increases during childhood, reaching a peak between 20 and 30 years of age. Males generally achieve a greater peak bone density than females. After peak bone mass attainment in women, there is a gradual decline until the menopause, then an accelerated phase of bone loss until 60 years of age, followed by a further steady decline until death, which leads to increasing fragility of the trabecular bone (**Figure 8.4**). After the age of 60 in women, the likelihood of osteoporotic fractures of the wrist, hip and spine increases.

Osteoporosis is defined as a skeletal disorder characterized by compromised bone strength predisposing to an increased risk of fracture. It is more frequent in women than men, with an approximate ratio of 4:1. Osteoporosis is a major health problem that will only worsen as the population ages. Identifying those most at risk (see **Box 8.2** 'Risk factors for osteoporosis') and determining targeted prevention strategies is required. Again, the menopause is an ideal time to assess this.

CARDIOVASCULAR SYSTEM

Approximately 30% of all deaths occur as a result of ischaemic heart disease and stroke. This makes cardiovascular disease (CVD) a condition that significantly burdens the global health system. While CVD is relatively uncommon before the menopause, this changes rapidly after the menopause and CVD becomes the leading cause of death among women over 60 years of age.

During the menopausal transition, there are several changes in the female physiology brought about by the loss of oestrogen that can influence individual risk of CVD. These include changes in the distribution in fat from more gynaecoid (fat on breasts and hips) to android (abdominal fat deposition); changes in serum lipid levels that include increases in triglycerides, total cholesterol and low-density lipoprotein cholesterol and a reduction in high-density lipoprotein cholesterol; and changes in blood vessel dynamics. Oestrogen has a supportive effect on the vessel wall that favours vasodilatation and prevents atherogenesis and these effects are reduced after the menopause.

Thus, while the management of CVD is not usually within the realms of the gynaecologist, it is important to recognize that, because many women seek the help of a gynaecologist during their life, and particularly around the menopause, there may be opportunities for the identification of, and improvement in, modifiable risk factors for CVD.

OTHER EFFECTS

Oestrogen receptors are distributed throughout the body, so the decline of oestrogen at the menopause can have widespread effects. These can have an impact on the skin, hair and joints and, long term, are associated with a reduction in muscle mass (sarcopenia). Although cognitive function can be affected, as discussed earlier, at present there is no clear evidence that menopause is associated with an acceleration of the onset or incidence of dementia.

ASSESSMENT OF THE MENOPAUSAL PATIENT

A menopause consultation should not only assess the impact of the menopause on the systems discussed previously, but should also take the opportunity to look for both modifiable and non-modifiable risk factors that may affect an individual's health and longevity (see **Box 8.3** 'Modifiable and non-modifiable risk factors affecting health and longevity').

There is rarely a need for investigations to confirm menopause. While a serum FSH level of more

---

BOX 8.3: Modifiable and non-modifiable risk factors affecting health and longevity

Relevant symptoms
- Vasomotor
- Urogenital tract, including sexual concerns
- Cognition
- Joint pains
- Vaginal bleeding (if relevant)

Signs
- Blood pressure
- BMI
- Vaginal assessment including cervical smear
- Breast examination if indicated

Lifestyle
- Exercise levels
- Nutrition
- Smoking and alcohol intake
- Relationship and sexual history
- Contraceptive needs

Personal medical/gynaecological history
- Obstetric history
- Administration of drugs that influence oestrogen levels
- Age of menopause
- History of cancer and cancer treatment
- Chronic disease and treatment
- Corticosteroid administration
- Fracture history

Family history
- CVD
- Osteoporosis
- Thromboembolic disease

---

than 30 IU/L is highly suspicious of menopause, the diagnosis can be confidently made in the majority of cases based on history alone, the key features being oligo/amenorrhoea, vasomotor symptoms, joint aches and minor cognitive changes.

The moment a perimenopausal woman presents for an assessment of whether they are menopausal or not gives an opportunity for preventative healthcare. It is important to address reasons for presentation, but also to appraise their compliance with various national screening programmes, their general health and their opportunities for improvement in health. Nationally, it is recognized that not all women spontaneously present for such advice, and there are currently national campaigns to educate women and to promote at least one such 'health check' around the time of the menopause.

MANAGEMENT

The menopause is a natural event, and many women have mild symptoms or no symptoms requiring intervention. The menopause is viewed differently in different cultures, and an empathy of the widely different experiences and symptoms around the menopause is important. Raising awareness of the long-term implications discussed previously, such as osteoporosis and CVD, should be part of good preventative medicine, even in those without significant symptoms.

The three main components of menopausal management are self-education, the treatment of troublesome symptoms and the prevention of longer-term risks.

DIET AND LIFESTYLE

The health benefits of regular exercise, weight management, smoking cessation and reducing alcohol consumption are well publicized and should help reduce an individual's risk of heart disease, lung cancer, diabetes and other conditions. However, the additional benefits of these actions are less well known and should be emphasized in the menopausal consultation (**Table 8.4**). Careful counselling around this is necessary, particularly with regard to weight gain. Women should be informed

121

Table 8.4 Beneficial effects of various lifestyle changes in postmenopausal women

Lifestyle change	Benefits
Stopping smoking	Prevention of lung cancer
	Reduction of CVD
	Beneficial effects on bone loss
Reducing alcohol consumption	Reduction of calorie intake
	Fewer, less severe vasomotor symptoms
	Beneficial effects on bone loss and falls
	Prevention of alcohol-related liver damage
	Reduction in incidence of breast cancer
	Reduction of CVD
Normalising BMI	Fewer, less severe vasomotor symptoms
	Beneficial effects on bone loss
	Reduction in incidence of breast cancer
	Reduction in incidence of endometrial cancer
	Reduction of CVD

BMI, body mass index; CVD, cardiovascular disease.

Table 8.5 Alternative and complementary treatments that are used to treat menopausal symptoms

Type	Treatment
Complementary drug-free therapies (delivered by a practitioner)	Acupuncture
	Reflexology
	Magnetism
	Reiki
	Hypnotism
Herbal/natural preparations (designed to be ingested)	Black cohosh (*Actaea racemosa*)
	Dong quai (*Angelica sinensis*)
	Evening primrose oil (*Oenothera biennis*)
	Gingko (*Gingko biloba*)
	Ginseng (*Panax ginseng*)
	Kava kava (*Piper methysticum*)
	St John's wort (*Hypericum perforatum*)
'Natural' hormones (designed to be ingested or applied to the skin)	Phytoestrogens such as isoflavones and red clover
	Natural progesterone gel
	Dehydroepiandrosterone (DHEA)

that average body weight increases by approximately 1 kg per year in the early postmenopause, and this, together with a more android fat distribution, contributes to a greater sensation of feeling overweight. HRT does not increase weight gain any further and may actually help by reversing the fat distribution changes.

NON-HORMONAL APPROACHES

Many women experiencing the early symptoms of menopause seek out advice and possible solutions from the wide range of alternative and 'natural' options available in pharmacies, supermarkets and health food shops and from online suppliers, with various levels of reliability. Patients often present for medical advice only after they have tried some of these measures. Women should be informed of the beneficial effects of lifestyle measures before exploring non-hormonal interventions. Cognitive behavioural therapy is a proven intervention that

can help in the management of some menopausal symptoms and should be considered before embarking on other treatments.

ALTERNATIVE AND COMPLEMENTARY TREATMENTS

These groups of treatments are widely available (**Table 8.5**) but are usually poorly researched, with limited evidence for their efficacy and safety. Any benefit is limited and of short duration, with the potential for adverse interactions with other pharmaceutical agents. Women should also be aware that products calling themselves 'natural' hormone products are usually unregulated and essentially a weak form of oestrogen, so they could be exposing themselves to the known risks of HRT.

NON-HORMONAL PRESCRIPTION TREATMENTS

This group of therapies (**Table 8.6**) may reduce hot flushes when hormones are not wanted or contraindicated, for example previous diagnoses

Table 8.6 Non-hormonal prescribed treatments for vasomotor symptoms

Type	Treatment
Alpha-adrenergic agonists	Clonidine
Beta-blockers	Propanolol
Modulators of central neurotransmission	Venlafaxine
	Fluoxetine
	Paroxetine
	Citalopram
	Gabapentin

of hormone-sensitive breast cancer. There is currently interest in the neurokinin pathway as a key controller of the hypothalamic thermoregulatory zone and a possible mechanism for vasomotor symptoms. Recent research has demonstrated that neurokinin 3 receptor antagonists are highly effective in relieving vasomotor symptoms and are well tolerated. Although these products are not yet available, this class of drug has the potential to be a practice-changing non-hormonal option for vasomotor symptoms.

Other issues specific to the menopause can also be treated without hormones. These include moisturizers and lubricants for vaginal dryness and bisphosphonates, raloxifene, denosumab and teriparatide for treating osteoporosis.

HORMONE REPLACEMENT THERAPY

HRT has been the mainstay of the treatment for menopausal symptoms for over 40 years. Its use has always attracted controversy, initially in its promotion as a drug with rejuvenating abilities and then during a period of widespread use when the long-term benefits in terms of osteoporosis and CVD prevention from large cohort studies were identified. In 2002, a large randomized trial highlighted a series of potential risks from HRT use. The surrounding media attention led many women to stop their HRT, and many doctors stopped prescribing it. Subsequent reanalyses of the data and new studies have either significantly reduced or removed many of the risks initially described and put them into context. Various authoritative reviews have

weighed up the benefits and risks of HRT and concluded that, for most postmenopausal women, HRT remains a safe and effective option to be considered.

HRT consists primarily of oestrogen and progesterone and a third hormone, testosterone, can sometimes be prescribed separately.

OESTROGENS

There are a variety of different oestrogen preparations available that are effective at relieving menopausal symptoms. Oestrogen given alone stimulates the endometrium, increasing the risk of endometrial hyperplasia and cancer. Thus, for all women with a uterus, progesterone is also recommended (combined HRT). Systemic oestrogen-only HRT is only suitable for women who no longer have a uterus following a hysterectomy.

Progestogen is given alongside oestrogen as part of HRT to protect the endometrium in women with an intact uterus. It is normally given cyclically over a 28-day cycle in which 14–18 days provide oestrogen alone and 10–14 days provide oestrogen and progestogen combined (cyclical HRT). This mimics the normal menstrual cycle and results in a regular monthly withdrawal bleed. It is suitable for women during the perimenopause or early postmenopausal years.

Oestrogen and progestogen may be given continuously (continuous combined HRT) to women who are known to be postmenopausal or over the age of 54 years. These are usually preparations with the same dose of daily oestrogen combined with a smaller dose of progestogen taken every day. These regimes normally result in about 90% of patients not experiencing vaginal bleeding.

There are several different types of progestogens used in HRT. A change of type, dose or route of progestogen may be required to reduce unwanted side effects or control bleeding patterns. Irregular bleeding should be investigated.

Vaginal oestrogens

Oestrogens can be given vaginally in very low doses to correct atrophic changes (see **Figure 8.2**) and improve vaginal and urinary symptoms. There is minimal systemic absorption and no endometrial stimulation, so no additional progestogen is required.

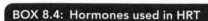

BOX 8.4: Hormones used in HRT

Oestrogens

- Oestradiol (the main physiological oestrogen)
- Oestradiol valerate
- Oestrone sulphate
- Oestriol
- Conjugated equine oestrogen

Progestogens

- Norethisterone
- Levonorgestrel
- Dydrogesterone
- Medroxyprogesterone acetate
- Drospirenone
- Dienogest
- Micronized progesterone

Note: Product availability may vary by country.

TESTOSTERONE

Half of testosterone production in women is from the ovaries (the rest is from the adrenals and peripheral conversion). There is evidence that testosterone replacement can help women with disorders of sexual desire that have failed to respond to normal HRT. The long-term safety of exogenous testosterone has not been reliably established in women. There are also no licensed testosterone preparations for women in the UK, so the only available preparations are those licensed for use in men. This usually means that testosterone needs to be instigated under the care of a doctor with specialist menopause knowledge.

ROUTES OF HORMONE THERAPY ADMINISTRATION

The two main routes of HRT delivery are oral and transdermal. The oral route is normally a daily tablet that contains the appropriate dose of oestrogen or a mix of oestrogen and progestogen, depending on the preparation. The oral route is convenient and cheap but does have the potential to influence lipid metabolism and the coagulation system through its effects on the liver during first-pass metabolism.

The transdermal route – given either as patches applied to the skin on the trunk or as measured amounts of gel or a measured spray on the forearm – is also effective, with the advantage of delivery of oestradiol directly into the circulation, avoiding the previously described potentially adverse effects on the liver and the coagulation system. This is particularly beneficial for those who are at an increased risk of complications, such as those with hypertension, obesity or a history of thrombosis.

Oestradiol is also available as small vaginal tablets and a vaginal ring, and oestriol is available as measured dose vaginal creams or pessaries that are important in the management of lower genital tract symptoms (as described previously).

Progestogen is usually given orally but can be given transdermally in a combined patch. It may also be administered in the form of levonorgestrel as an intrauterine releasing system (IUS). This device not only provides contraception and control of troublesome bleeding, but also provides endometrial protection for up to 5 years (see **Chapter 17**).

BENEFICIAL EFFECTS OF HORMONE THERAPY

Vasomotor symptoms

The principal reason for taking HRT is vasomotor symptom improvement. Well over 90% of patients note a significant improvement within 6 weeks, with reductions in frequency and severity of hot flushes and night sweats and consequent improvements in sleep and daytime energy levels, as well as concentration.

Skeleton

The protective effects of HRT on the skeleton include prevention of bone loss and the prevention of osteoporotic fractures of the hip and spine. The use of HRT is strongly recommended for patients with an early menopause, as they are at a much greater risk of osteoporosis. Most postmenopausal women should consider HRT as a means to prevent bone loss, especially if they require HRT for other symptomatology.

Lower genital tract

Both systemic and locally administered HRT have significant beneficial effects on the lower genital tract. There is good evidence that its administration

BOX 8.5: Key benefits of HRT

Symptoms improved

- Vasomotor symptoms
- Improved sleep patterns
- Improved other symptoms (e.g anxiety, joint aches)

Prevention of osteoporosis

- Maintenance of bone mineral density
- Reduced incidence of fragility fractures

Lower genital tract

- Improved vaginal dryness, soreness and dyspaerunia
- Improved urinary symptoms
- Reduced urinary tract infections

CVD

- Preventative effect if started early in menopause

improves vulvovaginal dryness, irritation, soreness and dyspareunia. There is also an improvement in symptoms of cystitis and occasionally dysuria. Local hormone therapy is unlikely to cure prolapse, but may improve some of the symptoms of prolapse. There is no evidence that local HRT improves incontinence. Many women considering local HRT are dissuaded from its use due to concerns about the published risks. However, they should be reassured that vaginal oestrogen preparations are considered very safe and are not associated with an increased risk of breast cancer.

Cardiovascular system

The cardiovascular benefits of HRT were first demonstrated in large observational cohort studies. The principal benefits were reductions in ischaemic heart disease and overall mortality. However, the large, randomized Women's Health Initiative (WHI) study demonstrated reductions in survival from CVD in women taking HRT. This study has been widely criticized due to the overweight and generally older population studied, a population probably at greater risk of CVD. Reanalysis for the appropriate age group and subsequent data have identified a 'window of opportunity' in the perimenopausal or early post-menopausal years during which the administration of HRT may reduce morbidity and mortality from CVD by prevention of atheroma formation.

While the prevention of CVD is not currently a licensed indication for HRT, the data are sufficient to include a discussion with patients that they should consider these benefits.

Colon

While the WHI study demonstrated a clear benefit of HRT on the incidence and mortality of colon cancer, the use of HRT to prevent this malignancy is not indicated.

PRESCRIBING AND SIDE EFFECTS OF HORMONE THERAPY

Prior to prescribing HRT, it is important to weigh up the indications, proposed benefits and potential risks for each individual patient. HRT is suitable for most women but there are certain situations when it may be contraindicated (e.g. a prior history of breast cancer or thromboembolic disease).

In general, side effects from HRT are few and minor. It is important before starting HRT to ensure that the patient has no contraindications and had no serious effects when on the contraceptive pill, such as venous thrombosis or migraine with aura.

Most side effects can be managed with a change in dose of oestrogen or a change in type of progestogen.

BOX 8.6: Contraindications of HRT

Absolute contraindications

- Suspected pregnancy
- Breast cancer
- Endometrial cancer
- Active liver disease
- Uncontrolled hypertension
- Known current venous thromboembolism (VTE)
- Known thrombophilia (e.g. factor V Leiden)
- Otosclerosis

Relative contraindications

- Uninvestigated abnormal bleeding
- Large uterine fibroids
- Past history of benign breast disease
- Unconfirmed personal history or a strong family history of VTE
- Chronic stable liver disease
- Migraine with aura

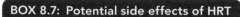

> **BOX 8.7: Potential side effects of HRT**
>
> **Side effects associated with oestrogen**
> - Breast tenderness or swelling
> - Nausea
> - Leg cramps
> - Headaches
>
> **Side effects associated with progestogen**
> - Fluid retention
> - Breast tenderness
> - Headaches
> - Mood swings
> - Depression
> - Acne

Some patients can also benefit from a switch of route. Many women find the IUS a useful device, as it delivers much less progestogen into the circulation than progestogens given systemically (i.e. all other routes), thus reducing progestogenic side effects.

There is no clear duration for which a woman should take HRT. Most women take it only for a few years, but there is no maximum age or duration after HRT should be stopped. The balance of risks and benefits should be reviewed regularly, as risks may change with age and duration of treatment and the indications for taking it may change.

RISKS OF HORMONE THERAPY

All treatments have risks and it is important that these are weighed up on an individual basis before initiating any intervention. The potential risks of HRT, particularly in relation to breast cancer, have attracted controversy and media attention over the years, which has caused alarm and confusion. Better ways of analysing and communicating the data have helped to rationalize this in recent years, but a full discussion of the potential risks is required before starting HRT.

Breast cancer

This is without doubt the cancer that attracts most concern from patients and most attention from the world's media. The relationship between HRT and breast cancer is complex, not least because breast cancer is relatively common in the age group concerned.

In summary, HRT taken for 5 years between the ages of 50 and 69 years is associated with a small increase in the risk of breast cancer, which varies depending on the type of HRT taken. Oestrogen-only HRT appears to have little or no risk, but combined HRT (oestrogen plus progestogen) is associated with a small increase in risk, which appears to be duration-dependent. Useful figures to quote are that, over a 7.5-year period, the background risk of breast cancer in the 50- to 59-year age group is 22.5 per 1,000 individuals. With 7.5 years' use of combined HRT, there will be an additional two to six cancers in a population of the same size (1,000 individuals), and this risk reduces after stopping HRT. Shorter durations of use are likely to have lower risks. Although the incidence of breast cancer may be higher with HRT, mortality from breast cancer is not increased. Recent data suggest that HRT may promote the growth of pre-existing malignant cells rather than initiate new tumours.

Other gynaecological cancers

Unopposed oestrogen replacement is associated with an increased endometrial cancer risk. This is largely eliminated if progestogens are prescribed appropriately. However, the background risk remains, particularly for those with additional risk factors, and abnormal bleeding requires appropriate investigation (see **Chapter 12**). There is a very small increase in the incidence of some types of ovarian cancer with more than 10 years of oestrogen-only HRT. This is not seen with combined HRT and, overall, these risks are very low. There is no association between HRT and cervical or vulval cancer.

Cardiovascular disease and stroke

Most of the effects of HRT on the cardiovascular system when given to younger women are beneficial. However, when given to older women (>65 years), the effects may become deleterious. The degree to which this happens is unclear, but is likely to be higher in women taking combined HRT.

Stroke incidence has a similar age-related effect, with the incidence increasing with age. The effect is small and is only on the incidence of ischaemic stroke, thought to be an increase of an additional two women per 10,000 women per year when on HRT, although this could be higher in those with additional risk factors.

Venous thromboembolism

The influence of HRT on the clotting system is similar to that of the oral contraceptive. The background incidence of all VTE in individuals over 50 years of age is low (approximately 15–20 per 10,000) and oral HRT doubles this risk. Transdermal HRT, through its avoidance of effects on the liver and coagulation factors, does not appear to increase VTE incidence so is the preferred option for those who are older or have thrombotic risk factors.

🔑 KEY LEARNING POINTS

- The menopause is a key time in the life of an individual.
- The physiological changes that occur have significant effects on the woman as a whole, affecting numerous body systems.
- The care of women during the post-reproductive years should be managed in a holistic fashion that addresses lifestyle and general health issues first. Using such an approach can address many elements of health, improving longevity and quality of life.

- HRT exists in a variety of forms and is the most effective treatment for improving menopausal symptoms.
- HRT is effective in helping prevent long-term conditions such as osteoporosis and CVD, and may become a cost-effective means of improving the lives of the expanding numbers of menopausal women globally.
- The potential risks of HRT need to be weighed up individually but, for the majority of symptomatic menopausal women under the age of 60, the benefits outweigh the risks.

FURTHER READING

Baber RJ, Panay N; IMS Writing Group (2016). 2016 IMS recommendations on women's midlife health and menopause hormone therapy. *Climacteric* 19(2): 109–115

Hamoda H, Panay N, Pedder H, Arya R, Savvas M (2020). The British Menopause Society and Women's Health Concern 2020 recommendations on hormone replacement therapy in menopausal women. *Post Reproductive Health*, 26(4): 181–209.

Hillard TC, Abernethy K, Hamoda H, Shaw I, Everett M, Ayres J, Currie H (2017). *Management of the Menopause*, 6th edn. British Menopause Society.

National Institute for Health and Care Excellence (NICE) (2015). *Menopause: Diagnosis and Management*. NICE guideline [NG23]. Last updated: 5 December 2019. https://www.nice.org.uk/guidance/ng23.

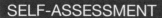

SELF-ASSESSMENT

For interactive SBAs and EMQs relating to this chapter, visit www.routledge.com/cw/crosbie.

CASE HISTORY 1

Mrs A is a 36-year-old woman. She had one child delivered normally 6 years previously after a brief period of subfertility. Following delivery of that child, she had 4 years of infrequent periods and, over the last 2 years, she has been amenorrhoeic and has had difficulty sleeping, often waking up feeling hot.

A What is the likely diagnosis?
B How would the diagnosis be confirmed?
C Following diagnosis, Mrs A asks what the immediate and long-term issues are and how they might be managed. Outline the key issues.

ANSWERS

A Premature Ovarian Insufficiency.
B A combination of the clinical picture and serum FSH levels are usually adequate to confirm the diagnosis. On receipt of one elevated FSH level (>30 IU/L), it is recommended that a repeat test no sooner than 6 weeks after the first is performed to confirm the diagnosis.

C Informing her of the likely diagnosis should be done sensitively, as it may cause distress, particularly if she was hoping to have more children. Conversely, she also needs to be informed that sporadic ovarian function may still occur and there is still an appreciable risk of pregnancy, so her contraceptive needs should also be discussed.

The importance of bone protection should be explained to her. With her prolonged entry into POI, she is at an increased risk of developing osteoporosis or osteopaenia over time. A bone densitometry scan should be arranged at some point and management with HRT should be considered.

The benefits of HRT should be explained to her. It is often helpful to highlight that, because she has lost her endogenous oestrogen at an early age in comparison with her peers, if she were to take HRT she would not be exposing herself to any appreciable excess risks from HRT until the age of natural menopause, approximately 51 years.

CASE HISTORY 2

Mrs M is a 49-year-old woman who has been complaining of poor sleep, difficulty concentrating at work and increased social anxiety for around 18 months. She was prescribed an anti-depressant a few months ago, but this has not helped. On close questioning, she is also experiencing some hot flushes and night sweats that are waking her up. Her periods are still fairly regular but have become much lighter recently. She has had two children, both born normally, and her partner has had a vasectomy. She is generally in good health, but her BMI is 30 and she is on anti-hypertensive medication. Her mother has recently been diagnosed with breast cancer at the age of 75.

A What is the likely diagnosis?
B What are her treatment options?
C Are there any specific concerns that would influence the type of treatment offered?
D Apart from treating her symptoms, what are the other main issues she should be made aware of?

ANSWERS

A Perimenopause. The combination of her age, the occurrence of typical menopausal symptoms and the change in her menstrual cycle is enough for the diagnosis. She does not need blood tests.

B HRT would be the most appropriate treatment, as her symptoms are clearly affecting her quality of life. Alternative options would be to offer cognitive behavioural therapy. Anti-depressants should not be given as the first-line treatment for low mood and anxiety secondary to menopause.

C Given her raised BMI and history of hypertension, transdermal oestrogen should be offered in preference to oral therapy, as it is less likely to raise her thrombotic risk or interfere with blood pressure control. A family history of breast cancer over the age of 70 is unlikely to have any particular genetic significance as far as Mrs M is concerned.

D Mrs M is overweight and hypertensive, both of which are significant risks for CVD. A high BMI is also associated with many other health risks. It is good professional practice to highlight these to her in a sensitive manner and recommend she seeks appropriate support and advice. She should also be encouraged to take up mammography screening when it is offered from 50 years of age.

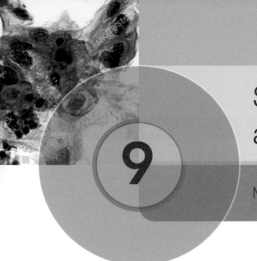

Sexually transmitted infections and related conditions

9

MARGARET KINGSTON

Learning Objectives
- Understand the importance of sexually transmitted infections and related conditions in gynaecology.
- Describe the testing, diagnosis and management of sexually transmitted infections and related conditions.
- Learn how to take a sexual history.
- Understand the diagnosis and principles of management and prevention of human immunodeficiency virus (HIV).
- Describe the management of a HIV-positive mother, their infant and family.
- Understand caring for transgender and non-binary individuals within gynaecology.

INTRODUCTION

An understanding of sexually transmitted infections (STIs) and related conditions is important in gynaecological practice. The subject is frequently misunderstood, with considerable consequences for patients, their partners and their children. STIs are often asymptomatic, but can still be transmitted to others and cause significant problems at the time of infection or in the future. STIs disproportionately affect younger people, but increasingly they are identified in older people, in whom the diagnosis is often not considered and therefore missed. STIs often coexist and, when one is found, screening for others is required.

Tests for STIs have hugely improved in recent years with the advent of highly sensitive and accurate tests that are very easy to use and can detect several infections on a single swab, urine or blood sample, including those taken by patients at home. Women are often diagnosed when they attend a clinic for reproductive healthcare and require support to inform partners, so they can also receive testing and treatment. Children require testing and treatment if they may have been exposed during

10.1201/9781003218036-9

pregnancy, birth or breastfeeding. This aspect of managing STIs can be very challenging but is important. It is important to consider the safeguarding of women and girls who may be exposed to sexual or domestic violence, abuse, coercion or exploitation, which may only become apparent in this context.

Human immunodeficiency virus (HIV) infection is a lifelong manageable condition that, when diagnosed and treated, has excellent outcomes. It is crucial to ensure screening in every pregnancy (along with screening for syphilis and hepatitis B) and to offer testing in those with conditions that indicate HIV infection; in gynaecology, this includes cervical neoplasia. Effective treatment prevents transmission to sexual partners, children and needlestick recipients. Post- and pre-exposure prophylaxis is effective and widely available for those at risk of infection.

Unfortunately, these remain stigmatizing conditions, and affected individuals may feel isolated and need additional support from their healthcare professionals and charitable organizations. Respecting confidentiality and dignity is vital.

TAKING A SEXUAL HISTORY

This allows healthcare professionals to identify which tests are required, offer contraception and STI prevention through vaccination and HIV prophylaxis, and offer opportunistic cervical screening for those who are overdue. In addition, this is an opportunity to identify possible abuse or exploitation. It is always important to consider if an individual is competent to make their own decisions, and, in children under the age of 16, this must be documented together with a safeguarding assessment. Sometimes, raising the issue of STIs may be unexpected, and it is important to start by ensuring privacy and to reassure the patient about confidentiality. Important points to cover are summarized in **Table 9.1**. Abuse, exploitation or coercion can happen to anyone, but young people and sexually active children especially so, and screening questions for this are also included in **Table 9.1**. This is also an opportunity for health promotion, brief intervention or signposting to other services when excessive alcohol, smoking or recreational drug use, especially sexualized use (the use

Table 9.1 Points to cover in a sexual history and screening questions for sexual exploitation

Rationale for questions	Points to cover in the questions
Assessment of clinical need and symptoms	Why the patient is attending
	If symptoms are present, explore their specific features
	History of past or current STIs, including HIV status
Sexual and other exposures to guide testing decisions	Sexual exposure: details of sex partners in the last 3 months and anatomical sexual exposure occurred in each case – were condoms used?
	Partner details: the gender of each partner, their country of origin, if they are contactable, if they had symptoms/are known to have any STIs and the nature of the relationship/if it is ongoing
	Other exposures: intravenous drug use, high-risk tattoos or piercings, or medical procedures
Contraception needs and pregnancy risk assessment	Last menstrual period, any current pregnancy risk and the need for a pregnancy test
	Opportunity to provide contraception
Other sexual health needs	Cervical screening – opportunity to provide if needed
	Vaccination: HPV or hepatitis B – opportunity to provide if appropriate
	Others, usually as raised by the patient (e.g. sexual function and satisfaction)
Assessment of risk behaviours open to health promotion	Alcohol, smoking, recreational drug use assessment, brief interventions or signpost to services

Rationale for questions	Points to cover in the questions
Assessment of exploitation/violence/abuse	Any forced sex or violence or other abuse from sex partners
	Domestic abuse
	Any coercive sex; is the woman in a vulnerable position from their sex partner or on occasion their family or friends?
	For younger people and all under 16 years, the age of their sex partner, if they receive presents for sex, if they attend school, if they have supportive family members and friends who know their partner(s), and any other vulnerability concerns

HIV, human immunodeficiency virus; HPV, human papillomavirus; STI, sexually transmitted infection.

of drugs to facilitate sexual experience), is identified. The methods for conveying results or any follow-up should be agreed.

Capacity assessment is crucial for those under the age of 16 seeking healthcare without the knowledge or consent of their parent(s). This is to ensure they are able to understand the healthcare they are accessing and the implications and consequences of the tests and treatment they are consenting to.

CARING FOR TRANSGENDER AND NON-BINARY INDIVIDUALS

Transgender is a term used to describe people whose gender is different from the sex they were assigned at birth, and cisgender describes those whose gender is congruent with the sex they were assigned at birth. Non-binary is a term people use to describe genders not identified as male or female. Trans people may or may not undergo medical transition, including the use of hormones and surgery. It is vitally important to ensure an inclusive and respectful healthcare environment for all, including those who are transgender, and appropriate equality and diversity training for all staff is required. Using an individual's preferred pronouns and name is crucial, and establishing their current anatomy, if they are taking hormones and the type of sexual activity they partake in will help inform appropriate management. Trans people experience increased rates of violence, including domestic violence and sexual abuse, and possibly drug or alcohol misuse.

Trans individuals who have a uterus require reproductive healthcare, including appropriate contraception, STI screening, vaccinations including human papillomavirus (HPV) in line with national recommendations, HIV prevention including pre- and post-exposure prophylaxis when needed and cervical screening.

TESTING FOR SEXUALLY TRANSMITTED INFECTIONS AND ASSOCIATED CONDITIONS

Accurate, non-invasive testing is widely available and are the first-line screening tests for most STIs. These include multiplex assays; however, it is important to use these appropriately, as many include inappropriate tests for commensal and organisms that may not be pathogenic. Point-of-care tests are available for many infections including HIV and, while helpful on occasions, may have suboptimal sensitivity and/or specificity, and it is important to be aware of these limitations. Close liaison with local laboratory staff is crucial to ensure the best available tests are used, appropriately interpreted and communicated in a timely fashion. **Table 9.2** summarizes appropriate screening and diagnostic tests.

INFECTIVE CAUSES OF VAGINAL DISCHARGE

BACTERIAL VAGINOSIS

The most common cause of abnormal vaginal discharge, bacterial vaginosis, has been reported in 5–55% of female cohorts worldwide, with both Black

131

Table 9.2 Tests for sexually transmitted infections and related conditions in women

Diagnosis	Tests
Bacterial vaginosis	Microscopy of vaginal discharge (not required if asymptomatic)
Candidiasis	Microscopy of vaginal discharge and/or culture (not required if asymptomatic)
Trichomoniasis	NAAT from vulvovaginal swab or, alternatively, culture or wet mount microscopy of vaginal discharge (not required if asymptomatic)
Chlamydia	NAAT from vulvovaginal swab If history of receptive oral or anal sex, swab from those sites
Gonorrhoea	NAAT from vulvovaginal swab Culture required if tested positive before treatment or as alternative test If history of receptive oral or anal sex, swab those sites
HIV	Serology for both HIV-1 and -2 antibodies, preferably in combination with HIV p24 antigen Tests also available on dried blood spot and saliva samples, some as near-patient tests
Syphilis	Serology for treponemal test (usually EIA); if positive, confirm with second treponemal test and non-treponemal test titre
Hepatitis B and C	Serology for hepatitis B core antibody or surface antigen or both and for hepatitis C antibody These tests should be done in women from high prevalence areas or at additional risk of infection (e.g. known or likely exposure, intravenous drug use, sex work)

EIA, enzyme immunoassay; HIV, human immunodeficiency virus; NAAT, nucleic acid amplification test.

women and women who have sex with women more frequently affected. While a definitive cause is not determined, depletion of the lactobacilli dominant in the healthy vaginal flora is observed, together with an elevation of vaginal pH to above 4.5. The existence of a vaginal epithelial biofilm consisting of *Gardnerella vaginalis* and other species has been more recently described. It is not presently considered an STI, and treatment of sexual partners is not currently recommended. However, it is associated with sexual activity and with a number of pathologies including pelvic inflammatory disease (PID), post-hysterectomy vaginal cuff cellulitis and, in pregnancy, preterm birth and rupture of membranes and miscarriage (although evidence does not support screening in pregnancy).

Symptoms include an offensive vaginal discharge that is often reported as having a 'fishy' malodour and, on examination, a homogeneous off-white vaginal discharge with a high pH is observed, but not vaginitis. Diagnosis is made by evaluating a Gram stain of the vaginal discharge using a validated method, such as the Hay–Ison criteria, the Nugent criteria or, less frequently in modern practice, the Amsel criteria (three of the following four

are required: homogeneous discharge, high pH, 'clue cells' on microscopy and a fishy odour when 10% potassium hydroxide is added to a sample of discharge; **Figure 9.1**). Bacterial vaginosis may resolve without treatment. Oral or intravaginal treatments with metronidazole or clindamycin are indicated in individuals with symptoms or those in whom it is diagnosed and elect for treatment – especially prior to gynaecological surgical procedures. Patients with bacterial vaginosis should be advised that vaginal douching or excessive genital washing should be avoided.

VULVOVAGINAL CANDIDIASIS

This condition occurs when yeast of the *Candida* species, most frequently *C. albicans*, causes vulval and vaginal inflammation. The majority of premenopausal women are colonized with *Candida* species, and around 75% will experience at least one episode of vulvovaginal candidiasis. When symptoms occur, they include itching, irritation and a typically white, curdy vaginal discharge. On examination, signs of inflammation – including erythema, oedema and fissuring of the vulva and vagina – together with the

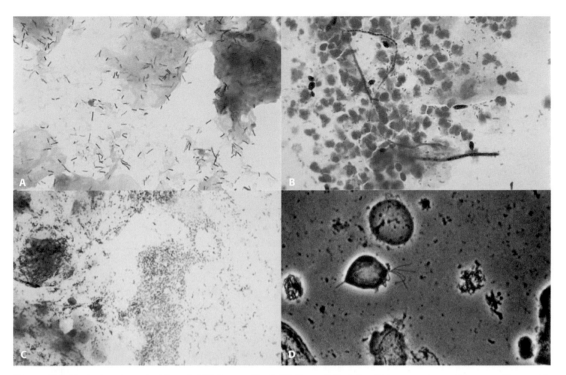

Figure 9.1 Vaginal and cervical flora (×1,000 magnified). (**A**) Normal: lactobacilli (seen as large Gram-positive rods) predominate. Squamous epithelial cells are Gram-negative with a large amount of cytoplasm. (**B**) Candidiasis: there are speckled Gram-positive spores and long pseudohyphae visible. There are numerous polymorphs present and the bacterial flora is abnormal, resembling bacterial vaginosis. (**C**) Bacterial vaginosis: there is an overgrowth of anaerobic organisms, including *Gardnerella vaginalis* (small Gram-variable cocci), and a decrease in the numbers of lactobacilli. A 'clue cell' is seen. This is an epithelial cell covered with small bacteria, so the edge of the cell is obscured. (**D**) Trichomoniasis: an unstained 'wet mount' of vaginal fluid from a woman with *Trichomonas vaginalis* infection. There is a cone-shaped, flagellated organism in the centre, with a terminal spike and four flagella visible. In practice, the organism is identified under the microscope by movement, with amoeboid motion and its flagella waving.

discharge described may be observed. Symptoms may be more frequent and persistent when the patient is diabetic, immunocompromised or in pregnancy. The diagnosis is made by taking a bacterial swab for microscopy and culture, and treatment with topical intravaginal pessaries or oral imidazoles is effective. Topical vulval antifungals and the use of a generic topical emollient and cleansing agent provide symptomatic relief. This is not an STI, and partners without symptoms do not require treatment.

TRICHOMONIASIS

Infection with the flagellate protozoan *Trichomonas vaginalis* results in symptoms of vaginal discharge with a variable appearance and symptoms and/or signs of vulvovaginitis. Asymptomatic colonization is observed in up to 50% of vulvo vaginal and most penile conditions. *T. vaginalis* is sexually transmitted, and simultaneous treatment of current sexual partners is required. There is some evidence of an association with pregnancy outcome: preterm birth, low birth weight and maternal post-partum sepsis. Testing is indicated in symptomatic women, and the gold standard is a nucleic acid amplification test (NAAT), which can also detect *Neisseria gonorrhoea* and *Chlamydia trachomatis*; for these, the optimal test is a vulvovaginal swab. Microscopy and culture of a sample of the vaginal discharge are also used, but are limited by reduced sensitivity. Treatment is with a systemic nitroimidazole (usually metronidazole) regime.

CERVICITIS AND PELVIC INFLAMMATORY DISEASE

GONORRHOEA

This condition is due to infection with the bacteria *N. gonorrhoea*, which occurs through sexual intimacy. Endocervical infection is asymptomatic in up to 50% of cases, with altered vaginal discharge the most common symptom and lower abdominal pain in up to 25% of cases. Rectal infection occurs through transmucosal spread and receptive anal sex, and pharyngeal infection occurs through receptive oral sex; the latter is nearly always asymptomatic. Examination is often normal, although cervicitis with or without a mucopurulent discharge may be seen (**Figure 9.2**). Ascending infection may result in PID and, rarely, haematogenous spread can cause disseminated gonococcal infection with a purpuric non-blanching rash and/or an arthralgia or arthritis that is typically monoarticular in a weight-bearing joint. Ophthalmic infection occurs due to inoculation from infected genital secretions, and neonatal infection occurs when the mother has endocervical infection at the time of delivery.

NAATs are highly sensitive and specific and, if *N. gonorrhoea* is identified, it is important to obtain

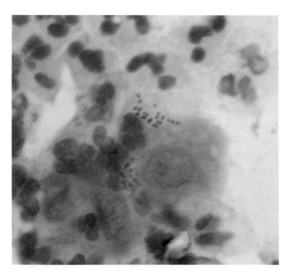

Figure 9.2 Gram-stained smear of cervical secretions showing polymorphs and Gram-negative intracellular diplococci (×1,000 magnified). This appearance is highly suggestive of gonorrhoea.

a sample for culture and sensitivity testing, as there has been a development of widespread anti-microbiological resistance that requires careful surveillance. First-line treatment includes a parenteral third-generation cephalosporin.

CHLAMYDIA

Chlamydial infection is the most common bacterial STI and is often asymptomatic, but it can still result in subclinical PID and subsequent complications. Testing is indicated in women with risk factors for an STI, such as a new sexual partner, or in those with symptoms that include altered vaginal discharge, intermenstrual or post-coital bleeding or abdominal pain. Examination is often normal, but cervicitis with mucopurulent discharge may be present. Infection at other mucosal sites occurs like in gonorrhoea and, similarly, neonates born to mothers with cervical infection may be infected during vaginal delivery and develop conjunctivitis. A reactive arthritis that is typically monoarticular affecting the weight-bearing joints may occur, and is more common in men.

NAATs are used to diagnose *C. trachomatis* infection, with most testing simultaneously for *N. gonorrhoea* with the option to add on testing for *T. vaginalis* in women with indicative symptoms. These tests offer high levels of sensitivity and specificity and, in women, the optimal genital specimen is a vulvovaginal swab that may be self-taken by the patient without compromising diagnostic accuracy. For uncomplicated genital chlamydia, the treatment of choice is doxycycline; for those who are pregnant, azithromycin with a test of cure is required. Simultaneous treatment of current sexual partners is necessary.

MYCOPLASMA GENITALIUM

Infection with *Mycoplasma genitalium* has been identified as a cause of cervicitis, endometritis and PID, and testing and appropriate treatment is indicated when these conditions are diagnosed. Infection is frequently asymptomatic and inconsequential, and treatment can be problematic due to established antimicrobial resistance and toxicity, so screening is not appropriate. Treatment of sexual partners when there is risk of reinfection is recommended. Diagnosis is by NAAT on vulvovaginal swabs, with testing for macrolide resistance where possible. Treatment regimens include doxycycline followed by azithromycin and moxifloxacin.

PELVIC INFLAMMATORY DISEASE

This occurs when there is ascending infection from the endocervix to the higher reproductive tract. It is a recognized complication of chlamydia, *M. genitalium* and, less frequently, gonorrhoea, but they are often not isolated and other implicated organisms include those in the vaginal microflora. The diagnosis of PID is usually made clinically, and symptoms typically include lower bilateral abdominal pain, dyspareunia, altered vaginal discharge and intermenstrual bleeding or post-coital bleeding. Systemic symptoms of infection may be present. Characteristic clinical findings include lower abdominal and cervical motion tenderness and cervicitis. Testing for all STIs is required, as is the exclusion of pregnancy. When PID is suspected, empirical treatment should be started immediately, as delay increases the risk of complications. These include the sequelae of endometrial and fallopian tube inflammation and damage such as subfertility, ectopic pregnancy and chronic pelvic pain. Right upper quadrant pain due to perihepatitis is an unusual complication called Fitz-Hugh–Curtis syndrome (**Figure 9.3**).

Laparoscopy in patients with established PID may reveal scarring and adhesion formation between the structures of the pelvis and the development of hydrosalpinges of the tubes. There is a subsequent increased risk of ectopic pregnancy (**Figure 9.4**). If an

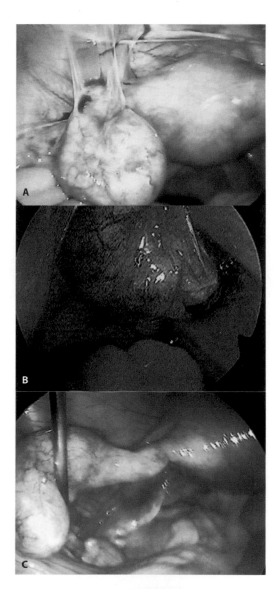

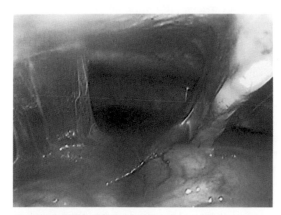

Figure 9.3 Fitz-Hugh–Curtis syndrome showing perihepatic adhesions (typical violin string appearance).

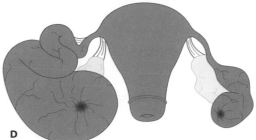

Figure 9.4 (**A**) Peritubal adhesions of the left fallopian tube. (**B**) Ectopic pregnancy within hydrosalpinx. (**C**) Left fallopian tube hydrosalpinx. (**D**) Large hydrosalpinx of the left fallopian tube with a smaller hydrosalpinx on the right side.

intrauterine device is in situ, consideration should be given to removing this, especially if initial treatment is not successful, and it is important to consider the risk of pregnancy if there has been unprotected sex in the last week. Treatment regimens should cover all common pathogens and are 2 weeks in duration; they usually include a macrolide or tetracycline plus metronidazole with a parenteral third-generation cephalosporin at the start. Sexual partners require simultaneous screening and empirical treatment. Patients require clear information regarding possible sequelae from their infection.

VIRAL SEXUALLY TRANSMITTED INFECTIONS AND SYSTEMIC MANIFESTATIONS

GENITAL HERPES

There are two types of herpes virus that cause this condition: herpes simplex virus (HSV) type 1 and type 2. HSV-1 also causes orolabial herpes and is often acquired in childhood; it is also a common cause of genital herpes alongside HSV-2. Following acquisition, the virus establishes latency in the local sensory ganglia and may reactivate, resulting in shedding of the virus, with or without symptoms. Most infections are asymptomatic, with asymptomatic shedding of the virus an important way in which the virus can be passed onto others, and subsequent recurrences may be asymptomatic. Recurrence rates are higher with HSV-2 and reduce in frequency with time.

Symptoms include genital pain and dysuria and, on examination, there are typically multiple superficial tender ulcers with regional lymphadenopathy in initial infection. Diagnosis is by detection of the virus from the genital lesions by gently taking a swab. The test of choice is a polymerase chain reaction (PCR) test that types the virus. Type-specific serology – testing for immunoglobulin (Ig)G and IgM to HSV-1 and -2 – can be helpful in establishing if the infection is primary or recurrent.

Neonatal herpes is a devastating infection with a mortality rate of up to 30% of cases and consequent lifelong neurological morbidity in up to 70% of cases. It is most often acquired during birth if the mother has primary infection within the third

trimester and especially during the last 6 weeks, when reported neonatal infection rates are as high as 41%. IgG to the virus crosses the placenta and provides neonatal protection from infection, and the risk of neonatal herpes when the mother has lesions of recurrent infection present at delivery is less than 3% of cases. The recommended mode of delivery for women with primary genital herpes in the third trimester is pre-labour caesarean section and, in those with proven recurrent lesions, vaginal birth may be anticipated.

Treatment of the symptoms of genital herpes is a course of aciclovir, which is very safe and effective. This is most effective when given as soon as possible after symptoms develop, and episodic and suppressive regimens are effective in managing symptoms from repeated recurrences. Information for patients, including the lifelong nature of the infection, asymptomatic shedding and antiviral treatment, is important.

GENITAL WARTS AND HUMAN PAPILLOMAVIRUS INFECTION

Warts are benign epithelial tumours caused by HPV infection. There are over 200 genotypes of HPV and types 6 and 11 cause around 90% of genital warts. Infection with HPV in the genital epithelium via sexual transmission is extremely common, with most cases being subclinical. Infection with the oncogenic genotypes 16 and 18 causes around 70% of cervical cancer and the majority of other HPV-related cancers, such as oropharyngeal, penile, anal, vaginal and vulval cancers. HPV vaccination is available as a bivalent (targeting types 16 and 18), quadrivalent (types 6, 11, 16 and 18) and nonavalent (types 6, 11, 16, 18, 31, 33, 45, 52 and 58) preparation. Data from clinical trials indicate that the cancers and pre-cancerous lesions caused by HPV infection are effectively prevented by HPV vaccination prior to sexual debut. Likewise, genital warts are effectively prevented in individuals vaccinated against HPV types 6 and 11 (recipients of quadrivalent and nonavalent vaccines). It is important to be clear for patients that the types of HPV that cause genital warts do not increase the risk of HPV-related cancers, and screening for those cancers in those with genital warts is the same as national screening recommendations.

Diagnosis of genital warts is by clinical examination and, as these are benign lesions, treatment is optional. Treatments include ablative therapies (such as application of liquid nitrogen or surgical techniques) or patient-applied topical therapies, including podophyllotoxin-containing preparations or the local immune modulator imiquimod. When genital warts are present in pregnancy, treatment is limited to ablative options. Rarely, warts may become very large and obstruct the birth canal, necessitating caesarean delivery. Very rarely, the neonate can develop respiratory papillomatosis, but the risk is extremely small and the benefit of caesarean delivery in preventing this is unproven.

SYPHILIS

Syphilis is caused by infection with the bacterium *Treponema pallidum* subspecies *pallidum*, which occurs through direct contact with secretions from an infective lesion or via transplacental passage of the bacteria during pregnancy. The infection is multisystem and has many clinical features (**Figure 9.5**); these may mimic other conditions and so syphilis is frequently misdiagnosed. Untreated, it can relapse and remit, and late complications can present many years after the original infection.

Infectivity declines with time, and treatment with penicillin-based regimens are curative, although reinfection may occur. Syphilis is most common in African and Asian countries and Eastern Europe, and in the last two decades there have been significant resurgences of infection in gay and bisexual men who have sex with men. There have been a number of cases identified in pregnant women and their babies, and screening during pregnancy and consideration of this infection is crucial in mothers and their children with any relevant symptoms or risk in all cases.

The infection is classified as congenital or acquired, and each of these as late or early. In acquired early syphilis, the initial manifestation is the chancre, which develops at the site of exposure. This is classically a single, painless genital lesion, but is increasingly seen at other sites such as the oral cavity and is often described as multiple and painful. Typically, the lesion exudes serous fluid containing *T. pallidum* and there is regional lymphadenopathy. This resolves within a few weeks and then, as the bacteria disseminate, a plethora of clinical symptoms and signs may be apparent. These include a widespread erythematous rash, typically including the palms and soles, and that can result in alopecia, oral and genital mucous lesions, and raised lesions, usually in the anogenital area, termed 'condylomata

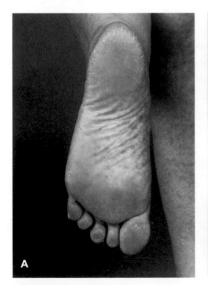
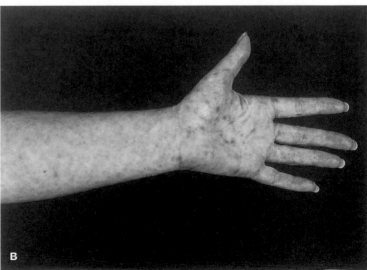

Figure 9.5 A typical rash of secondary syphilis: widespread and characteristically involving soles of feet (**A**) and/or palms of hands (**B**).

lata'. Complications include neurological involvement, resulting in meningovascular inflammation, ophthalmic involvement including visual loss, most often due to uveitis, and sensorineural deafness. This stage also spontaneously resolves, as the host immune response is often effective in controlling the infection, although relapse may occur for up to 2 years, the accepted time limit of early infection, and approximately two-thirds of infected individuals suffer no further ill effects.

Late complications include:

- gummatous lesions – granulomatous, locally destructive lesions typically affecting skin and bone
- cardiovascular involvement, usually affecting the ascending aorta, resulting in aortic valve incompetence
- neurological involvement, classified as meningovascular disease, tabes dorsalis and a progressive dementing illness, general paresis

The riskiest time for congenital infection is when syphilis is acquired either very soon before or during pregnancy. Screening for syphilis in pregnancy is well established, allowing effective treatment of most women, although infection occurring in pregnancy risks transmission to the infant; women who have screened negative for infections at the start of pregnancy should be made aware that they are negative at that point but may be at risk of infection later – the "negative now" message – and should be encouraged to rescreen for all STIs should that be appropriate for them or should they experience symptoms. The manifestations of congenital syphilis are summarized in **Table 9.3**.

Diagnosis is by serology and/or directly detecting *T. pallidum* in infectious lesions, usually by dark field microscopy or, more recently, by PCR testing, where available. Non-treponemal serological tests include the rapid plasma reagin test and the venereal disease research laboratory test, which demonstrate rising titres during acute, active infection that drop with time and following treatment, and so can be used to monitor treatment. They may be negative in early infection, falsely positive in other physiological (such as pregnancy) or disease (including several rheumatological conditions) states, and so

Table 9.3 Clinical features of congenital syphilis

Early (within 2 years)	Late
Common manifestations (one of these is noted in 40–60% of infants):	*These are termed the 'stigmata of congenital infection':*
Rash	Interstitial keratitis
Haemorrhagic rhinitis (bloody snuffles)	Clutton joints
Generalized lymphadenopathy/ hepatosplenomegaly	Dental abnormalities including 'Hutchinson incisors' and 'mulberry molars'
Skeletal abnormalities	High palatal arch
Other manifestations:	Rhagades
Condylomata lata	Sensineural deafness
Vesiculobullous lesions, osteochondritis	Fontal bossing
Periostitis	Short maxilla
Pseudoparalysis	Protuberance of mandible
Mucous patches	saddle nose deformity,
Perioral fissures	sternoclavicular
Non-immune hydrops	thickening, paroxysmal
Glomerulonephritis neurological ± ocular involvement	cold haemoglobinuria Neurological involvement including intellectual
Haemolysis and thrombocytopenia	disability, cranial nerve palsies

require confirmation by treponemal tests such as enzyme immunoassays or *T. pallidum* haemagglutination assays. These treponemal tests may also be negative in the very early stages of disease and should be repeated if negative 4–6 weeks later if this is suspected. Serological tests for syphilis are usually positive for life, even with curative treatment. Reinfection results in the non-treponemal titre rising rapidly. Different testing algorithms are applied according to locally available tests, and expertise is required together with a full clinical history to interpret their results adequately. Treatment is curative and involves depot preparations of penicillin; different regimes for differing stages of infection are the treatment of choice. Simultaneous testing and when-needed treatment of current sexual partners is required, certainly in early disease. Tracing and testing of previous partners and of children may be required.

HUMAN IMMUNODEFICIENCY VIRUS

NATURAL HISTORY, EPIDEMIOLOGY, TESTING AND TREATMENT

Infection with HIV results in an initial acute viral illness followed by a chronic decline in cellular immunity due to progressive depletion of CD4-positive T-lymphocytes, and eventually results in one or more illnesses defined as acquired immune deficiency syndrome (AIDS). These are listed in the box 'AIDS-defining illnesses' and, importantly in gynaecological practice, include cervical cancer. In addition, cervical pre-cancer is an HIV indicator condition, that is, a condition in which the prevalence of undiagnosed HIV is greater than 0.1%. HIV infection disproportionately affects those living in or originating from sub-Saharan Africa and their partners, gay and bisexual men who have sex with men and intravenous drug users without access to clean injecting equipment. The global burden of HIV infection is depicted in **Figure 9.6**. Highly active retroviral therapy (HAART) has transformed the lives of HIV-positive people and their families, making early diagnosis and treatment crucial to allow maintenance of that individual's own health and to protect their partners and children from infection. In addition to those with AIDS-defining or HIV indicator conditions, HIV testing should be recommended in those for whom missing infection would have a significant impact on management, such as in cancer, immunosuppressive treatments or transplantation. Screening adults in populations with an increased baseline prevalence is also recommended. For example, in the USA, national guidelines recommend offering HIV testing to all those aged 13–64 accessing medical care in areas where prevalence in their population is greater than 0.1%. In the UK, the recommendation is for testing in areas with rates above 0.2% in those aged 15–59. The notification of present and previous partners and, if applicable, children is crucial, as treatment in the earlier asymptomatic stages improves outcomes and prevents onward transmission. As routine HIV testing and care, including HAART for all those diagnosed, has become widely available, rates of new HIV diagnoses are falling in many areas (over 30% worldwide), and the elimination of new infections is an achievable aim. Ensuring all those who need HIV testing receive

Number of people living with HIV in 2020

East and Southern Africa	Western and Central Africa	Asia and Pacific	W. and C. Europe and N. America	Latin America	East Europe and Central Asia	Caribbean	Middle East and North Africa
20.6 million	4.7 million	5.8 million	2.2 million	2.1 million	1.6 million	330,000	230,000

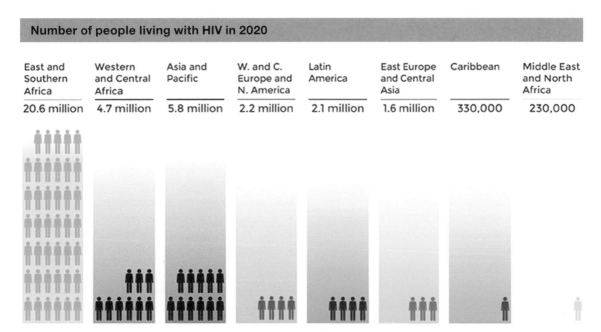

Figure 9.6 Global burden of HIV infection. (HIV, human immunodeficiency virus.)

it and supporting those in vulnerable or marginalized groups to engage in care is crucial. Unfortunately, as with all STIs, HIV remains a condition with much associated stigma, and non-statutory agencies such as charities and community groups can provide valuable support for those affected.

GYNAECOLOGICAL COMPLICATIONS IN HIV-POSITIVE WOMEN

Women with HIV infection are more likely to have persistent infection with oncogenic HPV and have a higher prevalence and incidence of cervical intraepithelial neoplasia/high-grade squamous intraepithelial lesion. For this reason, annual cervical screening is recommended, with most guidelines recommending subsequent management that is the same as in HIV-negative women. It is worth noting that other anogenital malignancies resulting from oncogenic HPV infection also occur more frequently and at a younger age in HIV-positive people.

CONTRACEPTION AND PRECONCEPTION MANAGEMENT

Several antiretrovirals interact with hormonal contraceptives and may reduce contraceptive efficacy. However, this is dependent on the combination of specific medicines, and a holistic assessment is required of the individual's suitability for, and the availability of, both treatments. The dynamic HIV drug interaction website from the University of Liverpool (see 'Further reading') provides accurate information on specific drug interactions. Non-hormonal contraception such as condoms and intrauterine devices are appropriate in most circumstances where they would otherwise be offered.

Preconception counselling includes standard health promotion and, for sero-discordant couples, advice regarding prevention of HIV transmission. This is achieved by optimal HIV control, as transmission between sexual partners does not occur when the positive partner has undetectable HIV ribonucleic acid (RNA) levels (termed the 'viral load' [VL])

BOX 9.1: AIDS-defining illnesses

- Bacterial infections, multiple or recurrent
- Candidiasis of bronchi, trachea or lungs
- Candidiasis of oesophagus
- Cervical cancer, invasive
- Coccidioidomycosis, disseminated or extrapulmonary
- Cryptococcosis, extrapulmonary
- Cryptosporidiosis, chronic intestinal (>1 month's duration)
- Cytomegalovirus disease (other than liver, spleen or nodes), onset at age >1 month
- Cytomegalovirus retinitis (with loss of vision)
- Encephalopathy, HIV-related
- Herpes simplex: chronic ulcers (>1 month's duration) or bronchitis, pneumonitis or oesophagitis (onset at age >1 month)
- Histoplasmosis, disseminated or extrapulmonary
- Isosporiasis, chronic intestinal (>1 month's duration)
- Kaposi sarcoma
- Lymphoid interstitial pneumonia or pulmonary lymphoid hyperplasia complex
- Lymphoma, Burkitt (or equivalent term)
- Lymphoma, immunoblastic (or equivalent term)
- Lymphoma, primary, of brain
- *Mycobacterium avium* complex or *Mycobacterium kansasii*, disseminated or extrapulmonary
- *Mycobacterium tuberculosis* of any site, pulmonary, disseminated or extrapulmonary
- *Mycobacterium*, other species or unidentified species, disseminated or extrapulmonary
- *Pneumocystis jirovecii* pneumonia
- Pneumonia, recurrent
- Progressive multifocal leucoencephalopathy
- *Salmonella* septicaemia, recurrent
- Toxoplasmosis of brain, onset at age >1 month
- Wasting syndrome attributed to HIV

Source: Centers for Disease Control and Prevention (2008). AIDS-defining conditions. http://www.cdc.gov/mmwr/preview/mmwrhtml/rr5710a2.htm (see source for notes on specific illnesses).

in the serum. If an individual is in a new partnership, screening for and treating coexistent STIs is good practice. It is appropriate to offer fertility treatment when this is indicated to couples when one is or both are HIV-positive, within regulatory frameworks.

MANAGEMENT OF THE HIV-POSITIVE MOTHER AND THEIR CHILD

All pregnant women must know their current HIV status, and those who are positive require access to high-quality medical and obstetric care. Effective antiretroviral therapy, ensuring an undetectable VL during pregnancy, is the first step after diagnosis. Most vertical transmission occurs during birth or breastfeeding. Intrauterine infection is unusual, and the risk of this is increased by an intervention that disrupts the placenta (e.g. amniocentesis). Delivery by pre-labour caesarean section further reduces vertical rates when the VL is detectable. Obstetric risk factors that increase the risk of transmission

in mothers with detectable VL include prolonged rupture of membranes, procedures that breach the infant's skin (such as fetal scalp electrodes) or increased maternal blood in the birth canal. With appropriate management, vertical HIV transmission can be brought to extremely low levels; **Figure 9.7** clearly demonstrates this.

Women with well-controlled HIV have very low rates of transmission to the infant. In studies from resource-poor settings where breastfeeding is the norm, transmission rates of up to 3% are observed, so, in circumstances in which formula feeding is safe, this is considered preferable. However, even when bottle feeding is safe, women who have well-controlled HIV are increasingly choosing to breastfeed, with support from their healthcare professionals. It is important that the babies are exclusively fed breast milk with rapid weaning so no mixed feeding occurs. Other strategies to safely breastfeed include ensuring there is no blood in the breast milk by not feeding an infant from a breast with mastitis or cracked nipples and instead expressing and discarding the milk until

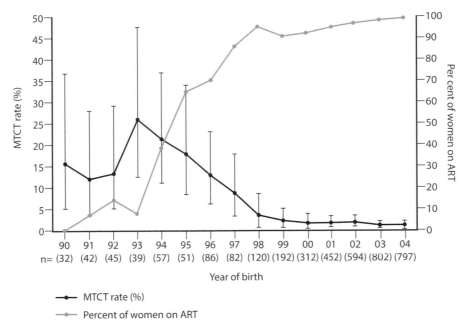

Figure 9.7 UK data from the Integrated Screening Outcomes Surveillance Service, demonstrating extremely low rates of vertical transmission of HIV due to screening and appropriate management. (ART, antiretroviral therapy; HIV, human immunodeficiency virus; MTCT, mother-to-child transmission.)

healing has occurred; optimizing the mouth health of the infant; and frequently monitoring the HIV VL of both the mother and infant, for example every month.

CONCLUSION

Current knowledge of the modern tests for and management of STIs and related conditions has been summarized in this chapter. This is important in gynaecological practice, as these conditions are common and have serious implications, but can be effectively managed to minimize the risk of complications and transmission. The management of HIV continues to improve with effective and safe treatments that are widely available for women and removes the worry of transmitting the infection to future partners and children. It is crucial to ensure that women receive appropriate testing for all STIs including HIV, especially when conditions that indicate possible infection are present.

FURTHER READING

British Association for Sexual Health and HIV (BASHH). https://www.bashh.org/guidelines.

BASHH (n.d.). *Spotting the Signs: A National Proforma for Identifying Risk of Child Sexual Exploitation in Sexual Health Services*. http://www.bashh.org/documents/Spotting-the-signs-A%20national%20proforma%20Apr2014.pdf.

British HIV Association (n.d.). Current guidelines. https://www.bhiva.org/guidelines.

Centers for Disease Control and Prevention (CDC) (2023). STI treatment guidelines. https://www.cdc.gov/std/treatment-guidelines/default.htm.

International Antiviral Society – USA (2022). Guidelines. https://www.iasusa.org/resources/guidelines/.

International Union against STIs (n.d.). Guidelines. https://iusti.org/regions/guidelines/.

University of Liverpool – HIV Drug Interactions. http://www.hiv-druginteractions.org/.

SELF-ASSESSMENT

For interactive SBAs and EMQs relating to this chapter, visit www.routledge.com/cw/crosbie.

CASE HISTORY 1

A 29-year-old woman presents to the emergency gynaecology unit with a 5-day history of lower abdominal and pelvic pain that has got progressively worse over the last 24 hours. She also feels generally unwell with chills and rigors.

On examination, she looks unwell. She has a raised temperature at 38°C and is tachycardic. She is very tender on abdominal examination with guarding. On speculum examination, the cervix appears inflamed with a profuse mucopurulent discharge. A vulvovaginal swab for chlamydia, gonorrhoea and trichomonas, plus a pregnancy test, is taken. On pelvic examination, there is marked cervical tenderness. She is also generally tender to palpate throughout the pelvis and is unable to tolerate the examination. The pregnancy test is negative.

A What is the diagnosis?
B What tests are required?
C What is the management?

ANSWERS

A The clinical diagnosis is suggestive of acute PID with pelvic peritonitis.
B Vulvovaginal, high vaginal and cervical swabs (as available depending on your local microbiology service) are taken, as well as a midstream urine sample, full blood count and C-reactive protein test. A pelvic ultrasound shows the possibility of an adnexal mass with some free fluid in the pelvis.
C She is admitted and started with intravenous antibiotics (ceftriaxone and metronidazole) and oral doxycycline. She is also supported with intravenous fluids, analgesics and regular paracetamol.

She continues to be unwell with a raised temperature even after 48 hours of antibiotics. Thus, a decision is taken to perform a laparoscopy. Usually, conservative management is preferred, but, when it is unsuccessful after 24–48 hours, laparoscopy is indicated. At the operation, she is found to have a 7 cm enlarged tubo-ovarian abscess and marked inflammation of the uterus and other tube. The abscess is drained and the patient markedly improves after the surgery. She is found to have chlamydia and gonorrhoea on the vulvovaginal and endocervical swabs with anaerobes on the high vaginal swab. She improves over the course of a few days and is treated with oral antibiotics for 2 weeks. She is counselled regarding the implications of the infection and is encouraged to contact her partner for testing and treatment. In the future, she would require referral to fertility services early if she failed to conceive. An early scan in pregnancy is indicated to confirm intrauterine pregnancy, as the risk of an ectopic pregnancy is increased.

CASE HISTORY 2

A 32-year-old woman is found to be HIV-positive at antenatal screening. She is 13 weeks' pregnant and has not disclosed a previous HIV diagnosis and attends for the result alone. She has two older children born elsewhere, and she tells you this pregnancy is with a new partner. She is well with no medical problems and takes no regular medication apart from multivitamins for pregnancy.

A What are the initial tests and treatment she needs?
B What are the implications for her wider family?
C How can she expect to safely deliver and feed her baby?

ANSWERS

A She needs a confirmatory HIV test as well as all routine baseline investigations, including a HIV genotypic resistance assay; human leucocyte antigen B5701 testing (to predict hypersensitivity to abacavir – a commonly used antiretroviral); serology for other infections such as hepatitis A, B, C, syphilis, rubella, measles and varicella; screening for other STIs; and routine bloods tests such as full blood count and renal, bone and liver profile. HIV treatment in line with national guidelines should be commenced as soon as possible, both for the mother's health and to prevent transmission to the fetus and sexual partner.

B Partner notification and testing should be sensitively discussed and progressed for both sexual partners and children – as appropriate. It is important to be mindful of safety and of the possible exploitation and vulnerabilities of all parties.

C If HIV treatment is started and virological control established quickly, then the risk of HIV transmission to the infant can be minimized. Achieving an HIV VL that is undetectable will minimize the risk of transmission to the infant and, if this is achieved within the 4 weeks prior to delivery, will mean that vaginal birth is as safe as caesarean birth in terms of HIV transmission. Interventions that breach the infant's or mother's skin, such as scalp electrodes and episiotomy, should be avoided, and a senior obstetrician should be involved in the delivery of the infant should interventions beyond normal birth be required. Prophylaxis for HIV is required for the infant at birth; the number of drugs and the length depends on maternal virological control before and at the time of birth. Formula feeding of the infant eliminates the risk of postnatal HIV transmission, but, for those with well-controlled HIV, exclusive breastfeeding carries minimal risk and should be supported, until weaning is required.

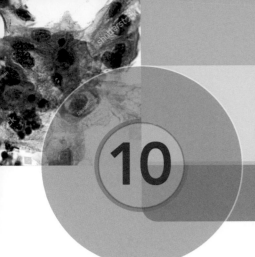

Urogynaecology and pelvic floor problems

10

RANEE THAKAR

Learning Objectives
- Understand the applied anatomy of the pelvic floor and related organs.
- Understand the mechanism of continence in women and how disorders of this can lead to symptoms.
- Learn how to clinically assess the patient with incontinence (urinary and anal) and/or pelvic organ prolapse.
- Understand the principles of treatment of incontinence and pelvic organ prolapse.

INTRODUCTION

Pelvic floor dysfunction is a condition in which the pelvic floor muscles around the bladder, anal canal and vagina do not work properly. Urinary incontinence, anal incontinence and pelvic organ prolapse are the three most common symptoms. Other symptoms include emptying disorders of the bladder and bowel, sexual dysfunction and chronic pelvic pain. One in four adult women have at least one pelvic floor disorder during their lifetime. Age has an important effect, as 6% of women in their 20s experience symptoms, with this increasing to 40% of women in their 60s.

APPLIED ANATOMY

The intimately related pelvic organs are supported by connective tissue attachments to the pelvic walls and the levator ani muscle (**Figure 10.1**). The levator ani is the most important muscle of the pelvic floor. It maintains a constant state of contraction, thus providing an active floor that supports the weight of the abdominopelvic contents against the forces of the intra-abdominal pressure. The puborectalis, pubococcygeus and iliococcygeus are the three components of the muscle. The pubococcygeus is further divided into the pubovaginalis, puboanalis and puboperineal muscles according to fibre attachments. They are attached on each side of the pelvic side wall from the pubic ramus anteriorly, over the obturator internus fascia to the ischial spine to form a bowl-shaped muscle filling the pelvic outlet and supporting the pelvic organs (see **Chapter 1**). There is a gap between the fibres of the puborectalis to allow passage of the urethra, vagina and rectum, called the urogenital hiatus. Uterovaginal prolapse is caused by failure of the interaction between the levator ani muscles and the ligaments and fascia that support the pelvic organs.

10.1201/9781003218036-10

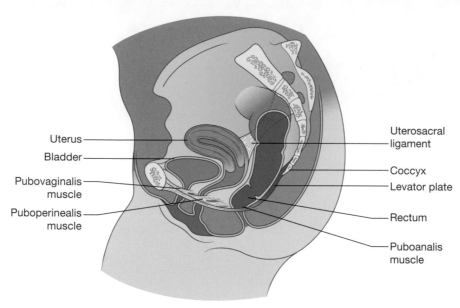

Figure 10.1 Female pelvic anatomy.

There are three levels of supporting ligaments and fascia, which work together to provide a global and dynamic system to support the uterus, vagina and associated organs (**Figure 10.2**). Level 1 (apical) support is provided by the uterosacral ligaments, which attach the cervix to the sacrum. Support at this level is crucial in contributing to support of the vaginal walls that are attached to the cervix. Defects in level 1 support can be seen on examination by the descent of the uterus within the vagina. Level 1 support remains critical, even after hysterectomy, and it is important during that procedure to reattach the uterosacral ligaments to the vaginal vault to prevent prolapse.

Level 2 support is provided by the fascia that surrounds the vagina, both anteriorly and posteriorly, lying between the vagina and the bladder (pubocervical fascia) or rectum (rectovaginal fascia). These fascial sheets fuse together at the vaginal edge and then are attached to the pelvic side wall, fusing to the fascia overlying obturator internus. Defects in the fascia providing level 2 support will lead to prolapse of the anterior vaginal wall into the vaginal lumen and stress urinary incontinence.

Level 3 support is provided by the fascia of the posterior vagina, which is attached at its caudal end to the perineal body. The perineal body is a dense connective tissue mass underneath the lower third of the posterior vaginal wall and is the insertion of the posterior vaginal fascia, fibres of levator ani and the transverse perineal muscles. Damage at this level leads to development of lower posterior vaginal wall prolapse.

URINARY SYMPTOMS

In a healthy individual, the bladder stores, and then voids, urine. This is known as the micturition cycle. Most of the time, the detrusor muscle of the bladder is relaxed, allowing storage of increasing urine volumes with no increase in pressure. As bladder capacity is reached, sensory signals from stretch receptors in the bladder wall send the sensation of bladder filling. The sphincter mechanism is closed. As an adult, voluntary delay of micturition until socially convenient is achieved by cortical inhibition of the spinal voiding reflex arc. Before voiding begins, this inhibition is removed and the pelvic floor and urethral sphincters relax in a coordinated fashion to allow detrusor contraction and bladder emptying. The detrusor muscle is innervated by muscarinic cholinergic nerves of the parasympathetic nervous system (causing detrusor muscle contraction) and the urethral sphincter

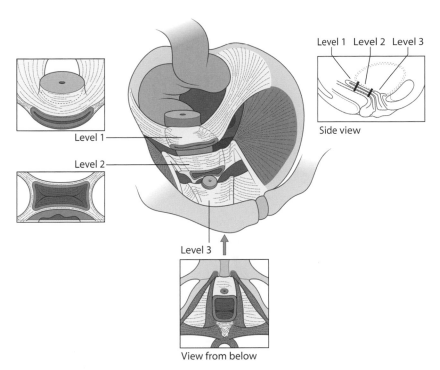

Figure 10.2 Fascial supports of the pelvic organs. Level 1 support is provided by the uterosacral ligaments, suspending the uterus and vaginal vault. Level 2 (mid-vagina) support is provided by the fascia lying between the vagina and the bladder or rectum that fuses laterally and runs to attach on the pelvic side wall. Level 3 support is provided by the perineal body, which has the posterior vaginal fascia fused to its upper surface.

is innervated by noradrenergic neurons of the sympathetic nervous system (sphincter contraction) and somatic fibres (voluntary contraction and relaxation) from the pudendal nerves.

In women, the urethral sphincter mechanism is a functional system that includes the internal (smooth muscle) and external (striated muscle) sphincters, the muscles of the pelvic floor and the pubourethral ligament supporting the urethra. Increases in abdominal pressure are transmitted equally to the bladder and bladder neck (**Figure 10.3**). In a premenopausal woman, the urethral epithelium has a rich blood supply and contributes to continence by acting as a seal. The mechanism of causation of stress incontinence and detrusor overactivity is shown in **Figure 10.3**.

URINARY SYMPTOM TERMINOLOGY

Urinary symptoms are categorized according to the time at which they are experienced in relation to

the micturition cycle. The presence of a symptom (severity) does not always lead to impact on quality of life (bother), and healthcare professionals should consider both severity and bother for a complete evaluation.

URINARY INCONTINENCE

Urinary incontinence is the complaint of involuntary leakage of urine associated with urgency and/or with exertion, effort, sneezing or coughing. It includes stress, urge and mixed incontinence.

STRESS INCONTINENCE

In isolation, the symptom of stress incontinence is a reasonably good predictor of the presence of an incompetent urethral sphincter. Urethral sphincter weakness in most cases is due to hypermobility, whereby the pelvic floor and ligaments cannot

147

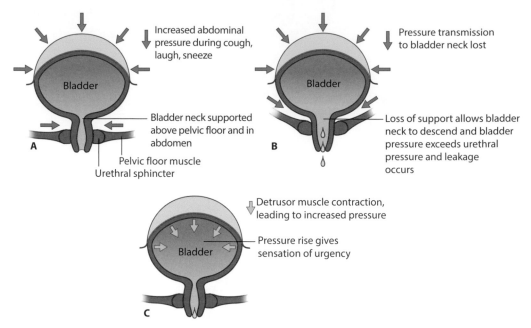

Figure 10.3 Mechanism of incontinence. In healthy women, the bladder neck is supported above the pelvic floor and increases in abdominal pressure are transmitted to the bladder neck (**A**). Loss of bladder neck support results in descent of the bladder neck and loss of pressure transmission, resulting in leaking when coughing, straining, etc. (stress incontinence) (**B**). Detrusor overactivity causes increased sensation; leakage occurs only if the contraction pressure exceeds the pelvic floor and sphincter pressure (**C**).

BOX 10.1: Urinary symptoms

Urine storage symptoms

- *Frequency*: patient considers they void too often by day
- *Nocturia*: waking at night one or more times to void
- *Urgency*: a sudden compelling desire to pass urine, which is difficult to defer
- *Urge incontinence*: involuntary leakage accompanied by or immediately preceded by urgency
- *Stress incontinence*: involuntary leakage on effort, exertion, sneezing or coughing
- *Nocturnal enuresis*: the loss of urine occurring during sleep

Urine voiding symptoms

- *Slow stream*: perception of reduced urine flow
- *Splitting or spraying*: the stream of urine is not a single flow
- *Intermittent stream*: urine flow that stops and starts
- *Hesitancy*: difficulty in initiating micturition resulting in a delay in the onset of voiding
- *Terminal dribble*: a prolonged final part of micturition, when the flow has slowed to a trickle or dribble

---

retain the urethra in position and it falls through the urogenital hiatus during increases in abdominal pressure, leading to loss of pressure transmission to the urethra and hence leakage of urine (see **Figure 10.3**).

Intrinsic sphincter deficiency is less common and occurs when urethral closure pressure is low without any urethral mobility. Intrinsic sphincter deficiency is due to weakness of the sphincter muscles and loss of the cushioning seal effect in the urethra.

Urethral sphincter weakness is associated strongly with a history of vaginal childbirth and various related risk factors, and with some non-obstetric factors. Obstetric risk factors act by a combination effect of stretching of the pudendal nerves and/or detachment of the pelvic floor muscles from their insertions on the pelvic side wall. Direct muscle damage results in loss of pelvic floor support and hence urethral hypermobility. Pudendal nerve damage causes both weakening of the pelvic floor muscles and urethral sphincter dysfunction.

Depending on age, the prevalence of stress incontinence ranges from 29% to 75%, with a mean of 48%.

> **BOX 10.2: Risk factors for stress urinary incontinence**
>
> - Multiparity (particularly vaginal births)
> - Forceps delivery
> - Perineal trauma
> - Long labour
> - Epidural analgesia
> - Birth weight >4 kg
> - Increasing age
> - Postmenopause
> - Connective tissue disease
> - Chronic cough (e.g. bronchiectasis or chronic obstructive pulmonary disease)
> - Doxazocin (alpha-adrenergic antagonist) for hypertension, which causes relaxation of the urethral sphincter
> - Obesity

OVERACTIVE BLADDER SYNDROME

Overactive bladder (OAB) syndrome is a collection of symptoms: urinary urgency, usually accompanied by urinary frequency and nocturia, with or without urinary incontinence, in the absence of urinary tract infection or other obvious pathology. It has a prevalence of 20% and is more common in women than men. Some risk factors are modifiable (noted by asterisks in **Box 10.3** 'Risk factors for OAB syndrome').

> **BOX 10.3: Risk factors for OAB syndrome**
>
> - Childhood bed-wetting
> - Obesity*
> - Alcohol*
> - Smoking*
> - Neurological factors (e.g. stroke, multiple sclerosis, diabetic neuropathy)
> - Previous hysterectomy
> - Previous surgery for urinary incontinence

CLINICAL ASSESSMENT OF INCONTINENCE

A detailed history should be taken to elicit the patient's presenting symptoms to identify whether the patient has only stress or urge incontinence symptoms or has a combination of the two. If there are mixed symptoms, an assessment should be made as to which predominates. It is useful to record measures of severity, including the number of episodes per day of frequency, urgency and leakage; whether continence pads are needed and, if so, how many and what size; whether the patient needs to change their underclothes or outer clothes because of leakage; and what behaviour changes have been employed. Commonly, patients will have reduced their fluid intake and may limit their social activities to places where they already know about the position and cleanliness of toilet facilities. Associated symptoms of prolapse, faecal incontinence and sexual difficulties should be sought, as well as a detailed medical history to identify potential predisposing factors and any ongoing medical conditions that may have an impact on treatment (including comorbidities that increase the risk of anaesthesia or present cautions or contraindications to drug therapy). A drug history (diuretics, narcotics, muscle relaxants, alpha-adrenergic antagonists) is important to elicit, as certain drugs may cause bladder symptoms. Remember to be alert for 'red flag' signs suggesting malignancy, such as haematuria, rectal bleeding or significant pain. Many clinicians will also ask patients to complete one of a range of disease-specific quality-of-life instruments to assess the impact of the patient's problem, and this can be repeated after treatment to allow collection of outcomes. This is useful for the purpose of service audit and for individual clinician appraisal and revalidation.

Physical examination should include general, abdominal and pelvic examinations. Abdominal examination will identify any surgical scars, evidence of obesity and the presence or absence of any pelvic mass that may be a factor in urinary frequency. A palpable bladder – which may be a feature of underactive bladder or outflow obstruction – should prompt further investigations for infection, cauda equina syndrome, pelvic organ prolapse or gynaecological malignancy. An abdominal mass (e.g. large fibroid uterus or ovarian cyst that increases intra-abdominal pressure) can produce symptoms like those of OAB.

Pelvic examination of the incontinent patient ideally should be done in the lithotomy position or left lateral position using a Sim's speculum (see **Chapter 2**: **Figure 2.4**) to assess each vaginal wall adequately for associated prolapse (see later sections in this chapter on prolapse) and/or atrophy in the postmenopausal woman. Pelvic floor muscle function can be qualitatively evaluated according to the tone at rest and the strength of a voluntary or reflex contraction. Visible leakage during coughing or Valsalva manoeuvre should be sought.

BASIC INVESTIGATIONS

All patients should be asked to provide a fresh, midstream specimen of urine to exclude overt infection or asymptomatic bacteriuria. Additional simple investigations include a patient bladder diary (3 days is usually adequate) to record the amount, type and frequency of drinks taken as well as the timing, frequency and volume of voids (**Figure 10.4**). This can be a useful exercise for the patient to take note of exactly what they are drinking and their voiding habits. The bladder diary will also allow the patient to record leakage episodes and urgency.

INVESTIGATIONS TO CONSIDER

POST-VOID RESIDUAL VOLUME

Post-void residual volume can be measured using a bladder scan when there is a history of voiding dysfunction or recurrent urinary tract infections.

PAD TEST

It is possible to obtain an objective measure of urine leak by conducting a pad test, although it is not routinely recommended. This is an investigation whereby the patient wears one or more pre-weighed sanitary pads for a variable length of time (between 1 hour in clinic and 24 hours at home) while performing specific provocation tests (e.g. hand washing, climbing stairs, coughing) or activities of daily living. The change in weight (g) is a measure of the amount of urine lost (mL).

PELVIC AND/OR RENAL TRACT ULTRASOUND

A pelvic and/or renal tract ultrasound may be indicated if there are symptoms of pelvic pain, clinical suspicion of a pelvic mass, haematuria, bladder pain or recurrent urinary tract infection.

URODYNAMIC STUDIES

Urodynamic testing in the form of multichannel filling and voiding cystometry is reserved for patients who fail to improve with conservative measures and/or those with complex histories or who have undergone previous surgery for incontinence or prolapse (**Figure 10.5**). For women with OAB syndrome, many clinicians perform this investigation only when considering second-line interventions (see **Box 10.5** 'Common urodynamic diagnoses') after medical treatment fails. The purpose of urodynamic testing is to reproduce a micturition cycle (bladder filling and voiding) while recording abdominal and bladder pressure and attempting to reproduce the patient's symptoms, to provide a diagnosis. A fine pressure catheter is placed in the bladder through the urethra and a second catheter is placed in the rectum; the bladder is then filled with warm saline while pressure recordings are made with the patient sitting on a commode that records leakage (**Figure 10.5A**). The pressure generated by any contraction of the detrusor can be inferred by subtraction (bladder pressure – abdominal pressure = detrusor pressure). During filling, the patient is asked to declare the onset of bladder filling sensation (usually around 150 mL volume), a strong desire to void (around 350 mL) and the onset of urgency (up to 500 mL, depending on bladder capacity) (**Figure 10.5B**).

Date: Sunday 27th November 2016

I got up at...7 am   I went to bed at...10.30 pm

Time	Record drinks taken (type and amount)	Volume of urine passed (mL)	Each time you leak, circle whether you were:	Each time you pass water, circle how severe the urgency was:
6 am			Almost Dry Damp Wet Soaked	None Mild Moderate Severe
7 am		400 mL	Almost Dry Damp Wet Soaked	None Mild Moderate Severe
8 am	1 cup of tea 200 mL		Almost Dry Damp Wet Soaked	None Mild Moderate Severe
9 am		200 mL	Almost Dry Damp Wet Soaked	None Mild Moderate Severe
10 am	1 cup of tea 200 mL		Almost Dry Damp Wet Soaked	None Mild Moderate Severe
11 am		200 mL	Almost Dry Damp Wet Soaked	None Mild Moderate Severe
Mid-day	1 glass of wine 150 mL 1 cup of coffee 200 mL	100 mL 150 mL	Almost Dry Damp Wet Soaked	None Mild Moderate Severe
1 pm			Almost Dry Damp Wet Soaked	None Mild Moderate Severe
2 pm	1 glass of orange 200 mL		Almost Dry Damp Wet Soaked	None Mild Moderate Severe
3 pm		250 mL	Almost Dry Damp Wet Soaked	None Mild Moderate Severe
4 pm		100 mL	Almost Dry Damp Wet Soaked	None Mild Moderate Severe
5 pm	1 cup of tea 200 mL		Almost Dry Damp Wet Soaked	None Mild Moderate Severe
6 pm		200 mL	Almost Dry Damp Wet Soaked	None Mild Moderate Severe
7 pm			Almost Dry Damp Wet Soaked	None Mild Moderate Severe
8 pm	1 can of coke 240 mL	100 mL	Almost Dry Damp Wet Soaked	None Mild Moderate Severe
9 pm		100 mL	Almost Dry Damp Wet Soaked	None Mild Moderate Severe
10 pm	1 cup of hot chocolate 150 mL	100 mL	Almost Dry Damp Wet Soaked	None Mild Moderate Severe
11 pm			Almost Dry Damp Wet Soaked	None Mild Moderate Severe
Mid-night			Almost Dry Damp Wet Soaked	None Mild Moderate Severe
1 am			Almost Dry Damp Wet Soaked	None Mild Moderate Severe
2 am			Almost Dry Damp Wet Soaked	None Mild Moderate Severe
3 am			Almost Dry Damp Wet Soaked	None Mild Moderate Severe
4 am			Almost Dry Damp Wet Soaked	None Mild Moderate Severe
5 am			Almost Dry Damp Wet Soaked	None Mild Moderate Severe

Reminders

1. Don't forget to record the time you woke up in the morning and the time you went to sleep
2. Don't forget to record what happened overnight
3. Try and make a record of things just after they happen
4. Record things to the nearest hour
5. Record type and amount of drinks taken (e.g. 2 cups of tea, 1 can of coke)

Urgency severity scale

NONE: no urgency

MILD: awareness of ugency but easily tolerated

MODERATE: enough urgency discomfort that it interferes with usual activities/tasks

SEVERE: extreme urgency discomfort that abruptly stops all activities/tasks

Figure 10.4 An example of a bladder diary, including columns for recording fluid intake (volume and amount), voided volume, the amount of leakage and the severity of urgency.

When urgency is reported (and functional bladder capacity is reached) filling is stopped and the patient performs various actions to provoke leakage and/or detrusor contractions (e.g. coughing, star jumps, listening to running water), before voiding while the pressure catheters remain in place. A urodynamic test will provide evidence of urethral sphincter weakness and/or detrusor overactivity (**Figure 10.5C**), as well as identifying normal or abnormal voiding function.

CYSTOURETHROSCOPY

Cystourethroscopy can aid in the diagnosis of patients with haematuria or a history of pelvic surgery and in those patients who have failed traditional treatments to determine normal anatomy or the presence of pathology including a vesicovaginal or urethrovaginal fistula, a foreign body or a tumour/mass.

For patients with mixed symptoms, or those with recurrent problems after previous treatment, it is good practice to discuss management plans within a multidisciplinary team meeting, including a gynaecologist, a urologist, a continence nurse, a physiotherapist and possibly an elderly care consultant.

🔑 KEY LEARNING POINTS

- Stress incontinence is typically a result of a weak urethral sphincter, often as a consequence of childbirth.
- OAB syndrome is a collection of symptoms, including urinary urgency, usually accompanied by urinary frequency and nocturia, with or without urgency urinary incontinence.
- Clinical examination should exclude pelvic masses (e.g. fibroid uterus) and assess the patient's ability to contract their pelvic floor muscles and the strength of that contraction.
- Patients with pain, haematuria or recurrent infections should have the renal tract investigated radiologically and by cystoscopy.

TREATMENT FOR INCONTINENCE

NON-SURGICAL MANAGEMENT

Non-surgical management is the preferred initial strategy for urinary incontinence. Women are encouraged to make lifestyle changes such as caffeine reduction and modification of their fluid intake (increasing if it is too low, decreasing if it is too high). Patients with urinary incontinence or OAB syndrome who have a body mass index greater than 30 are advised to lose weight.

BOX 10.4: Conservative treatment for urinary incontinence

- Advice about fluid balance
- Reduction of caffeine intake or drinks that may irritate the bladder (e.g. alcohol, carbonated drinks, fruit juices)
- Bladder retraining
- Pelvic floor muscle training

PELVIC FLOOR MUSCLE TRAINING

Pelvic floor muscle training (PFMT) works for both stress and mixed urinary incontinence. In the latter case, it is likely that the benefit is from improving muscle strength to give patients the confidence to resist the urge without fear of leakage and also by pelvic floor contraction having a reflex inhibition action on detrusor muscle contraction. A trial of supervised PFMT consisting of contraction performed three times per day for at least 3 months' duration should be offered as a first-line treatment to patients with stress or mixed urinary incontinence. For patients who are unable to perform an effective pelvic floor muscle contraction, supplementing PFMT with biofeedback techniques, electrical stimulation or vaginal cones should be considered. When supervised PFMT is not available, the NHS-approved Squeezy app can be recommended.

A Cochrane review comparing PFMT with no treatment or inactive control treatments found that women with stress urinary incontinence who were in the PFMT group were six times more likely to report cure or symptom improvement (74% versus 11%).

BLADDER RETRAINING

For women with OAB syndrome or mixed incontinence, PFMT is combined with a form of bladder drill or bladder retraining. Bladder training

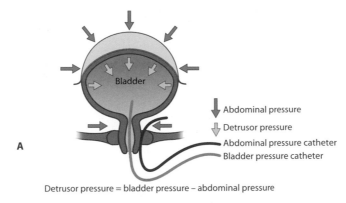

A

Detrusor pressure = bladder pressure − abdominal pressure

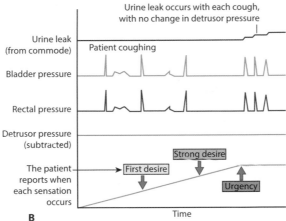

B

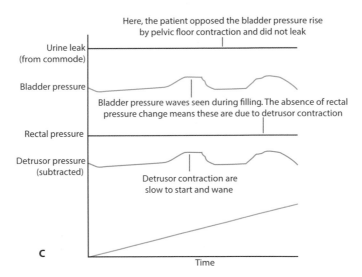

C

Figure 10.5 A urodynamic investigation (cystometry) records bladder pressure and abdominal pressure (usually via a rectal pressure catheter) and calculates detrusor pressure by subtraction (**A**). During filling, the patient is asked to report the occurrence of first desire to void (usually about 150 mL), strong desire and urgency (at functional bladder capacity) (**B**). With urodynamic stress incontinence, leakage is seen with increases in abdominal pressure (e.g. coughing) with no change in detrusor pressure (**C**). With detrusor overactivity, detrusor contractions are seen during the filling phase. These may or may not result in leakage, but normally will be associated with increased sensation.

requires the patient to resist the urge to urinate by 5–15 minutes before voiding and over a period of weeks. This time is gradually increased by a further 5–15 minutes until a patient can hold their urine for 2.5 hours. This can be explained at an initial consultation emphasizing that this discipline needs to be maintained over the long term for durable results. Bladder retraining can be very successful in reducing frequency and urgency but, like pelvic floor exercises, it requires perseverance and determination from the patient to succeed.

BOX 10.5: Common urodynamic diagnoses

- *Detrusor overactivity*: the presence of a detrusor contraction, with or without sensation, during the filling phase of urodynamics
- *Detrusor overactivity incontinence*: leakage from the urethra in association with a detrusor contraction and increase in bladder pressure
- *Urodynamic stress incontinence*: leakage from the urethra in association with a rise in abdominal pressure (e.g. coughing) without a detrusor contraction (a sign of urethral sphincter weakness)
- *Mixed incontinence*: the presence of both urodynamic stress incontinence and detrusor overactivity

---

🔑 KEY LEARNING POINTS

- Non-surgical treatment with fluid advice, pelvic floor exercises and bladder retraining is the first-line management strategy for all patients with incontinence or OAB syndrome.
- Patient motivation is important for success of conservative treatment.
- Urodynamic testing is reserved for patients who fail to improve with conservative measures, those with complex histories or those who have undergone previous surgery for incontinence or prolapse.

MEDICAL TREATMENT

Pharmacological treatment can be introduced if satisfactory symptom control is not achieved after 6 weeks of bladder training. Anticholinergic drugs are the most common treatment for OAB syndrome. They act by blocking the muscarinic receptors on the bladder, which are stimulated by acetylcholine released from activated cholinergic (parasympathetic) nerves. In this way, they inhibit the ability of the bladder to contract.

Counselling is important before starting medication to ensure compliance. Explain to the patient the likelihood of the medicine being successful, the common adverse effects, that some adverse effects (such as dry mouth and constipation) may indicate that the medicine is starting to have an effect and that substantial benefits may not be seen until they have been taking the medicine for at least 4 weeks. It is important to consider coexisting conditions (such as poor bladder emptying, cognitive impairment or dementia), the current use of other medicines that can affect total anticholinergic load and the risk of adverse effects, including cognitive impairment.

There are a number of medications available to treat OAB syndrome. If the first medicine for OAB or mixed urinary incontinence is not effective or well tolerated, another medicine with a low acquisition cost should be offered. Oxybutynin (immediate release) should not be offered to older women who may be at a higher risk of a sudden deterioration in their physical or mental health. Note that the contraindications to antimuscarinics include gastrointestinal obstruction, intestinal atony, myasthenia gravis, paralytic ileus, pyloric stenosis, severe ulcerative colitis, significant bladder outflow obstruction, toxic megacolon and urinary retention.

BOX 10.6: Drugs used for OAB syndrome

- *Oxybutynin*: 2.5–5 mg up to three times daily
- *Trospium chloride*: 20 mg twice daily
- *Tolterodine*: 2 mg twice daily (reduced to 1 mg in hepatic impairment); modified release preparation 4 mg once daily
- *Fesoterodine*: 4 mg once daily, maximum 8 mg once daily (fesoterodine is related to tolterodine)
- *Solifenacin*: 5 mg once daily; can be increased to 10 mg once daily

---

All drugs have similar efficacy, with published randomized studies demonstrating a decrease in urgency and a decrease in incontinence episodes in the range of one or two fewer episodes per day, compared with placebo. The side effect profile is similar across all drugs, with dry mouth, constipation and blurred vision being the most common.

Mirabegron is a more recently developed medication for OAB syndrome, which is a beta-3 adrenergic agonist. It acts upon the sympathetic neurones innervating the bladder to enhance relaxation of the detrusor. It acts on the storage function of the bladder, while antimuscarinic medications act by suppressing voiding.

In postmenopausal patients, topical vaginal oestrogen for 3 months can provide dramatic improvement in bladder sensation and associated urgency. Duloxetine is used very occasionally for stress incontinence. It is a combined serotonin and noradrenaline reuptake inhibitor also used for the treatment of depression in higher doses. Duloxetine acts at the micturition centre in the sacral spinal cord to increase the sympathetic nerve output to the urethral sphincter and increase sphincter tone. Randomized trials have shown a 50% or more improvement in leakage symptoms in over half of the patients treated. However, the side effects, including nausea, cause many women to stop treatment. **Figure 10.6** shows a suggested step-wise treatment pathway for women with OAB.

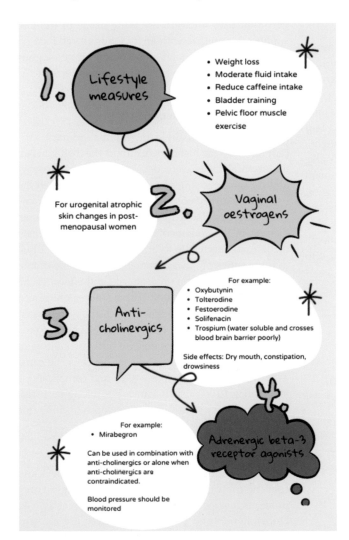

Figure 10.6 Treatment ladder for overactive bladder. Review the effects of conservative management (step 1) after 8–12 weeks and of medication (steps 2–4) after 4 weeks.

MECHANICAL DEVICES FOR URINARY INCONTINENCE

These are devices that are placed into the vagina to prevent urine leakage (e.g. continence ring, continence device, urethral plug).

SURGICAL TREATMENT

STRESS INCONTINENCE

Surgical options should be considered when non-surgical management fails. Procedures available include a midurethral sling, a pubovaginal sling, retropubic colposuspension and urethral bulking.

Midurethral and pubovaginal slings

There are several variations of midurethral tapes available, with the same underlying principle. A permanent, non-absorbable mesh of polypropylene woven into a tape approximately 1 cm wide is placed through a small vaginal incision under the midurethra and into a U-shape behind the pubic symphysis, via two small suprapubic incisions (a retropubic placement), or into a hammock shape behind the inferior pubic rami and through the obturator foramen, via a small incision in each groin (a transobturator placement) (**Figure 10.7**). The midurethral tapes have a cure rate for stress incontinence of 80–85%, and this high success rate persists in the long term (10 years or more). Complications specific to midurethral tapes relate to

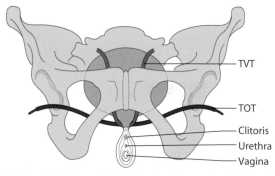

Figure 10.7 The position of tension-free vaginal (TVT) and transobturator (TOT) midurethral tapes. The TVT lies under the midurethra and in the retropubic space between the pelvis and bladder. The introducing trocars pass through the urogenital diaphragm and the rectus sheath. The TOT lies in a more horizontal position under the midurethra and exits through the obturator foramen, piercing the obturator muscle and the adductor longus tendon in the thigh.

the non-absorbable polypropylene they are manufactured from. There is a low rate of mesh exposure.

Common surgical complications include:

- voiding difficulty (usually short term) in 2–5%
- bladder perforation during the procedure (2–5%)
- the onset of new OAB symptoms after surgery (5%)

The use of surgical mesh/tape for urogynaecological conditions whereby the mesh is inserted through the vaginal wall is currently restricted in the UK following an independent review. In July 2018, NHS England advised that all cases should be postponed if it is clinically safe to do so.

A pubovaginal sling is an abdomino-vaginal surgery that uses a length of fascia, tissue or graft to support the urethra with an abdominal wall fixation site. The sling material is most commonly autologous and, therefore, the procedure has been referred to as a 'fascial' sling.

Retropubic colposuspension

Retropubic colposuspension was the primary procedure for stress incontinence until the 1990s, when midurethral tapes were developed. The controversy around synthetic slings has led to a resurgence in the use of colposuspension in recent years. At colposuspension, the retropubic space is opened via a Pfannenstiel incision in the abdomen and the bladder is reflected medially on each side to allow the placement of two or three sutures (either absorbable or permanent) into the paravaginal fascia on each side at the level of the bladder neck (**Figure 10.8**). These sutures are placed through the pectineal ligament on the pubic ramus on the same side and then tied to provide support to the bladder neck and prevent descent during coughing or straining. The cure rate for incontinence is the same as for midurethral tapes (80–85%) and complications are similar. Colposuspension carries a long-term risk of developing posterior vaginal prolapse (5–10%) due to lifting of the anterior vaginal wall.

Urethral bulking agents

Urethral bulking agents bulk up the bladder neck and coat the urethral mucosa to prevent leakage. Three products are widely available (Macroplastique®, Durasphere® and Bulkamid®). These are all synthetic polymer materials, either microscopic beads

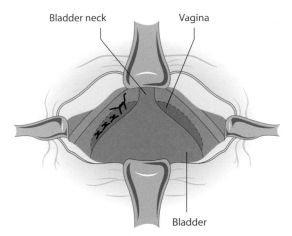

Figure 10.8 A sketch of a colposuspension through a Pfannenstiel incision. The patient's head is at the bottom of the picture, and interrupted sutures are being placed in the paravaginal fascia at the level of the bladder neck through the pectineal ligament on the posterior surface of the superior pubic ramus.

or viscous liquid. The procedure can be performed under local anaesthetic and is particularly suitable for patients deemed medically unfit or too frail for a general anaesthetic, or for patients with residual leakage after a tape or colposuspension (**Figure 10.9**). Cure rates after these procedures are in the order of 60–80%, but responses may be short lived and some patients require two or more treatments.

OVERACTIVE BLADDER

For OAB, a surgical option may be considered as second-line treatment. The neurotoxin botulinum toxin A (marketed as Botox® or Dysport®) has been shown in recent randomized trials to be a highly effective treatment. Botulinum toxin is a long-acting molecule that prevents the release of neurotransmitter vesicles from the motor end-plate and causes a flaccid paralysis in the treated muscle. A single intramuscular injection can last for 3–6 months. Botulinum toxin is administered via a flexible or rigid cystoscope and injected in multiple sites across the dome of the bladder to abolish the involuntary detrusor contractions that cause symptoms. Reduction of urgency and leakage episodes of over 50–80% have been reported and reduction in continence rates in excess of 40% have been reported. The major drawback of this treatment is a voiding difficulty rate of 8–15%, which may necessitate self-catheterization.

Sacral neuromodulation is also an effective surgical management option.

PELVIC ORGAN PROLAPSE

Pelvic organ prolapse can cause symptoms either directly due to the prolapsed organ or indirectly due to organ dysfunction secondary to displacement

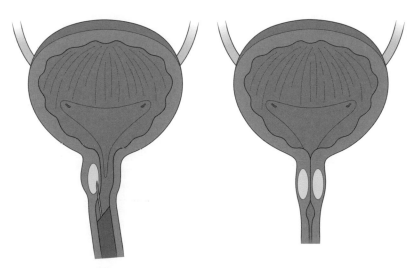

Figure 10.9 Urethral bulking agents reduce the calibre of the urethra and support the bladder neck to reduce urinary incontinence.

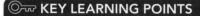
from its anatomical position. Pelvic organ prolapse symptoms include a sensation of vaginal bulge, heaviness or a visible protrusion at or beyond the introitus. Patients may also describe lower abdominal or back pain or a dragging discomfort relieved by lying or sitting.

Indirect symptoms will depend on which other organs are involved in the prolapse but may include difficulty in voiding urine or emptying the bowel (termed obstructive defaecation) and sensations of incomplete emptying of the bladder or rectum. Patients may have to support or reduce the prolapse with their fingers to be able to void or evacuate stool completely (termed digitation, distinct from manual evacuation of the rectum). Urinary or faecal incontinence may also be present. It is important to ask about sexual activity, even in older patients, and to enquire about difficulty achieving penetration, pain or discomfort during intercourse, a loss of sensation or difficulty achieving orgasm due to vaginal or introital laxity.

Patients may experience vaginal bleeding from a prolapse that is external and becomes ulcerated or abraded, but in women with a uterus, one must remember to exclude endometrial carcinoma by biopsy and ultrasound.

Risk factors predisposing to prolapse are very much similar to those predisposing to stress incontinence. Research has shown the pudendal nerves to be damaged after childbirth, with increased nerve

conduction times, and ultrasound studies of the pelvic anatomy of women with prolapse have demonstrated thinning or avulsion of the puborectalis muscle from its insertion on the pubic ramus, on either one or both sides in a high proportion of cases.

CLINICAL ASSESSMENT OF PROLAPSE

The history should elicit presenting symptom(s) and their severity and include questions to ascertain whether the patient has coexisting urinary, faecal or sexual symptoms. For women who are not sexually active, it should be discussed whether this is due to the prolapse symptoms or other personal or social issues (e.g. health of the partner). For some women, intercourse is avoided because of anxieties or embarrassment over the appearance of the genitalia and a loss of perceived attractiveness.

Clinical examination should ideally be done in the lithotomy position or left lateral position with a Sim's speculum (see **Chapter 2**: **Figure 2.4**). This allows retraction of the anterior and posterior vaginal wall in turn, to allow full assessment of the degree of prolapse and to assess how much descent of the cervix and uterus is present. Prolapse is described in four stages of descent, and a note should be made of whether it occurs at patient straining or at rest (**Figure 10.10**):

- *Stage 0* – no prolapse is demonstrated
- *Stage I* – the most distal portion of the prolapse is more than 1 cm above the level of the hymen
- *Stage II* – the most distal portion of the prolapse is 1 cm or less proximal to or distal to the plane of the hymen
- *Stage III* – the most distal portion of the prolapse is more than 1 cm below the plane of the hymen
- *Stage IV* – complete eversion of the total length of the lower genital tract is demonstrated

Vaginal prolapse of the anterior vagina (the anterior compartment) is also known as cystocele in the upper half or urethrocele in the lower half (**Figure 10.11A**). Posterior vaginal prolapse (the posterior compartment) is also known as enterocele in the upper third or rectocele below this (**Figure 10.11B**).

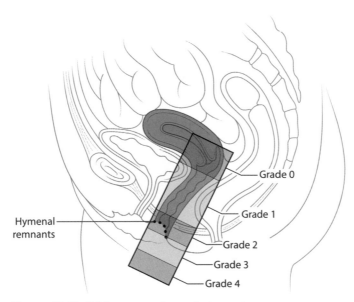

Figure 10.10 Pelvic organ prolapse staging system.

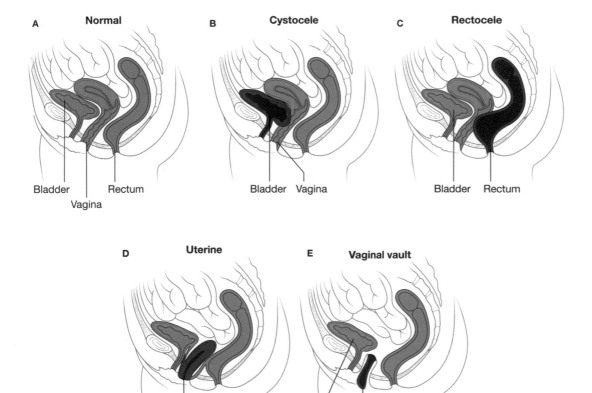

Figure 10.11 (**A**) Anterior vaginal wall prolapse. (**B**) Cystocele with Anterior vaginal wall prolapse. (**C**) Rectocele with Posterior vaginal wall prolapse. (**D**) Uterine prolapse. (**E**) Vaginal vault prolapse.

The uterus can prolapse (**Figure 10.11C**) and, in women who have undergone hysterectomy, vaginal vault prolapse may be seen (**Figure 10.11D**). The Pelvic Organ Prolapse Quantification system is recommended for clinicians dealing with patients with prolapse, as it uses a uniform characterization and recording method.

For women with symptoms of pressure or vaginal bulge only, there is rarely a need to arrange any investigations, other than those relating to anaesthetic preassessment (see **Chapter 17**). In view of the complex relationship between prolapse and bladder or bowel function, if patients have additional indirect symptoms, then it is prudent to arrange relevant investigations. Such patients should be reviewed with the completed investigations in a multidisciplinary team meeting, including a gynaecologist, a colorectal surgeon, a continence nurse and a physiotherapist.

TREATMENT FOR PROLAPSE

NON-SURGICAL MANAGEMENT

Non-surgical management of prolapse includes pelvic floor muscle exercises and the use of supportive vaginal pessaries. A programme of supervised PFMT for at least 4 months for individuals with symptomatic pelvic organ prolapse that does not extend greater than 1 cm beyond the hymen upon straining is recommended.

An alternative to this is to insert a vaginal pessary to reduce the prolapse, which leads to resolution of many of the symptoms. Pessary use can be very effective at relieving symptoms and has the advantage of avoiding surgery and the associated risks, which can be extremely useful in those who are medically unfit and elderly. A range of shapes of pessary is available (**Figure 10.12**). Ring pessaries are usually tried first, but an intact perineal body is necessary for these to be retained. Shelf pessaries, Gellhorn pessaries and others are useful for patients with deficient perineal bodies. It is usual practice to replace a pessary every 6 months and to examine the patient for signs of vaginal ulceration, although this frequency is traditional and not based on any evidence. Complications are uncommon and usually minor (bleeding, discharge), although rarely the pessary can become incarcerated,

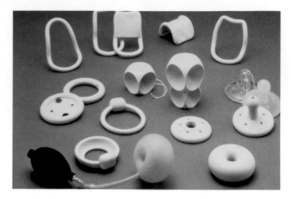

Figure 10.12 Various types of vaginal pessaries.

requiring general anaesthesia to remove, and rare cases of rectovaginal or vesicovaginal fistula formation have been reported. Sexual intercourse remains theoretically possible with a well-placed ring pessary, but not with the others, so would not generally be suitable for women who are sexually active. Motivated patients can be taught to insert and remove their own pessaries if they do wish to remain sexually active.

SURGERY FOR PELVIC ORGAN PROLAPSE

Surgical treatment can be offered if conservative treatments have failed or if the patient chooses surgery from the outset. There are a wide range of specific procedures that are described further in **Chapter 17**. The procedures can be reconstructive or obliterative. The procedure chosen depends on which compartment is affected, whether the patient wishes to retain their uterus, whether the patient is sexually active and whether the vaginal or abdominal route (laparoscopic or robotic) of surgery is chosen. The essential principles of prolapse surgery apply for all procedures. Prolapse surgery is performed through the vagina to restore the ligamentous tissue supports to the apex, anterior and posterior vagina (anterior repair, posterior repair) and repair of the perineal body. The vaginal route can also be used for post-hysterectomy vault prolapse, attaching the vaginal vault to the sacrospinous ligament with non-absorbable or slowly absorbable sutures, but here an abdominal approach to perform a sacrocolpopexy is an option that will provide an excellent, durable, long-term cure. The relative merits of abdominal compared with vaginal surgery and the usual recovery times are discussed in **Chapter 17**. In the last 3–5 years, there has been an increasing number of women wishing to avoid hysterectomy during prolapse surgery, so both sacrospinous fixation and sacrocolpopexy can be performed by attaching the cervix rather than the vaginal vault.

Obliterative procedures for pelvic organ prolapse, often termed colpocleisis, are defined as obliteration of the vaginal canal by removal of vaginal epithelium on the anterior and posterior vaginal walls and suturing together the fibromuscular layers of the anterior and posterior vaginal walls.

BOX 10.7: Principles of prolapse surgery

- Remove/reduce the vaginal bulge
- Restore the ligament/tissue supports to the apex, anterior and posterior vagina
- Replace associated organs in their correct positions
- Retain sufficient vaginal capacity to allow intercourse
- Restore the perineal body

Vaginal repair using mesh improves the anatomical outcome and reduces the risk of recurrent prolapse. However, the available long-term data do not demonstrate a difference in symptom relief between standard repair and mesh repair. Mesh repair carries the risk of later erosion and need for removal, which is challenging surgery. Vaginal mesh surgery for pelvic organ prolapse is not currently available in the UK following an independent review of complications affecting patients who had received vaginal mesh for this indication.

ANAL INCONTINENCE

Anal incontinence is the involuntary passage of flatus or faeces. Anal incontinence occurs when the normal anatomy or physiology that maintains the structure and function of the anorectal complex is disrupted. The anal sphincter complex consists of an internal anal sphincter made of smooth muscle and is responsible for 70% of the resting pressure of the anal sphincter complex. Damage to the internal anal sphincter gives rise to the symptom of flatus incontinence and passive faecal leakage. The external anal sphincter is made of striated muscle and is responsible for voluntary squeeze pressure. Damage to this muscle causes faecal incontinence associated with urge. The anal mucosal folds and the anal endovascular cushions also contribute to maintenance of continence.

The underlying aetiology is often complex, with multiple possible contributing factors. Anal incontinence affects up to 10% of adults and is more common in nursing home residents, the multiparous, patients with cognitive impairment or neurological

---
KEY LEARNING POINTS

- Uterovaginal prolapse causes troublesome symptoms but is not life threatening.
- A course of pelvic floor exercises can reduce symptoms and may reduce prolapse progression in women with mild/moderate prolapse.
- Vaginal pessaries are a useful conservative treatment.
- Surgery for prolapse is effective.
- It is not essential to perform hysterectomy for prolapse.
- Mesh complications are common and can be extremely difficult to manage.

KEY LEARNING POINTS

Causes of faecal incontinence
- Structural anorectal abnormalities (e.g. sphincter trauma, rectal prolapse)
- Neurological abnormalities (e.g. multiple sclerosis, stroke, pudendal neuropathy)
- Alterations in stool consistency (e.g. infectious diarrhoea, inflammatory bowel disease)
- Overflow (e.g. impaction)
- Cognitive/behavioural dysfunction (e.g. dementia, learning difficulties)
- General disability (e.g. age, acute illness)
- Iatrogenic factors (e.g. lateral sphincterotomy)
- Idiopathic factors
---

disorders, and older people. In women, obstetric injury due to direct muscle damage and/or neuropathy due to pelvic nerve stretching during vaginal birth is a common cause. Obstetric sphincter damage is the most common cause of incontinence in young women, and sphincter damage may occur in around 3.5% of vaginal deliveries. Risk factors include forceps delivery, larger babies, delayed second stage of labour and occipitoposterior presentation.

CLINICAL ASSESSMENT

Symptoms of faecal incontinence include urge, passive leakage or seepage, and flatal incontinence. It is often found in conjunction with urinary incontinence, as similar mechanisms underlie both. A detailed obstetric history and questions focused on exploring the causes are important. It is important to explore the severity and impact on quality of life. Various validated questionnaires (e.g. the Vaizey incontinence and Wexner constipation questionnaires) are available for assessment.

On examination, look for scarring around the anus. A digital rectal examination will help to assess sphincter tone and any anorectal pathology. Assess the pelvic floor tone and any evidence of concomitant prolapse. Investigations are carried out at specialist centres. Anal manometry allows measurement of anal pressure generated at rest and during squeeze. Endoanal ultrasound helps assess the integrity of the anal sphincter complex.

MANAGEMENT OF ANAL INCONTINENCE

Treatment is focussed on the underlying cause, and it is important to try conservative strategies first.

NON-SURGICAL MANAGEMENT

This consists of dietary modification and offering coping mechanisms such as the use of pads and anal plugs. Antidiarrhoeal agents such as loperamide or codeine may be useful. Pelvic floor muscle exercises, biofeedback and electrical stimulation are aimed at improving sensation, coordination and strength of the pelvic floor and should be offered in symptomatic patients, especially after childbirth injury to the pelvic floor.

SURGICAL MANAGEMENT

This depends on the underlying cause and includes repair of the anal sphincter, sacral nerve modulation and injections of bulking agents.

FURTHER READING

Brown S (2023). Faecal incontinence in adults. BMJ Best Practice. https://bestpractice.bmj.com/topics/en-gb/840.

Davila GW, Martin L (2023). Urinary incontinence in adults. BMJ Best Practice. https://bestpractice.bmj.com/topics/en-us/169.

Developed by the Joint Writing Group of the American Urogynecologic Society and the International Urogynecological Association (2020). Joint report on terminology for surgical procedures to treat pelvic organ prolapse. *International Urogynecology Journal*, 31(3): 429–463. https://doi.org/10.1007/s00192-020-04236-1.

NICE (2019). *Urinary Incontinence and Pelvic Organ Prolapse in Women: Management*. NICE guideline [NG123]. Last updated: 24 June 2019.

Wei JT, De Lancey JO (2004). Functional anatomy of the pelvic floor and lower urinary tract. *Clinical Obstetrics and Gynecology*, 47: 3–17.

SELF-ASSESSMENT

For interactive SBAs and EMQs relating to this chapter, visit www.routledge.com/cw/crosbie.

CASE HISTORY 1

A 47-year-old woman presents with symptoms of leaking urine on coughing, sneezing and exercise, and when she has the urge to pass urine.

A Describe the important parts of the history to be taken.
B Describe the investigations required.
C Describe the first line of treatment.

ANSWERS

A Take a detailed history of urinary symptoms: frequency, nocturia, urgency and voiding difficulties. Enquire about the severity and find out how bothersome the symptoms are. As she has mixed incontinence, find out which component is more bothersome. Find out if she has other pelvic floor symptoms, such as pelvic organ prolapse and/or constipation or faecal incontinence. Take a standard gynaecological history including menstrual history. Note number and mode of deliveries. Note any abdominal or vaginal surgery. Find out if she has any medical conditions and what drugs she is taking.

B A midstream urine sample should be taken to check for infection. The patient should be asked to keep a 3-day bladder diary.

C Lifestyle interventions should be instituted. The first line of management is supervised PFMT and bladder retraining. If the midstream urine sample shows infection, antibiotics should be prescribed.

CASE HISTORY 2

A 74-year-old woman presents with symptoms of passing urine 14 times a day and four times at night and experiences incontinence associated with severe urge.

A Describe the important parts of the history to be taken.
B Describe the investigations required.
C Describe the best treatment.

ANSWERS

A Take a detailed history of urinary symptoms: frequency, nocturia, urgency, voiding difficulties and haematuria. Enquire about the severity and find out how bothersome the symptoms are. As she has mixed incontinence, find out which component is more bothersome. Find out if she has other pelvic floor symptoms, such as pelvic organ prolapse and/or constipation or faecal incontinence. Take a standard gynaecological history including menstrual history. Note number and mode of deliveries. Note any abdominal or vaginal surgery. Find out if she has any medical conditions such as gastrointestinal obstruction, intestinal atony, myasthenia gravis, paralytic ileus, pyloric stenosis, severe ulcerative colitis, significant bladder outflow obstruction, toxic megacolon or urinary retention, as these are contraindications to antimuscarinics used for OAB not responding to bladder retraining. A history of drug intake should be taken to ensure that the patient is not subjected to an anticholinergic load.

B A midstream urine sample should be taken to check for infection. The patient should be asked to keep a 3-day bladder diary.

C Lifestyle interventions should be instituted. The first line of management is bladder retraining. If the midstream urine sample shows infection, antibiotics should be prescribed.

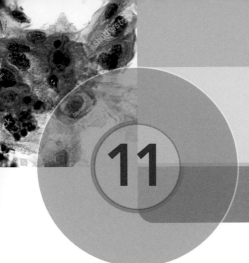

Benign conditions of the ovary and pelvis

11

T JUSTIN CLARK

Learning Objectives

- Describe the types of benign ovarian cysts and their symptoms, diagnosis and treatment.
- Describe the presentation and management of acute pelvic pain.
- Understand the pathology of endometriosis and recognize its involvement in chronic pelvic pain and subfertility.
- Understand how to diagnose and treat endometriosis.
- List potential causes of chronic pelvic pain.
- Appreciate the multifactorial nature of chronic pelvic pain and potential management options.

BENIGN DISEASES OF THE OVARY

Benign ovarian tumours are listed in **Table 11.1**. Most benign ovarian tumours will be diagnosed following investigation of women complaining of acute or chronic pelvic pain (CPP) or with the presence of an abdominal mass. Such tumours may also be found incidentally during a gynaecological examination or pelvic ultrasound scan (USS). The differential diagnosis of a pelvic mass includes tumours of adjacent structures (uterus, bladder and bowel) and pregnancy.

The presentation of different types of benign ovarian tumours varies with age. Functional cysts are common in young girls, adolescents and women in their reproductive years. Germ cell tumours occur more commonly in young women, whereas benign epithelial tumours are more prevalent in older and postmenopausal women.

BOX 11.1: The differential diagnosis of a pelvic mass

- *Gynaecological*: benign or malignant ovarian cyst, torsion, para-ovarian cyst, ectopic pregnancy, hydrosalpinx, pyosalpinx, tubo-ovarian abscess, tubal malignancy, pregnancy, fibroids, uterine malignancy
- *Gastrointestinal*: small or large bowel obstruction, diverticular/appendicular abscess, intussusception, malignancy
- *Urological*: hydronephrosis, pelvic kidney, renal/bladder malignancy
- *Other*: pelvic lymphocele, peritoneal cyst, psoas muscle abscess, lymphoma, neuroblastoma, aortic aneurism

10.1201/9781003218036-11

Table 11.1 Types of benign ovarian cysts

Type	Examples
Functional	Follicular cyst
	Corpus luteal cyst
	Theca luteal cyst
Inflammatory	Tubo-ovarian abscess
	Endometrioma
Germ cell	Benign teratoma (dermoid cyst)
Epithelial	Serous cystadenoma
	Mucinous cystadenoma
	Brenner tumour
Sex cord stromal	Fibroma
	Thecoma

Diagnosis may be made based on symptoms of pelvic discomfort or pressure on the bowel or bladder. Acute pain may represent torsion of a cyst, rupture or haemorrhage into it. Abdominal and bimanual pelvic examination may elicit a pelvic/abdominal mass that may be tender and will be separate from the uterus.

Table 11.2 Tumour markers used in the investigation and follow-up of ovarian cysts

Tumour marker	Ovarian tumour type	Uses
CA125	Epithelial ovarian cancer (serous), borderline ovarian tumours	Pre-operative, follow-up
CA19-9	Epithelial ovarian cancer (mucinous), borderline ovarian tumours	Pre-operative, follow-up
Inhibin	Granulosa cell tumours (type of sex cord stromal tumour)	Follow-up
Beta-hCG	Dysgerminoma, choriocarcinoma (germ cell tumours)	Pre-operative, follow-up
AFP	Endodermal yolk sac, immature teratoma (germ cell tumours)	Pre-operative, follow-up

AFP, alpha-fetoprotein; hCG, human chorionic gonadotrophin.

BOX 11.2: Ovarian torsion

- Torsion of an ovary refers to a situation in which there is rotation of the vascular pedicle supplying the ovary, which compresses and cuts its blood supply. Torsion is more likely with enlargement of the ovary as is seen in the presence of an ovarian cyst. Up to 15% of dermoid cysts present acutely with torsion.

- Presenting symptoms are usually acute onset of lower abdominal pain associated with nausea and vomiting. Pelvic USS with Doppler measurement of blood flow may be useful in the diagnosis to confirm the presence of a cyst and comment on blood flow to the ovary. Torsion of a normal ovary is very unlikely.

- Emergency surgical treatment to untwist the ovary and its attached pedicle is required to restore blood flow, and the ovarian cyst should then be removed. However, if this complication is not recognized within a few hours of presentation, infarction and gangrene may result, necessitating removal of the necrotic ovary. Decision-making to operate should be based on clinical findings, with transvaginal ultrasound scan (TVUSS) support.

The first-line investigation for women with a suspected pelvic mass or pelvic pain is an USS. A TVUSS has better resolution for pelvic masses. A transabdominal USS is indicated in women who have never been sexually active, or in combination with a TVUSS when large ovarian masses extending beyond the pelvis and into the abdomen are present. Additional imaging with computed tomography scanning or magnetic resonance imaging (MRI) can further characterize the nature of ovarian cysts, especially when they are thought to be potentially malignant. Serological tumour markers should also be measured to help determine the type of ovarian cyst and differentiate between a benign and a malignant neoplasm (**Table 11.2**; see also **Chapter 14**). A pregnancy test should be performed to exclude pregnancy. Inflammatory markers, such as C-reactive protein and white cell count, are important if the differential diagnosis includes appendicitis or a tubo-ovarian abscess.

FUNCTIONAL OVARIAN CYSTS

This group of ovarian cysts includes follicular, corpus luteal and theca luteal cysts. The risk of developing functional cysts is reduced by the use of the combined oral contraceptive pill (COCP). Little is known about their aetiology, but diagnosis is made when the cyst measures more than 3 cm (normal ovulatory follicles measure up to 2.5 cm). They rarely grow larger than 10 cm and appear as simple unilocular cysts on ultrasound (**Figure 11.1A**). Management depends on symptoms: if asymptomatic, the patient can be reassured and a repeat USS performed to check resolution or non-enlargement and thereafter the patient can be discharged; if

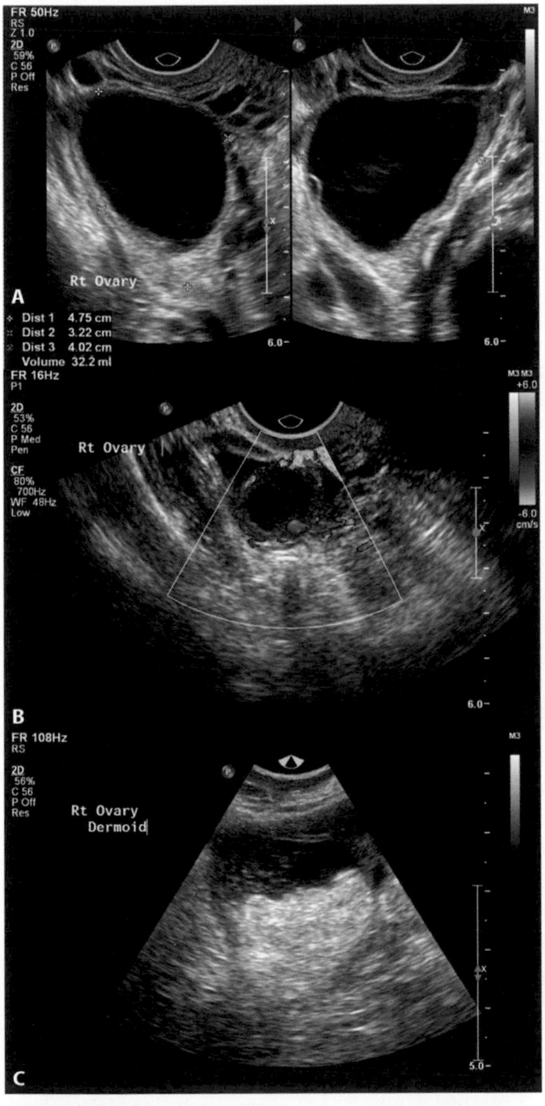

Figure 11.1 Transvaginal ultrasound scan. (**A**) Simple ovarian cyst. (**B**) Corpus luteal cyst. (**C**) Dermoid cyst.

symptomatic, the patient can be booked for laparoscopic cystectomy if necessary.

Corpus luteal cysts occur following ovulation and may present with pain due to rupture or haemorrhage, typically late in the menstrual cycle (**Figure 11.1B**). Treatment is expectant, with analgesia. Occasionally, surgery may be necessary if there has been significant bleeding to wash out the pelvis and perform an ovarian cystectomy.

Theca luteal cysts are associated with pregnancy, particularly multiple pregnancy, and are often diagnosed incidentally at routine ultrasound. They are often bilateral. Most resolve spontaneously during pregnancy.

INFLAMMATORY OVARIAN CYSTS

Inflammatory ovarian cysts are usually associated with pelvic inflammatory disease (PID) (see **Chapter 9**) and are most common in young women. The inflammatory mass may involve the fallopian tube, ovary and bowel and can be described on imaging as a mass or an abscess. Occasionally, the tubo-ovarian mass can develop from other infective causes, for example appendicitis or diverticular disease.

Diagnosis is similar to that for PID: inflammatory markers are helpful and initial treatment is with antibiotics and supportive measures such as fluid rehydration and the antipyretic paracetamol. Surgical drainage or excision is required if the patient remains unwell with malaise, pain and a continued pyrexia, which is typically a 'swinging pyrexia' – alternating between normal and elevated temperatures.

Patients may present with endometriomas, often known as 'chocolate cysts' due to the presence of altered blood within the ovary. They have a characteristic 'ground glass' appearance on USS. Further management of endometriosis is discussed in the section 'Endometriosis' later in this chapter.

GERM CELL TUMOURS

Germ cell tumours are the most common ovarian tumours in young women aged 20–40 years, accounting for more than 50% of ovarian tumours in this age group, with a peak incidence in those in their early 20s. The most common form of benign

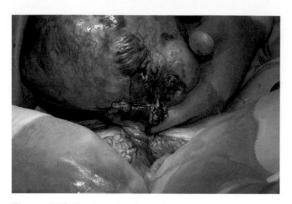

Figure 11.2 Torsion of a dermoid cyst at laparotomy.

germ cell tumour is the mature dermoid cyst (cystic teratoma), which contains fully differentiated tissue types derived from all three embryonic germ cell layers (mesenchymal, epithelial and stroma). Hair, teeth, fat, skin, muscle, cartilage, bone and endocrine tissue are frequently present. Up to 10% of dermoid cysts are bilateral. The risk of malignant transformation is rare (<2%), usually occurring in women over 40 years. Diagnosis is usually confirmed with a pelvic USS (**Figure 11.1C**) and, because of the high fat content in dermoid cysts, MRI may also be useful when there is uncertainty. In general, ovarian cystectomy is indicated because spontaneous resolution is unlikely. Surgery is indicated if the dermoid cyst is symptomatic (**Figure 11.2**), is more than 5 cm in diameter or is enlarging. Cystectomy will prevent ovarian torsion and provide tissue for histological analysis.

EPITHELIAL TUMOURS

Benign epithelial tumours increase in frequency with age and are most common in perimenopausal women. The most common epithelial tumours are serous cystadenomas, accounting for 20–30% of benign tumours in women under 40 years of age. Serous cystadenomas are typically unilocular and unilateral, whereas mucinous cystadenomas are large multiloculated cysts that are bilateral in 10% of cases.

Brenner tumours are small tumours often found incidentally within the ovary. They contain urothelial-like epithelium and may rarely secrete oestrogen.

SEX CORD STROMAL TUMOURS

Ovarian fibromas are the most common sex cord stromal tumours. They are solid ovarian tumours composed of stromal cells. They present in older women, often with torsion due to the heaviness of the ovary. Occasionally, patients may present with Meigs syndrome (pleural effusion, ascites and ovarian fibroma). Following removal of the ovarian fibroma, the pleural effusion will usually resolve.

Thecomas are benign oestrogen-secreting tumours. They often present after the menopause with manifestations of excess oestrogen production, usually postmenopausal bleeding. Although benign, they may induce an endometrial carcinoma.

OTHER OVARIAN CYSTS

Other non-ovarian cysts can occasionally present as ovarian tumours. Fimbrial cysts and paratubal cysts originate from the adjacent fallopian tube and broad ligament.

ENDOMETRIOSIS

Endometriosis is a common chronic inflammatory condition that is defined as endometrial tissue lying outside the uterine cavity. It is usually found within the pelvis, being commonly located on the peritoneum lining the pelvic side walls, pouch of Douglas, uterosacral ligaments and bladder. Three types of endometriosis are recognised: superficial, deep and endometriomas. Superficial endometriosis is found on the surface of pelvic structures. However, this 'ectopic' endometrial-like tissue can induce fibrosis and can be found infiltrating into deeper tissue such as the rectovaginal septum and bladder; this is known as deep endometriosis. When endometrial tissue is implanted into the ovary, an endometrioma forms. This cyst may be large and contains old, altered blood that has a thick brown appearance and, for this reason, is frequently referred to as a 'chocolate cyst'. Less commonly, endometriotic deposits can be found in other sites such as umbilicus, abdominal scars and the pleural cavity.

Endometriotic tissue responds to cyclical hormonal changes and therefore undergoes cyclical bleeding and local inflammatory reactions. These regularly repeated episodes of bleeding and healing lead to fibrosis and adhesion formation between pelvic organs, causing pain and infertility. In extreme cases, a 'frozen pelvis' results, where extensive adhesions tether the pelvic organs and obliterate normal pelvic anatomy.

Adenomyosis is a uterine condition often seen with endometriosis in which islands of endometrial tissue are found deep within the underlying myometrium (see **Chapter 12**).

INCIDENCE

Endometriosis occurs in approximately 10% of women of reproductive age and 10% of these will have deep endometriosis. The condition is found in at least one-third of women undergoing a diagnostic laparoscopy for pelvic pain or infertility. Endometriosis is oestrogen-dependent and therefore resolves after the menopause or when treatment induces a 'pseudomenopause' (i.e. suppression of ovarian oestradiol production).

AETIOLOGY

The aetiology of endometriosis is unknown, although there are several theories. There is unlikely to be a single explanation for its aetiology, but the two most commonly accepted theories are as follows.

1. *Sampson's implantation theory*: menstrual blood can be seen within the pelvis during laparoscopy at the time of menses. Sampson's implantation theory postulates that it is this retrograde menstrual regurgitation of viable endometrial glands and tissue along patent fallopian tubes, and subsequent implantation on the pelvic peritoneal surface, that causes endometriosis. Using animal/primate models, endometriosis has been induced with menstrual blood. Implantation of endometrium within human surgical scars after caesarean section or perineal repair following delivery lends support to this theory.

2. *Meyer's 'coelomic metaplasia' theory*: coelomic epithelium transformation describes the de-differentiation of peritoneal cells lining the Müllerian duct back to their primitive origin, which then transform into endometrial cells. This transformation into endometrial cells may be due to hormonal stimuli or inflammatory irritation.

GENETIC AND IMMUNOLOGICAL FACTORS

It has been suggested that genetic and immunological factors may alter the susceptibility of an individual and allow them to develop endometriosis. There appears to be an increased incidence in first-degree relatives of patients with the disorder. It is unclear if there are racial differences in the prevalance of endometriosis because of biases within studies investigating this area.

VASCULAR AND LYMPHATIC SPREAD

Vascular and lymphatic embolization to distant sites has been demonstrated and explains the rare findings of endometriosis in sites outside the peritoneal cavity, such as the lung.

CLINICAL FEATURES

Classical clinical features are severe cyclical pelvic pain around the time of menstruation, sometimes associated with heavy menstrual loss. Symptoms may begin a few days before the start of menses until the end of menses. However, patients often also complain of chronic non-cyclical pelvic pain and severe fatigue. It is well recognized that there is a lack of correlation between the extent of the disease and the intensity of symptoms.

Pelvic pain presenting with colicky pain throughout the menstrual cycle may be associated with irritable bowel syndrome symptoms. Deep pain with intercourse (deep dyspareunia) and on defaecation (dyschezia) are key indicators of the presence of endometriosis deep within the pouch of Douglas, otherwise known as rectovaginal endometriosis.

Table 11.3 Symptoms of endometriosis in relation to site of lesion

Site	Symptoms
Female reproductive tract	Cyclical pelvic pain (dysmenorrhoea) Non-cyclical pelvic pain Pain with intercourse (dyspareunia) Pain radiating to the lower back, legs and vagina Infertility
Urinary tract	Cyclical haematuria/dysuria Loin/flank pain (if ureteric obstruction)
Gastrointestinal tract	Dyschezia (pain on defaecation) Cyclical rectal bleeding Abdominal distension/colicky pain (obstruction)
Surgical scars/ umbilicus	Cyclical pain, swelling and bleeding
Thorax	Catamenial haemopneumothorax and haemoptysis Catamenial right upper abdominal or chest pain

Endometriosis can sometimes occur outside the pelvis, and the most common location is the thorax. Thoracic endometriosis represents a spectrum of disease, with endometriotic lesions being found on the diaphragm, pleural surfaces and/or lung parenchyma. The condition rarely occurs without pelvic disease. The other common extra-pelvic site where endometriosis is found is within scars after pelvic surgery, most commonly caesarean section, umbilical laparoscopic and appendix scars (**Table 11.3**).

DIAGNOSIS

PHYSICAL EXAMINATION

The accuracy of clinical examination in diagnosing endometriosis is limited and so the condition should be suspected even if vaginal examination is normal. Positive examination findings indicative of endometriosis include thickening or nodularity of the uterosacral ligaments, tenderness in the pouch of Douglas, an adnexal mass or a fixed retroverted uterus. However, pelvic tenderness alone is non-specific, and differential diagnoses for restricted mobility of the uterus include chronic PID and uterine, ovarian or cervical malignancy. In these conditions, other suggestive features are usually present, and imaging would rule out features of malignancy. In the presence of deep rectovaginal endometriosis, glandular and fibrotic endometrial lesions may be felt on digital bimanual examination and seen behind the cervix in the posterior vaginal fornix on speculum examination.

ULTRASOUND

TVUSS can detect endometriosis involving the ovaries (endometriomas or chocolate cysts) but its use in diagnosing smaller lesions is limited, although findings such as ovaries fixed together or to the back of the uterus (kissing ovaries) add strength to the diagnosis. In women with symptoms and signs of rectal endometriosis, TVUSS may be useful for identifying rectal disease, although again a negative scan does not exclude the disease.

MAGNETIC RESONANCE IMAGING

An MRI scan should be undertaken when deep endometriosis is suspected following clinical history taking and physical examination. This is because an MRI scan can detect lesions within deep tissues and organs, especially the rectovaginal septum and bowel. The information can allow careful pre-surgical planning.

LAPAROSCOPY

Visual diagnosis at laparoscopy remains the gold standard method of diagnosis. The endometriotic lesions can have a variety of appearances. They can appear as red glandular lesions; puckered, purple-black deposits; or white and fibrous (**Figure 11.3**). Often endometriotic deposits are surrounded by neovascularization. The advantage of laparoscopy is that it allows lesions to be biopsied for histological confirmation of diagnosis and it affords concurrent surgical diathermy ablation and/or excision of superficial endometriotic lesions. If deep endometriosis is seen, laparoscopy allows the assessment of the site and extent of the disease. This information – combined with radiological imaging, the clinical history and patient preferences – is important when planning further medical or surgical management.

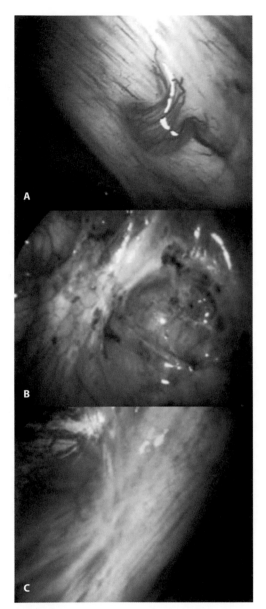

Figure 11.3 Laparoscopic view of endometriosis. (**A**) Red lesions on peritoneum. (**B**) Black 'matchstick' lesions. (**C**) White, fibrous lesion.

BIOMARKERS

There has been recent interest in the diagnosis of endometriosis using non-invasive biomarkers, such as CA125, and genetic biomarkers (e.g. looking for specific deoxyribonucleic acid [DNA] deletions), in plasma, urine or serum. However, to date, these non-invasive diagnostic approaches are too inaccurate for use in clinical practice. If accurate biomarkers can be developed, then unnecessary surgery can be avoided and tailored medical treatments can be initiated.

ENDOMETRIOSIS AND INFERTILITY

It is estimated that between 30% and 40% of patients with endometriosis complain of difficulty in conceiving. In many patients, there is a multifactorial pathogenesis to this subfertility (see **Chapter 7**). It is uncertain if and why minimal endometriotic deposits might render a patient subfertile. However, in the more severe stages of endometriosis, there is commonly anatomical distortion, with peri-adnexal adhesions and destruction of ovarian tissue when endometriomas develop.

From the balance of available evidence, medical treatment of endometriosis does not improve fertility and should not be given to patients wishing to conceive. However, surgical ablation/excision of minimal and mild endometriosis does improve fertility chances. It is uncertain whether surgical treatment of endometriomas increase spontaneous or in vitro fertilization (IVF) pregnancy rates, as the removal of the endometriomas must be balanced against damage to ovarian tissue. The consensus from fertility specialists at present is to leave endometriomas alone prior to IVF unless patients are symptomatic with pain or the endometrioma reduces access to the ovary for egg collection.

MANAGEMENT

Analgesics and hormonal ovarian suppression can be effective for treating cyclical and non-cyclical pelvic pain associated with endometriosis. Medical treatment of presumed endometriosis can be started if the clinical examination and TVUSS are normal, without the need for more invasive laparoscopy. However, if no symptom relief is obtained after 3–6 months of treatment, a laparoscopy should be considered. Patients with endometriosis are often difficult to treat, not only from a physical point of view, but also often because of associated psychological issues associated with their pain. Long-term therapeutic strategies should be formulated where possible. Coexisting additional diseases such as irritable bowel syndrome and constipation (present in up to

80% of cases) should also be treated to improve over-all success rates. Endometriosis is known to recur throughout reproductive life and it is impossible to guarantee complete cure. Treatment should there-fore be tailored for the individual according to their age and symptoms, the extent of the disease and the patient's desire to have children. In most women with superficial endometriosis, there is little pro-gression of their disease over time, and this may be reassuring. Owing to the variation in presentation, it has been shown that there is a significant delay to diagnosis – with research indicating around 7 years, on average – and some patients will be relieved by a positive laparoscopy that validates their symptoms.

MEDICAL THERAPY

Analgesics

Non-steroidal anti-inflammatory drugs (NSAIDs) are potent analgesics and are helpful in reducing the severity of dysmenorrhoea and pelvic pain. However, they have no specific impact on the disease and hence their use is for symptom control only. The additional use of codeine/opiates should be avoided if possible, as the coexisting irritable bowel symptoms can be worsened, exacerbating pelvic pain symptoms.

Combined oral contraceptives

In the absence of contraindications (see **Chapter 6**) or desire for pregnancy, the COCP should be considered because it has been shown to reduce endometriosis-associated dyspareunia, dysmenorrhoea and non-menstrual pain, as well as to provide cycle control and contraception. The COCP can be taken sequentially with the usual 7-day pill-free break, but may be more effective in alleviating pain symptoms, especially cyclical dysmenorrhoea, if it is tricycled (whereby three packets are taken back-to-back) or taken contin-uously without a break, inducing amenorrhoea. If the COCP achieves symptomatic relief, then this therapy can be continued for several years until pregnancy is intended. If symptoms persist, the diagnosis should be reviewed and common coexisting conditions such as irritable bowel disease and constipation treated (e.g. encouraging a high-fibre diet and adequate fluid intake). Alternative medical or surgical treatments should be discussed (see the following sections).

Progestogens

In those for whom there are risk factors for the use of a COCP, progestogens should be used to induce amenorrhoea. The long-acting reversible contra-ceptives depot medroxyprogesterone acetate and the levonorgestrel intrauterine system (LNG-IUS) (Mirena®) are useful in providing a long-term thera-peutic effect, particularly after surgical treatment. The effect is probably related to 100% compliance with treatment.

Gonadotrophin-releasing hormone agonists

Gonadotrophin-releasing hormone (GnRH) agonists are effective in relieving the severity and symptoms of endometriosis (see **Chapter 4** for a discussion of GnRH). Despite their side effects, the drugs are well tolerated by some and they have become established agents in the diagnosis (if CPP is of a gynaecological origin (e.g. endometriosis), then symptoms will be eradicated) and treatment of endometriosis. They are available as multiple, daily administered intranasal sprays, but are usually administered as slow-release depot formulations injected subcutaneously, each lasting for 1 month or more. Long-term use over 6 months is precluded because of drug-induced osteo-porosis. The recurrence of symptoms on cessation of therapy is usually rapid.

Other hormonal agents

There has been some interest in a newer class of drug called aromatase inhibitors; these inhibit the action of the enzyme aromatase, which converts androgens into oestrogens and is over expressed in endometri-otic tissue. Further research is ongoing for their use in refractory cases.

SURGICAL TREATMENT

Fertility-sparing surgery

Most surgery for endometriosis can be achieved laparoscopically. Symptomatic endometriotic choco-late cysts should not just be drained but the inner cyst lining should be excised or ablated to reduce the risk of recurrence; however, this will be associated with damage to functional ovarian tissue. Therefore, when drainage is performed as an adjunct to fertility treatment, drainage only may be considered. Deposits of superficial peritoneal endometriosis can be easily ablated or excised during laparoscopy using diathermy or laser energy.

Surgery in specialist endometriosis centres is needed to treat deep endometriosis in which the disease has caused extensive adhesions distorting normal pelvic anatomy or has involved other organs such as the rectum, large bowel or bladder, or when there are rectovaginal nodules of disease. This is because such surgery, while effective, can be associated with serious complications such as bowel and urinary tract injury.

The recurrence of pain symptoms following conservative surgery is as high as 30% and, therefore, concurrent long-term medical therapy is often necessary and may be started immediately after surgery.

Hysterectomy and oophorectomy

Hysterectomy with removal of the ovaries and all visible endometriosis lesions should be considered only in women who have completed their family and have failed to respond to more conservative treatments. Patients should be informed that hysterectomy with removal of the ovaries may not necessarily cure all endometriosis-related symptoms. Oestrogen-only hormone replacement therapy (HRT) will be required to offset menopausal symptoms. Occasionally, this hormone can reactivate residual endometriosis and so a combined

oestrogen- and progesterone-containing HRT can be used, because progesterone will inactivate endometrial glands and stroma.

CHRONIC PELVIC PAIN

CPP is a debilitating symptom among women, which has a major impact on health-related quality of life, work productivity and health care utilization. The Royal College of Obstetricians and Gynaecologists (RCOG) has defined CPP as 'intermittent or constant pain in the lower abdomen or pelvis of a woman of at least 6 months in duration, not occurring exclusively with menstruation (dysmenorrhoea) or intercourse and not associated with pregnancy'.

INCIDENCE

CPP presents in primary care as frequently as migraine, asthma or low back pain and accounts for 20% of all outpatient appointments in gynaecological secondary care. Estimates of prevalence vary widely but are thought to be between 10% and 20%.

AETIOLOGY

The potential causes of CPP are listed in **Table 11.4**. In contrast with acute pelvic pain, there is often more than one underlying cause contributing to CPP. The

Table 11.4 Causes of chronic pelvic pain

Type	Causes
Gynaecological	Endometriosis and adenomyosis* Adhesions including chronic PID* Uterine fibroids Ovarian cysts
Central and peripheral nervous system	Changes in both afferent and efferent nerve pathways in the central and peripheral nervous systems modifying pain perception (e.g. visceral hyperalgesia and neuropathic pain)
Gastrointestinal	Irritable bowel syndrome* (a functional bowel disorder characterized by the presence of a cluster of symptoms and signs that include cramping, abdominal pain, increased gas, altered bowel habits, food intolerance and bloating) Constipation Inflammatory bowel disease Coeliac disease (gluten sensitivity)

(Contd.)

(Contd.)

Type	Causes
Urological	Bladder pain syndrome (previously known as interstitial cystitis, consisting of pain, pressure or discomfort related to the bladder along with at least one other urinary symptom (e.g. urgency or frequency) in the absence of any other pathology) Recurrent urinary tract infections Urinary tract calculi
Musculoskeletal	Pain arising from the joints in the pelvis or from damage to the muscles in the abdominal wall or pelvic floor (e.g. degenerative joint disease, spondylolisthesis)
Nerve entrapment	Nerve entrapment within scar tissue, fascia or a narrow foramen may result in pain and dysfunction in the distribution of that nerve, which is highly localized and exacerbated by particular movements
Psychological and social issues	Depression, anxiety and sleep disorders are common in women with chronic pain and may be a consequence, rather than a cause, of pain Physical and sexual abuse

* Most commonly encountered.
PID, pelvic inflammatory disease.

experience of pain is affected by physical, psychological and social factors.

DIAGNOSIS

A thorough history should include questions about the pattern of the pain and its association with other problems, such as psychological, bladder and bowel symptoms, and the effect of movement and posture on the pain. An abdominal and pelvic examination should look for areas of tenderness and pelvic

masses, as well as distortion, tethering or prolapse of pelvic organs.

INVESTIGATIONS

The investigations that should be considered when evaluating patients with CPP are shown in **Table 11.5**. Findings from the history and examination will dictate the need for further testing; CPP refractory to medical treatment or associated with abnormal examination findings – such as enlargement, tenderness, irregularity

Table 11.5 Common investigations for chronic pelvic pain

Investigation	Indication	Potential diagnoses
Genital tract swabs	All sexually active women should be offered screening for STIs such as *Chlamydia trachomatis* or gonococcus	Pelvic infection/PID
Pelvic USS	Suspected pelvic masses	Adnexal masses – ovarian cysts including endometriomas, hydrosalpinges and tubo-ovarian abscesses Uterine pathology – adenomyosis, fibroids
MRI	Further assessment of pelvic masses or suspected deep infiltrating endometriosis	Further characterize masses seen on USS Deep rectovaginal/bowel endometriosis
Laparoscopy	When pelvic masses, endometriosis or adhesions are suspected	Superficial and deep endometriosis Abdominopelvic adhesions Pelvic masses

MRI, magnetic resonance imaging; PID, pelvic inflammatory disease; STI, sexually transmitted infection; USS, ultrasound scan.

or fixity of pelvic structures – would indicate the need for further investigation. TVUSS is the least invasive and first-line method of imaging the pelvis. Diagnostic laparoscopy is the most invasive test for evaluating the female pelvis and has been regarded as the 'gold standard' investigation for CPP. However, depending on the preceding clinical evaluation, 40% of diagnostic laparoscopies fail to show any cause for the CPP symptoms. Structural pathologies identified at laparoscopy can often be surgically treated at the same time.

MANAGEMENT

The multifactorial nature of CPP should be discussed and explored with the patient from the start. General health advice, including the importance of diet, hydration, exercise and sexual health, should be given. Analgesia such as NSAIDs, opiates and paracetamol to control pain should be discussed.

When clinical examination and USS are normal, patients with cyclical CPP should be offered a therapeutic trial using hormonal treatment to suppress ovarian function for a period of 3–6 months before having a diagnostic laparoscopy. Hormonal treatments include the COCP, systemic and local (LNG-IUS) progestogens, and GnRH analogues. Structural pathologies can be treated surgically, usually via laparoscopy, including the removal of adnexal masses, the treatment of endometriosis and adhesiolysis.

If the nature of the CPP is thought to be primarily non-gynaecological, then referral to the relevant healthcare professional, such as a gastroenterologist, urologist, genitourinary medicine physician, physiotherapist, psychologist or psychosexual counsellor, should be made. If, despite the above interventions, pain is not adequately controlled, referral to a pain management team or a specialist, multidisciplinary pelvic pain clinic should be considered.

⊙ KEY LEARNING POINTS

- Commonly encountered benign ovarian tumours include functional cysts, teratomas (dermoid cysts) and endometriomas.
- Ovarian cysts can be asymptomatic or can be present with pain or as an abdominal mass. Acute pain may arise because of an ovarian cyst 'accident' such as haemorrhage, rupture or torsion.
- TVUSS is the primary test used to diagnose different types of ovarian cyst. Along with the CA125 serological tumour marker, ultrasound can be used to help differentiate between benign and malignant ovarian tumours.
- Treatment is based on the symptoms and the size and type of cyst. Ovarian cystectomy or even oophorectomy may be required, and this is usually undertaken using a laparoscopic approach.
- Endometriosis refers to the finding of endometrial glands and stroma outside the uterus and is one of the most common conditions seen in gynaecology, affecting 5–10% of women of reproductive age.
- Endometriosis usually presents with cyclical pelvic pain around the time of menstruation and is sometimes associated with heavy menstrual loss. However, affected women may also complain of chronic non-cyclical pelvic pain, dyspareunia, dyschezia and severe fatigue.

- There are three types of endometriosis: superficial endometriosis (most common), deep endometriosis and ovarian endometriomas.
- Endometriosis is associated with tubal and ovarian damage and the formation of adhesions and can compromise fertility.
- Medical treatment of endometriosis involves suppressing oestrogen levels to induce amenorrhoea using the COCP, progestogens or GnRH agonists.
- Conservative laparoscopic surgical treatment of endometriosis involves excising or ablating visible lesions. More radical excisional laparoscopic surgery may be required for deep endometriosis involving the bowel and rectovaginal septum. Total hysterectomy and bilateral salpingo-oophorectomy is often undertaken for refractory symptoms.
- CPP is usually multifactorial involving physical, psychological and social factors. Management should be directed at the underlying causes and include general health advice, analgesics, hormonal therapies and surgery. Multidisciplinary pelvic pain clinics are necessary to manage severe, refractory cases.

FURTHER READING

European Society of Human Reproduction and Embryology (ESHRE) Endometriosis Guideline Development Group (2022). *Endometriosis. Guideline of European Society of Human Reproduction and Embryology*. https://www. eshre.eu/Guidelines-and-Legal/Guidelines/ Endometriosis-guideline. (*Note, in particular, the flow diagrams at the end of the document.*)

National Institute for Health and Care Excellence (NICE) (2017). *Endometriosis: Diagnosis and Management*. NICE guideline [NG73]. http://www. nice.org.uk/guidance/ng73. (*Note, in particular, the endometriosis algorithm on pages 17–18.*)

NICE Clinical Knowledge Summaries (2020). Scenario: Management of endometriosis. https://cks.nice.org.uk/topics/endometriosis/ management/management-of-endometriosis/.

RCOG (2012). Green-top guideline No. 41: The initial management of chronic pelvic pain. https://www.pelvicpain.org.uk/wp-content/uploads/2018/03/CPP_RCOG-Initial-management-CPP.2ndEdition230512-1.pdf.

RCOG (2016). Green-top guideline No. 34: Ovarian cysts in postmenopausal women. https://www. rcog.org.uk/en/guidelines-research-services/ guidelines/gtg34/.

SELF-ASSESSMENT

For interactive SBAs and EMQs relating to this chapter, visit www.routledge.com/cw/crosbie.

CASE HISTORY 1

A 26-year-old law student presents with a 2-year history of CPP. She admits to a poor diet but is otherwise fit and healthy. She contracted genital chlamydial infection from a previous relationship 3 years ago, but is currently in a new and stable relationship. A urinary pregnancy test has been performed and the result is negative.

A What questions would you ask about the presenting complaint?

B What features of the history would suggest a gynaecological cause for the pain?

C What features from a bimanual pelvic examination would suggest a gynaecological cause for the pain?

D List likely gynaecological causes of CPP.

E List likely non-gynaecological causes of CPP.

F Suggest diagnostic tests that you would perform.

G How might you manage this patient?

ANSWERS

A Establish the nature of the pain, such as by using SOCRATES – site, onset (e.g. relationship to chlamydial infection), character, radiation (gynaecological pain may be bilateral and into the back, groin and vagina), associations, time course (especially relationship to the menstrual cycle), exacerbating/relieving factors (e.g. sexual intercourse,

voiding and defaecation), severity (e.g. effect on activities of daily living, use of analgesics, etc.).

B Onset or exacerbation in relation to the menstrual cycle along with deep dyspareunia is suggestive of a gynaecological origin for the pain, although CPP is often multifactorial.

C The presence of a pelvic mass may suggest the presence of an adnexal mass (e.g. ovarian cyst, hydrosalpinx) or enlarged uterus (e.g. fibroids, adenomyosis). Tenderness, fixed, immobile pelvic organs (suggestive of adhesions secondary to endometriosis or infection) and nodularity of the uterosacral ligaments (indicative of deep endometriosis) are other features to assess.

D Chronic PID causing adhesions and/or a chronic tubo-ovarian abscess should be considered given the history of a sexually transmitted infection. Endometriosis is common in women of reproductive age and usually presents in the second or third decade. An ovarian cyst should form part of the differential diagnosis.

E Gastrointestinal causes such as irritable bowel syndrome or constipation should be considered in the light of her poor diet. A negative pregnancy test excludes an ectopic pregnancy. Genitourinary problems such as bladder pain syndrome, musculoskeletal causes, neuropathic pain and psychological contributors should be evaluated depending on the history and examination.

F Genital tract swabs and a midstream urine specimen (if there are symptoms) should be taken. First-line imaging should be a pelvic USS in order to identify uterine and adnexal masses. Laparoscopy should be undertaken to detect adhesions and endometriosis if the pain is resistant to medical treatment or the gynaecological examination is abnormal.

G Management depends on the cause. The patient should be given general health advice, analgesics and hormonal treatments (e.g. the COCP or systemic and local [LNG-IUS] progestogens) to suppress ovulation for at least 3–6 months assuming a likely gynaecological origin for the chronic pain and the absence of an adnexal mass requiring surgical removal. Laparoscopic surgery should be considered in the presence of adhesions (adhesiolysis), endometriosis (excision or ablation of endometriotic deposits) or adnexal pathology (removal of adnexal masses [e.g. ovarian cystectomy]).

CASE HISTORY 2

A fit and well 26-year-old woman complains of CPP and deep pain with sex. She also reports pain and bleeding on opening her bowels during her period. She is using condoms for contraception but would like to try for a pregnancy in 2 years' time.

A What diagnosis do you suspect from this history?

B What would you expect to find on pelvic examination?

C What investigations would you arrange?

D Is medical treatment indicated and if so what?

E What non-hormonal and non-surgical treatments would you consider?

F Is radical surgical treatment indicated?

G Does surgery usually prevent the need for ongoing medical treatments?

ANSWERS

A Deep endometriosis affecting the rectovaginal septum is the most likely diagnosis because she complains of deep pain with sex and cyclical pain and bleeding on opening her bowels – symptoms that suggest active endometriotic disease infiltrating the posterior vaginal fornix and rectum. Rectal bleeding can occur for a variety of gastrointestinal reasons, but such causes are not usually cyclical and may not be associated with pain on evacuation or with sexual intercourse.

B A vaginal speculum examination may reveal red/ purple visible deposits of endometriosis typically in the posterior vaginal fornix (i.e. behind the cervix). On bimanual palpation, these deposits can be easily felt as firm, irregular lesions. Nodules of endometriosis may be felt over the uterosacral ligaments, and the uterus/ovaries are often fixed and immobile, suggesting dense associated adhesions.

Pelvic tenderness is usually elicited during examination.

C A pelvic USS (transabdominal and transvaginal) is the first-line imaging test for most women presenting with pelvic pain. However, if deep endometriosis is detected or suspected on clinical history and examination, then MRI is a better imaging modality because it can provide information about the location and degree of infiltration of deep endometriotic lesions in the vagina, rectum and elsewhere in the large bowel. This information is important for planning potential surgical excision. With higher resolution USS and better training of practitioners, TVUSS is increasingly being used for evaluating deep endometriosis, but, currently, MRI is more widely used. A preliminary diagnostic laparoscopy to 'stage' is often undertaken in addition to imaging to better understand the extent of the endometriosis and to plan future excisional surgery.

D Yes, medical treatment is indicated. In general, women of reproductive age with pelvic pain are initially managed medically unless there are abnormal findings on clinical examination requiring a laparoscopy or abnormalities seen on a pelvic USS (e.g. a significant ovarian cyst requiring surgical removal). In this case, deep endometriosis has been detected clinically and is likely to be confirmed on MRI. Conventional medical treatments used for treating superficial endometriosis and CPP can be effective in the presence of symptomatic deep endometriosis and are less invasive and are associated with fewer side effects/risks than laparoscopic surgery. Medical treatments include analgesics, especially NSAIDs and paracetamol, which do not induce constipation. However, many women with severe disease have significantly

(Contd.)

(Contd.)

impaired quality of life and require stronger opiate analgesia. Hormonal contraceptives should be used first line unless desirous of pregnancy (which is not the case here) or if this has previously been tried and failed, in which case treatment should be escalated to the use of GnRH analogues with add-back HRT for refractory cases. Neuromodulators such as amitriptyline and gabapentin can also be considered.

E Some women find interventions such as physiotherapy, acupuncture, mindfulness, transcutaneous electrical nerve stimulation (TENS) machines and psychological therapy (e.g. cognitive behavioural therapy) to be useful in managing their symptoms.

F Yes, radical surgical treatment is indicated if the patient does not want medical treatment.

We know that laparoscopic surgery performed in specialist centres is efficacious but can be associated with serious complications such as bowel and urinary tract injury. Patients need to be thoroughly counselled about the relative risks and benefits before undergoing surgery. This complex laparoscopic surgery needs to be undertaken in specialist surgical centres and often the gynaecological surgeon operates in tandem with a colorectal surgeon.

G No, surgery does not usually prevent the need for ongoing medical treatments. While this is the aim of surgery, in reality, many women, while deriving significant symptomatic relief, still require medical treatments such as analgesics and hormonal contraceptives due to ongoing pain or recurrence of pain.

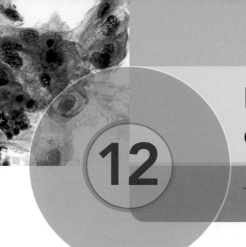

12

Benign conditions of the uterus, cervix and endometrium

T JUSTIN CLARK

Learning Objectives
- Describe the common benign conditions that affect the uterus according to their tissue of origin: the cervix, the endometrium and the myometrium.
- Understand the presenting symptoms and examination findings associated with benign uterine pathology.
- Describe the common tests used to evaluate the uterus and endometrial cavity.
- Explain the available treatment options for uterine fibroids and adenomyosis and the rationale for selection.

UTERINE CERVIX

The cervix is the cylindrical lower extremity of the uterus and consists mainly of collagen fibres. The vaginal part of the cervix, called the ectocervix, is lined with thick non-keratinized stratified squamous epithelium and has a pink appearance. The external os is visible in the centre of the ectocervix as a dark circular or slit-like area and is the opening to the endocervical canal, which is lined by simple columnar epithelium. There is a clear demarcation of this transformation between the two types of epithelium, called the squamocolumnar junction. This anatomical junction fluctuates under hormonal influence as described further in **Chapters 1** and **16**. Benign lesions can occur on the surface or within the cervix.

BENIGN CERVICAL SURFACE LESIONS

CERVICAL ECTROPION

In women of reproductive age, the columnar epithelium is visible on the ectocervix as a circular, red area surrounding the external cervical os (**Figure 12.1A**). This is a normal finding and should not be called 'cervical erosion', because this erroneously implies that it is an ulcer. An ectropion or 'ectopy' commonly develops under the influence of the 'three Ps': puberty, pill and pregnancy. The fragile, glandular columnar epithelium of a large cervical ectropion may predispose to intermenstrual bleeding (IMB) and post-coital bleeding (PCB). Some

10.1201/9781003218036-12

women may present with an excessive, clear, odourless, mucus-type discharge. To reduce the ectropion and associated symptoms, affected individuals should be changed from oestrogen-based hormonal contraceptives. The other option is cervical ablation, whereby the visible glandular producing columnar cells are ablated, usually with cryocautery, as an outpatient treatment. Prior to treatment, endocervical and lower genital tract swabs are taken to exclude chlamydia and other sexually transmitted infections, and normal cervical cytology should be confirmed to exclude cervical premalignancy and malignancy (see **Chapter 16**).

NABOTHIAN FOLLICLES

Sometimes the columnar glands within the transformation zone become sealed over, forming small, mucus-filled cysts visible on the ectocervix. These are termed Nabothian follicles and are of no pathological significance. No treatment is usually required, although extremely large ones can be drained using a large-bore needle (**Figure 12.1B**).

CERVICAL POLYPS

Cervical polyps are benign tumours arising from the endocervical epithelium and may be seen as smooth, reddish protrusions. They are usually asymptomatic, being identified incidentally during a routine cervical smear, but as with a cervical ectropion they can cause vaginal discharge, IMB and PCB. They are easily removed by avulsion with polyp forceps as an outpatient treatment.

CERVICAL STENOSIS

Cervical stenosis refers to pathological narrowing of the endocervical canal and is usually an iatrogenic phenomenon caused by a surgical event. Treatment of premalignant disease of the cervix using a cone biopsy or loop diathermy can cause cervical stenosis, as can endometrial ablation affecting the cervical canal. The ensuing trapped blood in the uterus (haematometra) causes cyclical dysmenorrhoea with no associated menstrual bleeding. Treatment is by surgical dilatation of the cervix under ultrasound or hysteroscopic guidance.

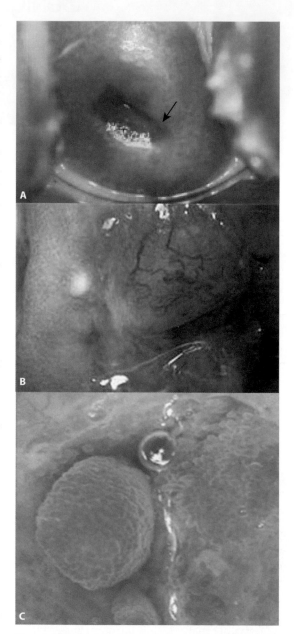

Figure 12.1 Benign changes in the cervix. (**A**) Cervical ectropion. (**B**) Nabothian follicle. (**C**) Cervical polyp.

BENIGN ENDOMETRIAL LESIONS

ENDOMETRIAL POLYPS

Endometrial polyps are focal endometrial outgrowths containing a variable number of glands, stroma and blood vessels, which influence their macroscopic appearance. Endometrial polyps may be asymptomatic but can cause abnormal uterine bleeding (AUB) (i.e. heavy menstrual bleeding [HMB], IMB or postmenopausal bleeding [PMB]) and can have an adverse impact on fertility. They are common and estimated to be present in around 10–20% of patients with AUB and 10% of patients with subfertility. Risk factors for endometrial polyp development include obesity, late menopause, the use of the partial oestrogen agonist tamoxifen and possibly the use of hormone replacement therapy (HRT). Most polyps do not appear to be subject to the normal cellular mechanisms that regulate the endometrium. Consequently, they are relatively insensitive to cyclical hormonal changes, leading them to persist and cause unscheduled vaginal bleeding. Endometrial polyps contain hyperplastic foci in 10–25% of symptomatic cases and 1% are frankly malignant. The risk of polyps harbouring serious endometrial disease is increased after the menopause and with the use of tamoxifen. Endometrial polyps may be pedunculated or sessile, single or multiple, and vary in size (0.5–4 cm).

Endometrial polyps can be diagnosed by transvaginal ultrasound scan (TVUSS) but, because they have focal, intracavity pathologies, the most accurate tests are outpatient hysteroscopy and saline infusion sonography (SIS), because these investigations involve distending the uterine cavity with fluid, thereby aiding detection (**Figure 12.2**). Smaller endometrial polyps can spontaneously resolve but most persist such that, once diagnosed, removal is

indicated (polypectomy) to alleviate AUB symptoms, optimize fertility and exclude hyperplasia or cancer. Polypectomy is a simple procedure that can be performed as day-case surgery under general anaesthesia, but is now increasingly performed as an outpatient treatment with or without local anaesthesia. A hysteroscope is used to visualize the polyp(s) and to allow miniature instruments to be passed down its operating channel in order to remove the polyp with scissors, electrodes or mechanical hysteroscopic tissue resection systems.

ASHERMAN SYNDROME

Irreversible damage to the single layer thick basal endometrium does not allow normal regeneration of the endometrium. The endometrial cavity undergoes fibrosis and adhesion formation, termed Asherman syndrome. The result is reduced, or absent, menstrual shedding and subfertility. This usually occurs after pregnancy when there has been uterine infection (endometritis) or following overzealous curettage of the uterine cavity during surgical management of miscarriage or following secondary post-partum haemorrhage. In this 'soft' uterine state, the myometrium (including the basal layer) can be inadvertently excavated while attempting to evacuate these retained products of conception using metal instruments or suction cannulae. Prevention of uterine scarring by adopting expectant, medical or less traumatic surgical approaches to managing retained products of conception and preventing endometritis is important, given its adverse impact on fertility. To treat Asherman syndrome, hysteroscopic surgical techniques are needed to manually break down the intrauterine adhesions (adhesiolysis). However, treatment can be difficult and risks further uterine trauma.

Surgical treatments to deliberately destroy the basal layer have been developed for the treatment of HMB, called endometrial ablation (see **Chapter 4**).

BENIGN LESIONS OF THE MYOMETRIUM

Uterine fibroids and adenomyosis are the two most prevalent conditions affecting the myometrium.

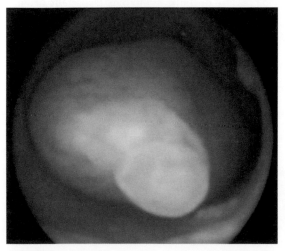

Figure 12.2 A hysteroscopic view of an endometrial polyp.

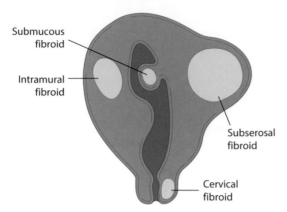

Submucous fibroid

Intramural fibroid

Subserosal fibroid

Cervical fibroid

Figure 12.3 Diagram showing the typical sites of uterine fibroids.

FIBROIDS

CLASSIFICATION

A fibroid is a benign tumour of uterine smooth muscle termed a leiomyoma. The gross appearance is of a well-demarcated, firm, whorled tumour. Such fibroids are highly prevalent, being found in approximately 40% of women overall, and are more common in those who are nulliparous, obese, have a family history or are of African descent. They are usually multiple and can substantially increase the size of the uterus. Fibroids are classified according to their location in relation to the uterine wall (**Figure 12.3**).

BOX 12.1: Symptoms caused by fibroids

Most fibroids are small and asymptomatic, but they can be associated with the following conditions:

- AUB (usually HMB and IMB)
- Reproductive failure
- Subfertility
- Recurrent pregnancy loss
- Bulk effects on adjacent structures in the pelvis
- Pressure and pain
- Bladder and bowel dysfunction
- Abdominal distension

NATURAL HISTORY

Fibroids are benign, oestrogen-dependent tumours that can enlarge during pregnancy in response to the hyperoestrogenic state, become common with advancing reproductive age and shrink after the menopause when ovarian oestrogen production ceases. They can undergo degenerative change, usually in response to outgrowing their blood supply. Three forms of degeneration are recognized:

1. *Red* – haemorrhage and necrosis occurs within the fibroid, typically presenting in the second trimester of pregnancy with acute pain
2. *Hyaline* – asymptomatic softening and liquefaction of the fibroid
3. *Cystic* – asymptomatic central necrosis leaving cystic spaces at the centre.

Degenerative changes can initiate calcium deposition leading to calcification. Rarely, malignant or sarcomatous degeneration can occur but the incidence of this is 1 in 350 cases or less. The suspicion is greatest in the postmenopausal period when a fibroid rapidly increases in size, is seen to be highly vascular or associated with PMB.

CLINICAL FEATURES

Fibroids can cause several gynaecological complaints and are one of the most common indications for hysterectomy. However, the vast majority of fibroids are asymptomatic. Abdominal examination might indicate the presence of a firm mass arising from the pelvis. Unless fibroids cause symptoms, they do not require any treatment. Common presenting symptoms include menstrual disturbance and pelvic pressure or 'bulk' symptoms (especially urinary frequency) and infertility. Pain is unusual, except in the special circumstance of acute red degeneration or torsion of a pedunculated fibroid (**Figure 12.4**).

Subfertility may result from mechanical distortion or occlusion of the fallopian tubes, and an endometrial cavity grossly distorted by submucous fibroids may prevent implantation of a fertilized ovum. Removal of submucosal fibroids may enhance fertility and outcomes with assisted reproductive techniques such as in vitro fertilization (IVF). However, the effectiveness of surgically removing the other types of fibroids is less clear and risks hysterectomy in 1% of cases because of significant intraoperative bleeding. Thus, these fibroids should be removed only if symptomatic and when there is proven, otherwise unexplained infertility. Once a pregnancy is established, however, the risk

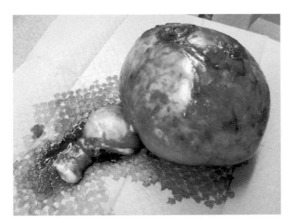

Figure 12.4 Pedunculated, subserosal fibroid on a hysterectomy specimen.

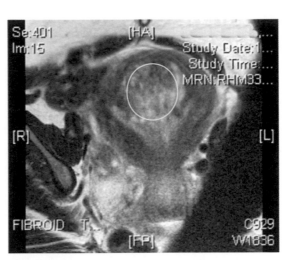

Figure 12.5 Magnetic resonance imaging of an enlarged fibroid uterus.

of miscarriage does not appear to be increased. In late pregnancy, fibroids located in the cervix or lower uterine segment may cause an abnormal fetal lie. After delivery, post-partum haemorrhage may occur due to inefficient uterine contraction.

Magnetic resonance imaging (MRI) is occasionally used to demarcate the morphology, size and location of uterine fibroids prior to radiological or surgical intervention (**Figure 12.5**).

BOX 12.2: Examination findings suggestive of uterine fibroids

- *General*: signs of anaemia
- *Abdominal examination*: visible and/or palpable abdominal mass arising from the pelvis
- *Bimanual examination*: enlarged, firm, smooth or irregular, non-tender uterus palpable (tenderness may suggest red degeneration)

DIAGNOSIS

Often, the clinical features obtained from the history and examination alone will be sufficient to establish the diagnosis. A full blood count should be taken in patients with HMB; severe anaemia associated with HMB invariably indicates the presence of significant fibroids.

Abdomino-pelvic ultrasound (transabdominal ultrasound scan and TVUSS) is the mainstay of diagnosis and helps delineate the origin of a clinically detected pelvic mass (i.e. distinguishing between a uterine fibroid and an ovarian tumour, and locating the position and size of fibroids). In the presence of large fibroids, ultrasonography is also helpful to exclude hydronephrosis from pressure on the ureters.

BOX 12.3: Useful tests where uterine fibroids are suspected

- *TVUSS*: good for detecting and locating submucous fibroids and small intramural fibroids
- *Transabdominal ultrasound scan*: good for detecting larger intramural and subserosal fibroids and excluding hydronephrosis secondary to pressure from fibroids obstructing the ureters
- *SIS*: good for detecting and locating submucosal fibroids and endometrial polyps.
- *Hysteroscopy*:
  - good for detecting submucosal fibroids and endometrial polyps
  - good for planning subsequent hysteroscopic surgical treatment
  - operative hysteroscopy can remove polyps, adhesions and submucosal fibroids
- *MRI*:
  - good for describing the morphology and location of fibroids
  - indicated prior to uterine artery embolization and to monitor treatment response

TREATMENT

Medical treatment

Conservative management is appropriate when asymptomatic fibroids are detected incidentally. The main types of medical treatment for HMB (see **Chapter 4**) – namely the levonorgestrel intrauterine system (LNG-IUS), tranexamic acid, mefenamic acid and the combined oral contraceptive pill (COCP) – tend to be less effective in the presence of a submucous fibroid or any fibroid(s) more than 3 cm in size, which equates to an enlarged uterus that is palpable abdominally (>12 weeks' size). The only effective medical treatment is to use injectable gonadotrophin-releasing hormone (GnRH) agonists, which induce a menopausal state by shutting down ovarian oestradiol production. This leads to a reduction in the size of fibroids (they are oestrogen-dependent benign tumours) and amenorrhoea. However, GnRH treatment is not tolerated by all patients because of severe menopausal symptoms. Add-back HRT is required for longer-term use to abate menopausal symptoms and prevent osteoporosis. Oral GnRH treatments have just been developed, and some also include HRT in one convenient daily tablet. Reassuringly, bone mineral density appears to be protected after 1 year of use (see **Chapter 8**).

The selective progesterone receptor modulator ulipristal acetate has been shown to be as effective as GnRH agonists in reducing fibroid volume and alleviating HMB symptoms, but use is restricted to patients for whom other treatment options for HMB associated with fibroids have failed, are contraindicated or are unacceptable because drug-induced liver impairment has been reported in a minority of users. It should be noted that, when GnRH analogues or ulipristal treatment is stopped, ovarian function will return, leading to regrowth of fibroids.

The treatment algorithms for HMB recommended by the National Institute for Health and Care Excellence (NICE) differ if diagnostic testing shows the presence of at least one fibroid greater than 3 cm in diameter.

Surgical treatment

The choice of surgical treatment is determined by the presenting complaint and the patient's aspirations for menstrual function and fertility. Minimally invasive hysteroscopic surgery can be used to remove a submucous fibroid using electro-surgical instruments or mechanical hysteroscopic tissue resection systems, helping to resolve HMB symptoms even in the presence of other types of fibroid (see **Chapters 4** and **17**).

When a bulky fibroid uterus causes pressure symptoms or when HMB is refractory to medical interventions, the options are myomectomy to surgically remove fibroids with uterine conservation or hysterectomy. Myomectomy will be the preferred option when preservation of fertility is required, and this procedure can be performed through a laparotomy incision or, increasingly, laparoscopically, whereby 'power morcellation' of the removed fibroids is required to debulk the tumour to facilitate removal through a small 15 mm laparoscopic port site. An important point for the pre-operative discussion during the consent process for myomectomy is that there is a small but significant risk of uncontrolled life-threatening bleeding during myomectomy, which could lead to hysterectomy. Furthermore, the small risk of disseminating occult – that is, malignant sarcomatous change in a fibroid during laparoscopic myomectomy when power morcellation is used – should be discussed. Specially designed containment bags have now been introduced to minimize this risk.

Hysterectomy and myomectomy may be facilitated by GnRH agonist pretreatment over a 3-month period to reduce the bulk and vascularity of the fibroids. Useful benefits of this approach include reduced operative blood loss and the need for transfusion. This approach also enables a suprapubic (low transverse), rather than a midline, abdominal incision and can facilitate laparoscopic or vaginal (rather than abdominal) hysterectomy, with laparoscopic and vaginal hysterectomy both conducive to a more rapid recovery and fewer post-operative complications.

Radiological treatment

Uterine artery embolization (UAE) is a technique performed by interventional radiologists. It involves embolization of both uterine arteries under radiological guidance. A small incision is made in the groin under local anaesthesia and a cannula placed into the femoral artery and guided into the uterine arteries. Embolization particles are then injected, reducing the blood supply to the uterus, which induces infarction and degeneration of fibroids such that the overall reduction in fibroid volume is around 50%. Following UAE, patients usually require admission overnight because of pain following arterial occlusion, requiring opiate analgesia. Complications include fever, infection, fibroid expulsion and potential ovarian failure.

Women wishing to retain their fertility should be counselled carefully before undergoing UAE, as the effects on subsequent reproductive function are uncertain. Pregnancies have been reported in the literature, but concerns remain over premature ovarian failure and effects on the endometrium that may lead to abnormal placentation. Moreover, one-third of patients subsequently require further medical, radiological or surgical intervention within 5 years of UAE. Thus, when counselling patients about treatment options for symptomatic fibroids, it is important to balance the less invasive nature of UAE compared with surgical myomectomy against the much higher likelihood of needing further treatments.

ADENOMYOSIS

The endometrium is usually well demarcated from the underlying myometrium. Adenomyosis is a disorder in which endometrial glands and stroma are found deep within the myometrium. Adenomyosis can be diagnosed definitively only following histopathological examination of a hysterectomy specimen, where it is identified in 40% of uteri from a general female population of reproductive age. This ectopic endometrium is responsive to cyclical hormonal changes that result in bleeding within the myometrium, leading to increasingly severe secondary dysmenorrhoea (pain throughout menses), uterine enlargement and HMB.

Patients with adenomyosis are usually multiparous and diagnosed in their late 30s or early 40s. Examination may reveal a bulky and sometimes tender 'boggy' uterus, particularly if examined perimenstrually. Ultrasound examination of the uterus may be helpful for diagnosis when adenomyosis is particularly localized, showing

---

BOX 12.4: Relative advantages and disadvantages of treatments for symptomatic uterine fibroids

Medical

- Tranexamic acid, non-steroidal anti-inflammatory drugs, COCP and LNG-IUS (Mirena®): all of these are simple and fertility sparing (although COCP and LNG-IUS are contraceptive) options that avoid more invasive interventions, but they are generally less effective in the presence of submucosal fibroids or fibroid(s) >3 cm in diameter/a uterus >12 weeks' size, when an enlarged uterine cavity can be expected.
- COCP: contains oestrogen, which may increase the growth of oestrogen-dependent fibroids.
- LNG-IUS: there is an increased likelihood of expulsion if the cavity is enlarged or distorted by submucosal fibroids.
- GnRH agonists: these reduce fibroid volume prior to surgery and induce amenorrhoea and cause a temporary oestrogen-deficient 'menopausal' state precluding long-term use without add-back HRT. A new generation of oral GnRH analogues has been developed, some of which contain HRT, allowing longer-term use.
- Ulipristal acetate (selective progesterone receptor modulator): this oral medication reduces menstrual bleeding and fibroids, but concerns over drug-induced liver impairment restrict its use to refractory cases.

Surgical

- Hysteroscopic myomectomy: this minimally invasive, day-case procedure for submucous fibroids avoids surgical incisions and is effective in resolving HMB and improving fertility. However, it will not treat other types of fibroid.
- Myomectomy: this fertility-sparing procedure will treat HMB and bulk symptoms. It usually requires a laparotomy, but a less invasive laparoscopic approach is possible with smaller and fewer fibroids. It is associated with intraoperative bleeding from vascular fibroids, a 1% risk of unplanned hysterectomy and post-operative intra-abdominal adhesions.

(Contd.)

(Contd.)

- Hysterectomy: this procedure is indicated for patients with no future fertility desires. It may be achieved vaginally, laparoscopically or via open surgery depending on the size of the uterus. It is definitive, guaranteeing amenorrhoea, but it is as invasive as myomectomy.

Radiological

- UAE: this procedure is minimally invasive and avoids general anaesthesia and surgery. Although it is fertility sparing, there are concerns over its effect on subsequent reproductive function.
- Novel radiological treatments are currently being explored to destroy fibroids through thermal ablation. These include MRI-guided transcutaneous focused ultrasound and laparoscopic and transcervical intrauterine ultrasound-guided radiofrequency ablation. However, the effectiveness and safety of these interventions need further study before they can be considered for use in routine clinical practice.

🔑 KEY LEARNING POINTS

- A cervical ectropion is a normal finding in women of reproductive age and is usually due to hormonal influence – the 'three Ps': puberty, pill and pregnancy.
- Tests to evaluate the uterus include TVUSS, SIS, MRI, hysteroscopy and endometrial biopsy.
- Endometrial polyps are common, usually benign, focal lesions arising from the endometrium. They can cause abnormal patterns of uterine bleeding including HMB, IMB and PMB.
- Surgical removal of endometrial polyps, known as polypectomy, is a simple procedure usually performed under direct vision with the aid of a hysteroscope as an outpatient or day-case procedure.
- Fibroids (leiomyomas) are common, oestrogen-dependent, benign tumours of the myometrium and are estimated to be present in about 40% of women over 30 years of age. Fibroids undergo shrinkage after the menopause. Malignant change to leiomyosarcomas occurs

in 1 in 350 fibroids and is usually associated with rapid fibroid growth and AUB in a postmenopausal woman.

- Fibroids are classified according to their relationship to the uterine wall, being described as submucosal or intramural and subserosal. Fibroids can be detected on abdominal and/or bimanual pelvic examination as an enlarged pelvic mass of uterine origin.
- Fibroids can cause HMB and pressure 'bulk'-related abdominal symptoms and, in some cases, subfertility. However, the vast majority of fibroids are asymptomatic. Treatment is indicated for symptomatic fibroids. Surgical or radiological intervention is often required because medical treatments are generally less effective.
- Surgical removal of fibroids is termed myomectomy. Submucous fibroids protrude into the uterine cavity and so can be removed using hysteroscopic techniques. Intramural and subserosal fibroids are removed via a laparotomy incision or laparoscopically depending on their size, location and number.
- Adenomyosis is a disorder in which endometrial glands and stroma are found deep within the myometrium, which can cause dysmenorrhoea, HMB and uterine enlargement. The mechanism through which fibroids affect fertility is unclear.
- Medical treatments, such as the LNG-IUS (Mirena®), that can induce amenorrhoea will alleviate symptoms associated with adenomyosis, but hysterectomy remains the only definitive treatment.

haemorrhage-filled, distended endometrial glands. Sometimes this may give an irregular nodular development within the uterus, very similar to that of uterine fibroids. MRI is the investigation of choice, although expensive, as it provides excellent images of the myometrium, endometrium and areas of adenomyosis (**Figure 12.6**).

In general, any treatment that induces amenorrhoea will be helpful, as it will render the ectopic endometrium quiescent, relieving pain and excessive bleeding. Thus, the use of progestin-containing

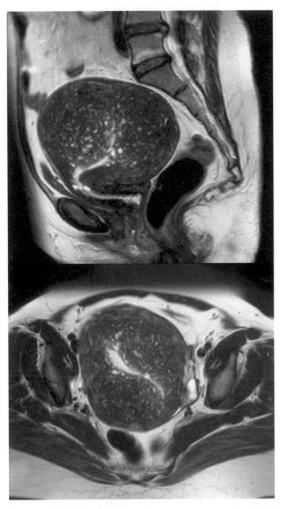

Figure 12.6 MRI showing adenomyosis – note the bright reflections of the central endometrium and flecks of ectopic endometrium in the underlying myometrium.

long-acting reversible contraceptives (see **Chapter 6**), such as the LNG-IUS and depot medroxyprogesterone acetate, and short-term GnRH agonists should be considered. On ceasing treatment, however, symptoms rapidly return in the majority of patients, and hysterectomy remains the only definitive treatment.

FURTHER READING

Al-Hendy A, Lukes AS, Poindexter AN III, et al. (2021). Treatment of uterine fibroid symptoms with relugolix combination therapy. *New England Journal of Medicine*, 384:630–642. https://doi.org/10.1056/NEJMoa2008283.

Brito LG, Stewart EA, Olivi Chaim SO, Martins WP, Farquhar C (2019). Interventions for uterine fibroids: An overview of Cochrane Reviews. *Cochrane Database of Systematic Reviews*, 9: CD013426. https://doi.org/10.1002/14651858.CD013426.

Munro MG, Critchley HOD, Fraser IS (2012). The FIGO systems for nomenclature and classification of causes of abnormal uterine bleeding in the reproductive years: Who needs them? *American Journal of Obstetrics and Gynecology*, 207: 259–265.

NICE (2018). *Heavy Menstrual Bleeding: Assessment and Management.* NICE guideline [NG88]. https://pathways.nice.org.uk/pathways/heavy-menstrual-bleeding.

Owen C, Armstrong AY (2015). Clinical management of leiomyoma. *Obstetrics and Gynecology Clinics of North America*, 42: 67–85.

SELF-ASSESSMENT

For interactive SBAs and EMQs relating to this chapter, visit www.routledge.com/cw/crosbie.

CASE HISTORY 1

A 34-year-old woman presents with increasingly heavy menstrual periods and an abdominal mass. She is known to have uterine fibroids. She is due to get married next month and plans to start a family soon. Several hormonal and non-hormonal medical treatments prescribed by her general practitioner (GP) have failed in the past 5 years.

A What questions would you ask in order to further explore the presenting complaint?

B What examination would you perform and what diagnostic tests would you perform or request?

C What medical treatments would you consider and why?

D What surgical or radiological treatments would you consider and why?

E Do you think she may be worried about anything in relation to her presenting complaint?

ANSWERS

A Assess the nature and severity of the menstrual bleeding (e.g. the chronicity of the symptoms, duration, regularity and amount [e.g. 'flooding' through sanitary protection] of menstrual loss and the adverse impact on health-related quality of life [e.g. the impact on work, social and emotional relationships, and physical and sexual functioning]). Establish whether there is any IMB or PCB that may indicate cervical pathology. Enquire about dysmenorrhoea and whether this is primary, spasmodic and short-lived at the onset of menses or secondary lasting throughout the period, which may suggest other gynaecological pathologies, especially if there is associated chronic pelvic pain. Information relating to the pelvic mass should be obtained (e.g. when was it first noticed and how is it enlarging and/or causing bulk or pressure symptoms and how were uterine fibroids diagnosed?). Fertility plans/desires should be established from the outset in addition to past 'failed' treatments, as this information will influence suitable management options.

B A gynaecological examination should be undertaken to better characterize the nature and origin of the mass; the size, regularity, mobility and tenderness of the mass should be determined. Investigations to consider include a pelvic ultrasound scan and possibly an MRI scan if the fibroids are large, rapidly enlarging or morphologically abnormal on ultrasound. An endometrial biopsy is generally unnecessary in patients under 45 years of age unless they have risk factors for endometrial hyperplasia (e.g. erratic cycles, obesity or polycystic ovaries). An outpatient hysteroscopy may be indicated if submucosal fibroids are suspected or seen on radiological imaging.

C As she plans to start a family soon, contraceptive hormonal treatments should be avoided, although may be used in the short term. Tranexamic acid and non-steroidal anti-inflammatory drugs are good options, although it is likely that these have already been tried, given the long-standing history. HMB in the presence of substantial uterine fibroids are more resistant to medical treatments and so surgery should be considered.

D In this instance, treatment should be fertility conserving, so hysterectomy and endometrial ablation are contraindicated. Myomectomy can be performed but, as there is a small risk of emergency hysterectomy because of severe intraoperative bleeding, this should probably be avoided unless she is unable to conceive within a year of trying. In contrast, hysteroscopic myomectomy is indicated if submucosal fibroids are detected, as the operation is minimally invasive, can treat HMB and can optimize subsequent fertility. UAE is another option, although the impact on subsequent reproductive function remains unclear.

E She may be worried about the effect of fibroids on her fertility and subsequent pregnancy in view of her forthcoming marriage. She may also be worried about the possibility of cancerous change if she feels the uterine mass has increased in size.

CASE HISTORY 2

A 45-year-old woman complains of regular, heavy and painful periods. She is having to take days off work every month because of her symptoms, and these absences are putting her job at risk. She has no medical problems, but has had three previous caesarean sections and has a body mass index of 35 kg/m². She has been sterilized and is reluctant to take hormones because they have affected her mood in the past. An ultrasound scan arranged by her GP has reported adenomyosis and she is worried about this diagnosis and wonders if it is a type of cancer.

A How would you explain in simple terms what adenomyosis is?

B How would you alleviate her concerns about the condition?

C What factors should you consider when formulating a management plan for this woman?

D Which medical treatments would you recommend?

E What are the advantages and disadvantages of hormonal medical treatments?

F Would you recommend a hysterectomy?

ANSWERS

A Adenomyosis is a benign condition in which the tissue that normally lines the uterus, called the endometrium, is found in the muscular wall of the uterus. This displaced tissue continues to act normally, thickening, breaking down and bleeding during each menstrual cycle causing heavy periods, menstrual cramps and lower abdominal pressure.

B She should be aware that adenomyosis is common, affecting 10–50% of women. It is not cancerous. The associated symptoms usually respond to the common treatments available for heavy periods and period pain.

C Her symptoms are significant because they are interfering with her health-related quality of life, especially her professional life. Thus, treatment is required. She has a preference to avoid hormonal therapies, but surgery in the form of hysterectomy is potentially hazardous because she has had three caesarean sections, which are likely to have caused bladder adhesions, and she is overweight.

D The antifibrinolytic tranexamic acid is safe, is well tolerated and may reduce the amount of menstrual bleeding by up to 50%. However, for many patients, tranexamic acid is not effective, and progestin-containing long-acting reversible contraceptives (especially the LNG-IUS or GnRH analogues) with add-back HRT should be considered to suppress endometrial tissue proliferation and reduce pain and bleeding symptoms.

E Long-acting reversible contraceptives are safe and well tolerated but can cause initial breakthrough bleeding and, in some women, this persists. She should be reassured that the mood disturbance she has experienced with hormonal contraceptives in the past is less likely to occur with the LNG-IUS, as it is locally acting contraceptive and only small amounts of the hormone enter the systemic circulation compared with oral or transdermal hormonal treatments. GnRH analogues with add-back HRT are effective, but regular injections are required and long-term HRT plus monitoring of bone mineral density using periodic dual X-ray absorptiometry scans are needed if used beyond 2 years.

F In the light of her risk factors for surgery, hormonal intervention in the form of an LNG-IUS is safer, less invasive and likely to be effective. However, if, despite counselling about the pros and cons of surgery (including potential complications compared with the use of the LNG-IUS or GnRH analogues), she still prefers surgery, then a hysterectomy should be offered.

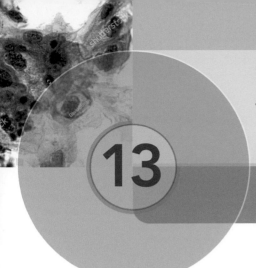

13

Benign conditions of the vulva and vagina, psychosexual disorders and female genital mutilation

LEILA CG FRODSHAM

Learning Objectives

- Describe the presentation and management of common benign conditions of the vulva and vagina.
- Describe the causes of superficial and deep dyspareunia.
- Understand the impact of vulval and vaginal conditions on sexual function.
- Understand the definition of psychosexual disorders.
- Describe the diagnosis, impact and management of psychosexual disorders.

ANATOMY AND HISTOLOGY

Vulva is the term used to describe the external female genitalia – the sexual organs. It includes the labia majora and minora, the clitoris and the fourchette. The vulval vestibule is defined anatomically as the area between the lower end of the vaginal canal at the hymenal ring and the labia minora. The different anatomical areas of the external genitalia have different histological characteristics and embryological origins. Both the labia minora and the labia majora are covered with keratinized, pigmented, squamous epithelium. The labia majora are two large folds of adipose tissue covered by skin containing hair follicles and sebaceous and sweat glands. In contrast, the labia minora are devoid of adipose tissue and hair follicles, but contain sebaceous follicles. The normal vulval vestibule is covered with non-keratinized, non-pigmented squamous epithelium and is devoid of skin adnexa. Within the vulval vestibule are the ducts of the minor vestibular glands, the periurethral glands of Skene, the urethral meatus and the ducts

of the Bartholin's glands. The Bartholin's glands are the major glands of the vestibule and lie deep within the perineum. Both the major and the minor vestibular glands contain mucus-secreting acini with ducts lined by transitional epithelium. The ducts of the Bartholin's glands exit at the introitus just above the fourchette at approximately five and seven o'clock on the perineum, and those of the minor vestibular glands are distributed throughout the vulval vestibule. The vagina and vulva are commonly known as the lower genital tract, with the vagina leading to the upper genital tract (uterus, cervix, fallopian tubes and ovaries). The vagina is a tubular structure but has anterior and posterior walls that lie in opposition.

Vulval skin has different physiological properties from other regions of the body, such as the forearm. Transepidermal water loss is twice the amount in vulval skin than in forearm skin. This suggests that the stratum corneum, the protective layer of vulval skin, functions poorly as a skin barrier compared with other skin areas and may explain why vulval skin is more prone to irritancy.

191

VULVAL OVERVIEW

Benign vulval conditions have a far-ranging impact on a person's health and lifestyle and yet there is a dearth of clinicians who are able to provide a holistic approach to care. Approximately 20% of women will have vulval symptoms such as itching, skin changes or pain at any time. Effective management of vulval diseases incorporates skills in dermatology, oncology, infectious disease and psychosexual medicine. Current training in these areas for gynaecologists is scanty and so patients are, at best, seen in vulval clinics with a multidisciplinary team approach. At worst, they may be passed between primary, secondary and tertiary care, feeling increasingly frustrated and disgruntled that no one seems to understand or be able to help them. In turn, this can make the speciality less appealing to clinicians. The recent survey entitled Tomorrow's Specialist by the Royal College of Obstetricians and Gynaecologists suggests that women expect psychosexual, dermatological and surgical skills from their gynaecologist and, while this chapter does not aim to cover all of these areas in detail, the intention is to give an overview of the management of these cases so that a sole clinician could manage most of these cases themselves. Of course, there will always be cases in which tertiary care is required, but the bulk of cases should remain in primary and secondary care.

ASSESSMENT

A full history and clinical examination (with optional vaginal swabs and biopsies) are essential to make a diagnosis. Vulval skin is an extension of general skin surfaces and it is important in the history to ask about general skin problems, as this might point towards the diagnosis; for example, psoriasis or eczema can synchronously affect the vulva and the limbs. The history should focus on the presenting complaint. It is important to discuss current methods of skincare (e.g. use of scented products that can aggravate symptoms), which topical treatments are being used (e.g. some creams such as antifungals can aggravate the problem) and the impact of the symptoms on sexual functioning. The clinical examination should include all skin

Table 13.1 Differential diagnoses of vulval complaints

Vulval pruritus	Vulval pain	Superficial dyspareunia
Infections (e.g. candidiasis, *Trichomonas vaginalis*)	Infections (e.g. candidiasis)	Skin conditions (e.g. lichen sclerosus [causes vulval splitting])
Skin conditions (e.g. lichen sclerosus, eczema, VIN)	Skin conditions (e.g. lichen sclerosus, eczema, VIN)	Vulvodynia
Contact dermatitis	Vulvodynia	Vulval fissures
	Bartholin's gland infection	Skin bridges of the vulva

VIN, vulval intraepithelial neoplasia.

surfaces, and the vulval area should be examined systematically with a good light source.

Vulval pruritus, pain and superficial dyspareunia are common symptoms, and **Table 13.1** illustrates the differential diagnoses of various symptoms, although this is not an exhaustive list. Confusingly for the clinician, most patients have more than one symptom.

VULVAL ITCHING (PRURITIS) AND DISCOMFORT

The most common presenting symptoms of benign vulval conditions are itching, discomfort, pain, discharge and dyspareunia (painful sex). Vulval disease can present at all ages, but there is a preponderance of benign dermatological conditions in the postmenopausal population. This group particularly lend themselves to a polypharmacy, as pathology may have multiple aetiologies (e.g. atrophic vaginitis and vulvitis or lichen sclerosus), and to a more holistic approach. Older individuals who are postmenopausal may be disinclined to seek advice early, and sexual dysfunction is already more common in this age group, among both patients and their partners. Additionally, individuals in this patient group can feel very 'alone' with their disease and can benefit significantly from joining support groups such as the Vulval Pain Society, which runs regular educational workshops.

Older individual can be particularly distressed by pruritis and can be mortified to find that they have woken up their partners with their nocturnal involuntary itching. As a result of nocturnal itching, some women can present with dysuria, as urine burns their excoriated vulval skin and the gross pathology can look alarming. It is also important to consider the effects of both urinary and faecal incontinence, as this can damage the skin barrier function and form vulval dermatitis.

REDUCTION IN ALLERGENS

The appearance of vulval dermatitis is often not specific and is strongly associated with a history of atopy and other dermatoses. It is therefore prudent to reduce allergens in all patients presenting with symptoms of vulval pruritis.

It is advisable to discourage washing with any soaps or detergents (including feminine washes), which disrupt the bacterial balance of the vagina and can cause vulval dermatitis. Water is preferable, but some patients find that olive/coconut (or other natural and unperfumed) oils offer moisturization and a better clean. Women who wish to have a scented, moisturizing bath can use similar oils with a few drops of tea tree oil.

Wearing cotton underwear (with minimal dyes) and washing clothing with an unperfumed, non-biological washing powder/fabric conditioner should be advised. It is also worth considering the effect of sanitary protection/pads for urinary incontinence. It is not uncommon to see marked vulval dermatitis from popular sanitary brands (particularly the super-thin gel-filled variety of sanitary towel), and these patients may benefit from sourcing unbleached, organic protection, washable pads or a menstrual cup (e.g. the Mooncup®).

RECURRENT USE OF ANTIFUNGALS

Women will frequently both self-source and be prescribed multiple courses of antifungals such as clotrimazole cream and pessaries, often without examination. While this can soothe in the initial stages, it can precipitate a hypersensitivity reaction that increases symptoms, and yet patients often feel obliged to use what is offered, as the 'doctor is the expert' and their symptoms are so distressing.

The vulval and vaginal condition of candidal infection or 'thrush' is common and particularly affects the reproductive-age population in whom oestrogen levels are high. There is an increased prevalence in pregnancy, but it is uncommon in prepubescent children and in the postmenopausal population, in whom other causes for irritation should be sought rather than relying on readily available antifungals. Hypo-oestrogenic women should therefore be checked for other causes of itching and should be examined before antifungals are prescribed. It is very important to consider diabetes as a cause of recurrent thrush. Oral fluconazole is a second-line treatment after clotrimazole. If courses of both clotrimazole and fluconazole are ineffective, a course of 150 mg econazole nitrate nightly over three consecutive nights can help some affected individuals. In menstruating women, this is most useful postmenstrually, when candida is more common due to alteration of the vaginal pH. A combination of a reduction of allergens and the above is sufficient in most cases. It is unnecessary to treat partners unless they have symptoms themselves, and there is no proven benefit in doing so. A referral to genitourinary medicine (sexual health) can be of great benefit in recurrent cases of treatment-resistant candida.

LOW FERRITIN

About 5% of women with vulval pruritis may have low ferritin, and the correction of this will improve symptoms, so it should always be checked in the early stages.

VULVOVAGINAL ATROPHY

Women who are perimenopausal, menopausal, breastfeeding or using progesterone-only contraceptives are at risk of vulvovaginal atrophy. In such cases, a reduction in oestrogen causes vulvovaginal atrophy, loss of rugae (wrinkles in the vaginal wall) and elasticity. Diagnosis is based on symptoms rather than clinical appearances, as these develop later and may be irreversible, despite topical vaginal oestrogen replacement. Many women describe discomfort not only during sex, but also when exercising, and many have concurrent bladder symptoms such as frequency, urgency and leakage. All (peri) menopausal individuals should be asked about sex, as many will not voluntarily disclose genitourinary symptoms to healthcare professionals.

Topical vaginal oestrogens have negligible systemic absorption (1 mg oral equivalent per annum), do not increase rates of endometrial hyperplasia or cancers, and should be used lifelong (in menopausal women) to prevent recurrence of symptoms. They can also be safely used in breastfeeding and do not affect lactation. If women present with superficial dyspareunia on progesterone-only contraception, topical vaginal oestrogens should be trialled before considering a change of contraception, if not contraindicated.

BIOPSY IN VULVAL DISEASE

Biopsy should be performed as first-line treatment only if there is a concern regarding malignancy. If there is a diffuse leukoplakia or erythema, treatment with steroids and emollients is recommended and, if symptoms do not resolve, biopsy should be considered. The Keyes punch biopsy is a 4 mm sample of skin that can be taken under local anaesthetic in the clinic (**Figure 13.1**). A pathology sample allows an accurate diagnosis to be made and the correct treatment to be instigated. Biopsies should be carried out when there is a pigmented lesion, a raised or indurated area, and a persistent ulcer.

LICHEN PLANUS

Lichen planus is an autoimmune disorder affecting 1–2% of the population (particularly in people

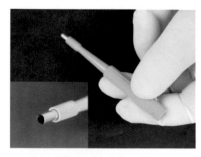

Figure 13.1 Keyes punch biopsy.

over 40 years of age) and affects the skin, genitalia, and oral and gastrointestinal mucosa. There is no known precipitating factor, although pressure can increase symptoms (e.g. restrictive underwear), but symptoms are often pruritis and/or superficial dyspareunia. Lesions in the mouth may be reticular-like cobwebs, and oral inspection should be performed if the diagnosis is suspected. Lesions can occur on the shins and there can be characteristic appearances to the nail bed such as longitudinal ridging and a sandpaper effect.

Genital lesions can be longitudinal, annular, ulcerative, hyperpigmented or bullous and may cause vaginal stenosis and resulting sexual dysfunction. Treatment is by high-dose topical steroids. Sexual dysfunction is common due to pain and stenosis. If there is a vaginal stenosis, it is preferable to try dilatation with manual means (fingers or dilators) rather than surgical means in the first instance.

LICHEN SCLEROSUS

Lichen sclerosus is a destructive inflammatory skin condition that affects mainly the anogenital area of women. It is believed to affect 1 in 300 women and the cause is believed to be autoimmune. Many patients have other autoimmune conditions, such as thyroid disease and pernicious anaemia. The destructive nature of the condition is due to underlying inflammation in the subdermal layers of the skin, which results in hyalinization of the skin. This leads to a fragility and white 'parchment paper' appearance of the skin and a loss of vulval anatomy. The condition can involve the foreskin of men to produce a phimosis. Lichen sclerosus is evident elsewhere on the body in 15% of patients. The main symptoms on the vulva are itching and subsequent soreness of the vulva, usually due to scratching. A biopsy can confirm the diagnosis, and treatment is a combination of good skincare and strong steroid ointments such as those containing clobetasol. Many patients with vulval cancer have lichen sclerosus at the time of diagnosis, and it is estimated that there is a low risk of cancer developing in a patient with lichen sclerosus (around 3–5%).

Lichen sclerosus characteristically presents in a 'figure of 8' pattern around the vulva and anus. There is frequently hypopigmentation, loss of anatomy,

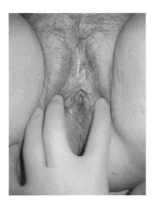

Figure 13.2 Lichen sclerosus.

vaginal stenosis and cracking (particularly in the posterior fourchette), but appearances can be subtle in early-stage disease (**Figure 13.2**). Treatment of both lichen planus and lichen sclerosus is by high-dose topical steroids (clobetasol proprionate): applying a pea-sized amount daily for 1 month then on alternate days for the second month and twice a week for the third month. If there is not complete resolution of symptoms, biopsy is indicated. Patients should be advised to seek advice if the lesions become raised or resistant to treatment. Once the course of treatment is completed, the steroid cream can be used by patients as and when required with the proviso that they seek review if symptoms don't start to settle within a week of daily use.

VULVAL CYSTS

Bartholin's cysts, Skene gland cysts and mucous inclusion cysts can affect the vulval area and cause a lump with or without vulval discomfort. If they do not cause the patient any problem, they can be either monitored or excised. A Bartholin's cyst is the most common type of cyst and develops in the region of the Bartholin's gland (**Figure 13.3**). The Bartholin's gland has a long duct that, when blocked, causes fluid to build up and eventually forms a cyst. It is not uncommon for these cysts to get infected and cause a Bartholin's abscess, which usually presents acutely and may require incision and drainage. Marsupialization of the cyst is the term used when the internal aspect of the cyst is sutured to the outside of the cyst to create a window so that the cyst does not reform. Marsupialization of Bartholin's

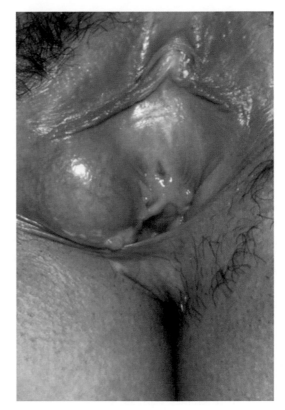

Figure 13.3 Bartholin's cyst.

cysts is usually an elective procedure under general or spinal anaesthesia. Outpatient drainage is also possible, sometimes followed by the insertion of a tiny catheter into the incision, which remains in place for several weeks to maintain its patency.

VULVODYNIA

Vulvodynia is the condition of pain on the vulva most often described as a burning pain, occurring in the absence of skin disease or infection. It is akin to a neuropathic pain syndrome. The pain can be further classified by the anatomical site (e.g. generalized, localized or clitoral) and also by whether pain is provoked or unprovoked. Vulvodynia can occur at any age and causes huge distress to sufferers. It is essential to exclude physical causes such as dermatitis. The Vulval Pain Society can be an invaluable source of information and support for sufferers. There is recent evidence that neuromodulators are of limited benefit in vulvodynia, but some patients find them useful (particularly if pain inhibits sleep, when a sedative neuromodulator such as amitriptyline can be used).

It is important to take a detailed history about the onset of symptoms and the timing and relation to the patient's sexual history. Patients with vulvodynia may have primary or secondary psychosexual dysfunction as described in the section 'Psychosexual medicine' later in this chapter. Vulvodynia usually coexists with vaginismus, as pain causes involuntary contraction of the pelvic floor to guard against further pain. Some patients can benefit from perineal massage, which may aid vulval desensitization, reduce muscular spasm and reassociate the patient with their own genitalia. Oils (such as coconut) may act as a barrier to precipitating factors (allergens or chafing from sports or clothing) and enable better lubrication for sexual function. While this can be initiated on guidance from a gynaecologist, highly specialized pelvic floor physiotherapists are doing invaluable work and research in this area, and there should be a low threshold for referral in this patient group.

Many patients with vulvodynia will see multiple clinicians and will have tried conventional and alternative therapies with no resolution of symptoms. Often it is a combination of perineal massage and a consideration of the patient's feelings regarding the diagnosis and their relationships that has the biggest impact. Patients need support to regain their sex lives. Ideally, this should be from someone who appreciates the physical and psychosexual aspects of their pain – not a 'specialist' but a healthcare professional with an empathetic ear who is able to work with the patient. The management of symptoms, rather than a complete resolution of pain, is the most realistic outcome. Many patients find that more satisfying sleep, mindfulness, and yoga or Pilates can really help.

Patient insight: Vulvodynia sufferer

For 8 years I have felt that I am not living my life but managing my pain on a daily basis. I have seen numerous specialists, used every possible cream and tablet and felt like a disappointment to doctors who want to help me to get better but can't. In recent months my pain patch has reduced, my sex life improved and I can see that one day, like a butterfly, it will just fly away.

DYSPAREUNIA

Dyspareunia is defined as pain during sexual intercourse. Dyspareunia may be associated with many gynaecological problems and is described as either superficial or deep, with the latter sometimes associated with pathology such as endometriosis or pelvic inflammatory disease. Deep dyspareunia is most commonly associated with pelvic pathology, while superficial is more likely to be labelled as psychosexual.

BOX 13.1: Dyspareunia

Definition: pain during or after sexual intercourse, which can be classified as superficial (affecting the vagina, clitoris or labia) or deep (pain experienced within the pelvis).

Epidemiology: the estimated prevalence is between 10% and 20%, although this may be an underestimate, as many affected individuals remain undiagnosed. Risk factors include female genital mutilation (FGM), suspected pelvic inflammatory disease and endometriosis, peri-/postmenopausal status, depression or anxiety states, and a history of sexual assault.

Clinical evaluation

- If pain is superficial and there are no concurrent symptoms, consider delaying speculum examination to avoid unnecessary pain. Topical lidocaine gel can be used vaginally a few minutes before examination to reduce discomfort.
- The clinical history should explore the nature and onset of pain, the relationship to intercourse, associated chronic pelvic pain symptoms, and the reproductive and past medical history. A psychosexual history should be considered, especially for superficial dyspareunia.
- Abdominal and pelvic examination should look for lower genital tract lesions (e.g. skin disorder, scarring, anatomical anomalies), vaginismus (involuntary contraction of vaginal muscles during vaginal examination), areas of tenderness within the lower and upper genital tract and evidence of pelvic disease (masses, tenderness or fixity of organs).

Investigations

- Superficial dyspareunia: consider vulval dermatoses/vulvovaginal atrophy – both need treatment before biopsy unless malignancy is suspected.
- Deep dyspareunia: consider transvaginal ultrasound scan, swabs and laparoscopy.

Treatment

- Superficial dyspareunia: treat any identifiable cause.
- Deep dyspareunia: treat in the same way as chronic pelvic pain.

PSYCHOSEXUAL MEDICINE

Psychosexual problems may be primary or secondary.

BOX 13.2: Psychosexual dysfunction

- Primary psychosexual dysfunction describes sexual difficulties in which there may be psychosomatic pain.
- Secondary psychosexual dysfunction describes sexual difficulties resulting from pain or emotional issues.

HOW TO APPROACH CONSULTATIONS

Vulval disorders are invariably linked with female (and occasionally secondary male) sexual dysfunction. Whether primary or secondary, and regardless of the aetiology, it is important to explore this in the consultation.

The Institute of Psychosexual Medicine uses the LOFTI model to aid with consultation.

VAGINISMUS AND NON-CONSUMMATION

Vaginismus is a debilitating condition that involves involuntary contraction of the pelvic floor either causing pain or making penetrative sex impossible. Patients often describe themselves as abnormal or broken and can take many years to present. More

---

BOX 13.3: LOFTI model

Listening

- Open questions and periods of silence allow the patient to divulge and elaborate on essential information.
- What is their tone/style of language?
- What is/is not said? How and when?

Observing

- Patterns of behaviour (e.g. frequent cancellations/avoidance of appointments).
- Urgency, demeanour, style of dress and mannerisms.
- Referral letters from the general practitioner (GP) may be detailed and pressurized, emphasizing the urgency of the referral (this is an example of transference: the unconscious redirection of feelings from the patient to the GP).

Feelings

- Be aware of feelings in the room.
- How does the patient make you feel?
- Feelings aroused in any doctor by the patient's language, behaviour and the attitude of the doctor to the patient are seen as possible evidence of the patient's own, less than conscious feelings.

Thinking

- Note what sort of doctor you are being in the consultation. A parent? A teacher?
- Why is the patient presenting now? How did the patient come to have the consultation/what is their motivation?
- Note how you feel before and after the consultation.

Interpreting

- Assess the overall picture – is the patient displaying certain types of behaviour or attitudes as a defence mechanism or as a means of hiding anxiety or fear such as tears or anger?
- Defence mechanisms include regression, dissociation, introjection, sublimation and denial.
- What do you notice from genital examination? Is there avoidance (i.e. patients menstruating at every appointment or always having difficulties with smears)?

---

recently, affected individuals are beginning to feel they can speak up, and there are patient support groups online such as the Vaginismus Network that are sharing individuals' stories and helping other sufferers to seek help/recover.

There is often a pressure of time (fertility or relationship issues), in addition to patients' concerns about a physical anomaly, that may lead the gynaecologist to a physical intervention such as a Fenton's procedure. While this may satisfy a short-term desire for a patient to widen what appears to be an impossibly small hole, it very rarely succeeds in resolving the issue of non-consummation, as the underlying vaginismus will continue to present an issue for penetration, as muscles will still contract without coexisting support.

Patient insight: Patient with non-consummation

Please will you just drive something through the blockage whilst I'm asleep so my husband can get in there?

Traditionally, both doctors and sex therapists have used vaginal dilators to enable the patient to 'overcome her/their blockage'. However, although patients often become very adept at going up the sizes, this may not translate into sexual activity, as noted anecdotally. Although frequently prescribed, the use of dilators has no proven benefit; the evidence in favour of their use remains anecdotal and evidence of efficacy is lacking in cases in which there is no physical pathology. More research is needed in this area.

Patient insight: Vaginismus patient

He gave me vaginal dilators, but when I used them it felt like an extension on the doctors fingers and got me no closer to having sex with my husband.

Practitioners undertaking psychosexual training will begin to recognize the transference of the patient's feelings onto themselves, and may notice the drive to open the vagina and achieve penetration exhibiting in themselves, subconsciously, as frustration and irritation with the patient. Additionally,

practitioners may feel inhibited from examining a patient with vaginismus and so may willingly accept patients' 'everlasting period' excuse as a means of avoiding examination. This may further lead to a temptation to provide an examination under anaesthesia and manual dilation, which may positively reinforce the patient's perception of a physical issue that might eventually lead to further unnecessary surgery.

Patients with vaginismus may make the most progress with a professional who is able to practice mind and body medicine, that is, by considering the impact on patients both physically and psychologically. Instead of responding to the patient's issue of being 'too small' by using the small speculum – and thereby positively reinforcing the phantasy – examination might be performed with the patient involved, for example using a mirror, allowing them control during the examination and encouraging self-exploration at home with perineal massage and stretching of the vagina with their or their partner's fingers. The practitioner should always question a patient's reluctance to engage with their own genitalia, because ultimately this might precipitate disclosure of a phantasy (physical fantasy) that is blocking exploration/penetration. Genital examination may lead to the 'moment of truth' in consultation, with the patient recognizing the influence of the mind over the body in their sexual problem. It is often tempting to reassure patients that their anatomy is normal, but it is more powerful to encourage them to see and feel that themselves.

Additionally, women with vaginismus are covertly in control of their sex lives (although this is largely subconscious in both partners). Empowering them to recognize this and take overt control, by encouraging them to tell their partners that penetrative sex is banned for a specified period of time, can be therapeutic. This is called modified sensate focus, and might help them to enable penetration through a combination of perineal massage and exploration of their subconscious defences (e.g. always wearing fleece pyjamas to bed or avoiding the same bedtime).

In summary, it is advisable to use the consultation to recognize and reflect the patient's anxieties and consider carefully whether surgery is the best option. The Institute of Psychosexual Medicine trains doctors and allied healthcare professionals in skills to enable them to see that the patient is the expert who has the answers, but requires a 'professional mirror' to see them. All health professionals act as chameleons in consultation (e.g. by adapting their tone of voice, body language or demeanour), but those trained in psychosexual medicine are able to recognize what is coming from the patient and reflect it back to them.

FEMALE GENITAL MUTILATION

There are four degrees of FGM/cutting (cutting is now the favoured term by survivors) (**Figure 13.4**) that are practised in different geographical areas, as shown in **Figure 13.5**. Although cutting is widely regarded in Western countries as a barbaric and unacceptable procedure, the prevalence remains extremely high, with physical, psychological and social ramifications. The World Health Organization (WHO) defines FGM as follows:

> Any procedure involving partial or total removal of the external genitalia and/or injury to the female genital organs whether for cultural, religious or other non-therapeutic reasons.
>
> (WHO, 2023)

FGM is frequently performed in girls from the age of 8 onwards without analgesia or adequate sterility. FGM is a practice that has far-reaching implications in both the acute and the chronic time frames. The implications are physical, psychological and psychosexual and may, in the worst-case scenario, lead to renal failure from urinary obstruction and infection. There is now a legal obligation in the UK to document all cases in the medical notes and report all cases through the safeguarding team in NHS Trusts to reduce the incidence of this practice in young girls and women in the UK. In cases in which FGM is suspected in minors, this is classified as child sexual abuse, and social services and the police should be involved.

The four main types of FGM are as follows (**Figure 13.4**):

1. Clitoridectomy: excision of the prepuce (clitoral hood) with or without the removal of the clitoris.
2. Excision of the clitoris and partial or total removal of the labia minora.
3. Excision of part or all of the external genitalia and stitching/narrowing of the vagina – infundibulation.
4. Piercing of the clitoris, cauterization, cutting the vagina or inserting corrosive substances. This also includes any plastic surgery procedures done as an adult.

There is often an extremely fine line between cosmetic surgery on the vulva (such as labioplasty) and FGM, and the gynaecologist must seek advice before considering such procedures. The prevalence of requests for labioplasty procedures has risen dramatically in recent years (possibly as a result of the accessibility of pornography and 'photoshopping' online), and many healthcare providers have withdrawn funding for such procedures on the NHS. This has, in turn, increased private practice in this area, which may offer less rigorous support

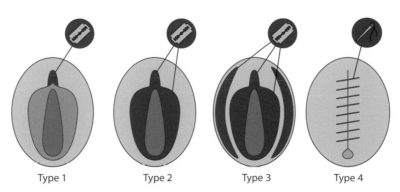

Figure 13.4 Types of female genital mutilation.

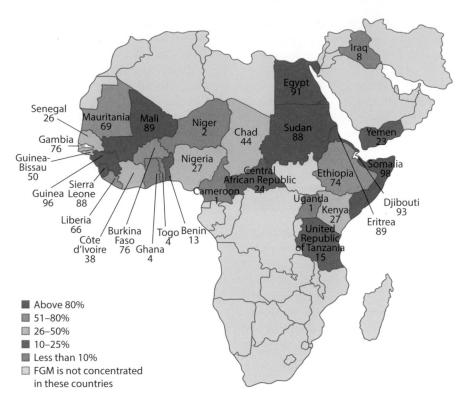

Figure 13.5 Geographical distribution of female genital mutilation. (Adapted from UNICEF 2013 data.)

for the emotionally vulnerable patient. Pre- and post-surgery patients are now attending NHS psychosexual medicine clinics for help with sexual dysfunction either related to body dysmorphia or side effects of the surgery. A useful tool for women to use is the artwork *The Great Wall of Vagina* by Jamie McCartney, a British artist who has taken hundreds of plaster casts of vulvas. Viewers are often pleasantly surprised to see how 'normal' their vulva is after looking at this.

It is difficult for UK gynaecologists to appreciate the cultural context of FGM, particularly when working in areas where it is infrequently seen. The novel *Possessing the Secret of Joy* by Alice Walker is an essential read for gynaecologists who are interested in the impact of FGM on women and the cultural influences behind the practice. The main character chooses FGM after puberty to feel more 'in tune with' her culture and eloquently describes the emotional and physical impact of her decision.

The obstetrician must be alert to this issue and must form a plan for such patients in labour; in such cases, birthing in hospital is usually advised and a detailed plan of care is needed. From the evidence to date, it is not fully known whether labour is obstructed in these patients, but obstructed labour is certainly a possibility in type 3 FGM. Depending on the type of FGM, it may be necessary to perform midline episiotomy for safe delivery. However, it is far more preferable to enquire early in the pregnancy and refer the patient to a specialist centre for deinfundibulation. It is illegal to re-suture (which many women request for fear of rejection by their partner or community) an FGM.

REVERSAL OF INFUNDIBULATION (DEINFUNDIBULATION)

Ideally, women should be identified preconceptually and sent to a specialist centre, but they can be managed antenatally. It should be rare that patients are managed on the labour ward, as all who are felt to be at risk should be identified by their booking midwives and, if this is the case, a senior obstetrician should be present.

Deinfundibulation should be performed with adequate analgesia to avoid flashbacks to the FGM/cutting procedure (local anaesthetic can be used but may distort anatomy). The incision should be made along the vulval incision scar and the urethra should be identified before surgery commences to reduce damage. All patients should have prior urinary infection screening and should be given appropriate antibiotic therapy, as bladder obstruction and urinary infection rates are high. A fine absorbable suture should be used and prophylactic antibiotics should be considered.

It should not be assumed that both sexual dysfunction and emotional distress are resolved by deinfundibulation, and specialist centres will be more adequately placed to access specialist services and support groups for affected women.

FURTHER READING

British Association for Sexual Health and HIV (2014). *2014 UK National Guideline on the Management of Vulval Conditions*.

Brough P, Denman E (2019). *Introduction to Psychosexual Medicine*, 3rd ed. Routledge.

Lee NMW (2018). Dyspareunia. *BMJ*, 361: k2341. https://doi.org/10.1136/bmj.k2341.

McEwan I (2007). *On Chesil Beach*. Jonathan Cape.

Royal College of Gynaecologists and Obstetricians (2015). Green-top guideline No. 53: Female genital mutilation and its management.

Rullo JE, Lorenz T, Ziegelmann MJ, Meihofer L, Herbenick D, Faubion SS (2018). Genital vibration for sexual function and enhancement: a review of evidence. *Sexual and Relationship Therapy*, 33: 263–274.

Walker A (1992). *Possessing the Secret of Joy*. Harcourt Brace Jovanovich.

WHO (2023). Female genital mutilation. https://www.who.int/news-room/fact-sheets/detail/female-genital-mutilation.

KEY LEARNING POINTS

- Women with vulval disease often present late, with extensive and debilitating disease that affects their daily lives and intimate relationships.
- Vulval disease may cause pruritis – good skin care and steroid treatment may help.
- Biopsy is indicated when there is suspicion of malignancy or failure to respond to treatment.
- Dyspareunia is described as either deep or superficial.
- Patients with psychosexual disorders are often frustrated and angry and so, as a practitioner, you may feel that they are 'difficult' to manage. However, these patients are rarely 'difficult' if they are listened to and a plan is formulated together with patient and practitioner. People with psychosexual problems are the experts in their condition, but need an empathetic approach to unlock unconcious feelings.
- FGM/cutting is frequently performed on girls worldwide, and it is essential to recognize and offer deinfundibulation.

Useful websites, podcasts and online resources

- *The Guardian* (2019). The problem with sex – Science Weekly podcast. https://www.the-guardian.com/science/audio/2019/may/10/.the-problem-with-sex-science-weekly-podcast.
- The diagnosis and treatment of dyspareunia. *BMJ* talk medicine. https://soundcloud.com/bmjpodcasts/dysparenuia-mixdown?in=mustafa-hizmah/sets/psychosexuality.
- BBC (2019). Vaginismus: 'My body won't let me have sex'. https://www.bbc.co.uk/news/av/world-europe-49695670.
- College of Sexual and Relationship Therapies. www.cosrt.co.uk.
- The Institute of Psychosexual Medicine. www.ipm.org.uk.
- The Vaginismus Network. https://www.thevaginismusnetwork.com/.
- Vagina Museum. https://www.vaginamuseum.co.uk/.

SELF-ASSESSMENT

For interactive SBAs and EMQs relating to this chapter, visit www.routledge.com/cw/crosbie.

CASE HISTORY 1

A 25-year-old woman has been seen by her community midwife and disclosed previous 'cutting'. The midwife has urgently referred her to your antenatal clinic. She is now 28 weeks' pregnant. What are the next steps that you should take?

ANSWER

Initial examination is helpful to determine the degree of FGM (type 1–4), as this will affect the management now and for labour. The safeguarding team must be made aware, and it is essential that documentation that is dated and timed is present in the notes. These are legal requirements. Ensure that a translator is available if necessary for all visits. Depending on the type of FGM, midline episiotomy in labour may be necessary. Early deinfundibulation is preferable. Suturing post-delivery should be performed by a senior obstetrician. In the UK, it is illegal to perform restoration of the FGM, even on request.

CASE HISTORY 2

Elizabeth is a 45-year-old who has recently noticed difficulty concentrating at work, increased irritability and a reduced desire to have sex and, when she does have sex, it is extremely sore. She denies any dryness during intercourse but describes it as feeling too tight and 'like paper cuts'. She is dealing with an extraordinary amount of stress with a senior managerial job and is caring for her mother who was recently bereaved and has multiple health problems. How might you assess her and consider treatment options?

ANSWER

A careful history and examination here is essential. There are a number of possible physical and psychological triggers for her difficulties.

1. *Perimenopause*: even if women still have normal menstrual cycles, they can experience menopausal symptoms. Only 75% of women will have flushes, so the absence of flushes does not exclude perimenopause. It is reasonable, even if examination appears normal, to try a course of topical vaginal oestrogens. Dyspareunia is a common presenting complaint in perimenopause/menopause, particularly if women are also using progesterone-only contraceptives, as these can reduce oestrogen levels further. If they respond well to this, it is worth discussing systemic hormone replacement therapy to manage their other menopausal symptoms. A Greene Climacteric scale can be used to assess symptoms. There is no need to check follicle-stimulating hormone/luteinizing hormone in those over the age of 45 to diagnose perimenopause. Both vulvovaginal atrophy/genital syndrome of menopause and systemic symptoms of menopause should be judged by clinical symptoms rather than blood tests or examination.

2. *Genital dermatoses*: examination should be performed to identify any genital skin conditions – the most common being atopic vulvitis, which may respond to barrier creams and a reduction in allergens. Any woman with superficial dyspareunia should be advised about allergen reduction and the use of massage (vibratory is best) of the pelvic floor. Lichen sclerosus should be excluded – clinical signs include hypopigmentation, loss of anatomy and leukoplakia. These are typically in a 'figure of 8' pattern. Treatment is with potent topical steroids at a reducing dose over 3 months.

3. *Psychosocial stressors*: women in middle age are often juggling careers, teenagers and increasingly dependent parents. It is important to explore these issues and consider potential support with the patient. It is also important to take a careful history to exclude signs of clinical depression. It should always be remembered that falling oestrogen will exacerbate the impact of external stressors, so the two often coexist.

CASE HISTORY 3

Penny is 24 years old and unable to have penetrative sex. She has had a boyfriend for 6 years, since university, where they met in the Christian Union. They had decided to wait until marriage to have penis in vagina sex, but she has noticed a difficulty inserting tampons and she freezes whenever he tries to insert a finger. It is acutely painful and feels like there is a blockage. They are marrying soon and she wants to be sure that she is 'anatomically normal' for their wedding night. They are both worried that there is an obstruction. She has normal regular periods. How might you assess her and consider treatment options?

ANSWER

Often, women in this position (with likely vaginismus) have strong and difficult feelings about being abnormal and are fearful that their problem will never resolve. Partners can feel very protective, and it may be difficult to gain a clear history, as patients can be very anxious about not upsetting their partner. Partners can often start to feel as fearful about the vagina being fragile and easily broken as the patient does.

It is equally important to consider how women will feel about examination and you should state that the woman is in control of what occurs and that you will stop at any time.

If there are no other gynaecological symptoms, it is better not to penetrate the vagina with digits or a speculum. Many doctors feel that demonstrating that the space is there will enable the couple to achieve penetration themselves; however, in the main, this further reinforces worries about pain and reinforces the feeling that any vaginal penetration is painful.

Examination should be taken slowly, with more observation than touch. Examination of the vaginal introitus can be achieved by parting the vulval lips to see the introitus by gently pulling the inner thighs laterally. If the patients is comfortable, you can palpate the pelvic floor or insert a single digit. Occasionally, a partially perforate hymen will allow for menstruation, but the perforation will be too small for the naked eye. This is very rare and can usually be managed with lacrimal/cercal dilator in an outpatient setting. Exceedingly rarely, a formal hymenoplasty is required. There is no evidence to support the use of Fenton's procedure for vaginismus. The pelvic floor is dynamic, so cutting part of a muscle will not stop the remainder of it contracting.

There is no evidence to support the use of vaginal trainers but, for women who experience pain, vibratory massage can be beneficial. Pelvic floor massage with psychosexual support can help some patients to overcome vaginismus.

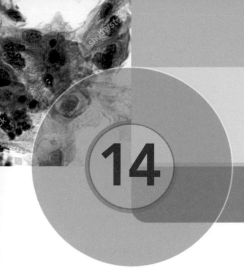

Malignant disease of the ovary

14

EMMA J CROSBIE

> **Learning Objectives**
> - Learn how malignant disease of the ovary, fallopian tube and peritoneum presents.
> - Learn how ovarian cancer is investigated and staged.
> - Learn how ovarian cancer is managed.

INTRODUCTION

Ovarian cancer is the second most common gynaecological malignancy and the primary cause of death from gynaecological cancer in the UK: there are approximately 7,500 new cases and 4,200 deaths from ovarian cancer every year. When detected in its early stages, ovarian cancer has an excellent prognosis. The dismal overall survival rates from ovarian cancer reflect the advanced stage at which most patients present. Screening has not been shown to be effective and, until recently, there have been few advances in the development of targeted treatments for advanced disease.

OVARIAN CANCER

INCIDENCE

The lifetime risk of developing ovarian cancer in the general population is 2% (1 in 50), and the mean age of presentation is 64 years. Ovarian cancer is more prevalent in high-income countries. There are variations in incidence with ethnicity; White women have the highest incidence at approximately 18 per 100,000, whereas Asian and Black women have a lower incidence at 12 per 100,000 and 9 per 100,000, respectively. Ovarian cancer is rare in young women and only 3% of ovarian cancers occur in patients under 35 years of age. It is now increasingly accepted that many ovarian cancers originate in the fallopian tube, rather than in the ovarian surface epithelium as previously thought. There is a significant genetic aspect to ovarian cancer (see the section 'Genetic factors in ovarian cancer' later in this chapter), and women with hereditary cancer present early, with a mean age at diagnosis of 54 years.

CLASSIFICATION OF OVARIAN CANCER

Primary ovarian cancers are epithelial (80%), sex cord stromal (10%) or germ cell (10%) tumours. The ovary is also a common site for metastatic

10.1201/9781003218036-14

Table 14.1 Histological classification of malignant ovarian tumours

Category	Histological subtype
Epithelial ovarian tumours (80%)	High-grade serous Endometrioid Clear cell Mucinous Low-grade serous (Borderline)
Sex cord stromal tumours (10%)	Granulosa cell Sertoli–Leydig Gynandroblastoma
Germ cell tumours (10%)	Dysgerminoma Endodermal sinus (yolk sac) Teratoma Choriocarcinoma Mixed
Metastatic (including Krukenberg) tumours	

spread; Krukenberg tumours are ovarian metastases associated with primary cancers of the colon, stomach and breast. **Table 14.1** shows a histological classification of ovarian tumours.

EPITHELIAL OVARIAN TUMOURS

Epithelial tumours of the ovary can be benign, malignant or borderline. Approximately 10% of epithelial tumours are classified as borderline ovarian tumours (BOTs). These tumours are well differentiated and have some features of malignancy (nuclear pleomorphism, cellular atypia), but do not invade the basement membrane. BOTs spread to other abdominopelvic structures (peritoneum, omentum) but do not often recur following initial surgery. The majority of BOTs are serous tumours. Mucinous BOTs may arise from appendiceal carcinomas of low malignant potential and can be associated with pseudomyxoma peritoneii.

High-grade serous carcinomas account for around 75% of all epithelial ovarian cancers; mucinous and endometrioid tumours are less common, together accounting for 10%, followed by clear cell carcinomas. High-grade serous tumours are characterized histologically by concentric rings of calcification known as psammoma bodies. Mucinous carcinomas are generally large, multiloculated tumours associated with pseudomyxoma peritoneii. Endometrioid carcinomas are similar in histological appearance to endometrial cancer and are associated with endometriosis in approximately 10% of cases, with a synchronous separate endometrial cancer in 10–15%. They tend to be well differentiated and are associated with a better survival than high-grade serous carcinomas. Clear cell carcinomas can also arise from endometriosis and are characterized histologically by cells with abundant clear cytoplasm, much like renal cancer.

AETIOLOGY AND RISK FACTORS

Epithelial ovarian cancers include a heterogeneous group of tumours of different histological subtypes and aetiologies that affect the ovary, fallopian tube and peritoneum.

HIGH-GRADE PELVIC SEROUS CARCINOMAS

Because most high-grade pelvic serous carcinomas present with advanced disease involving the ovary, fallopian tube and peritoneal surfaces, it is often impossible to establish the anatomical site of origin. Assigning primary tumour site is of little clinical relevance anyway, as the behaviour, prognosis and treatment of these tumours are identical wherever the tumour originated. Thus, the term 'high-grade pelvic serous carcinoma' has been coined to incorporate all high-grade serous tumours arising from the ovary, fallopian tube and/or peritoneum. Data from women with germline pathogenic variants in the breast ovarian cancer syndrome (*BRCA*) gene who have undergone risk-reducing prophylactic bilateral salpingo-oophorectomy (BSO) suggest a fallopian tubal precursor lesion for high-grade pelvic serous tumours. These precursors are called serous tubal intraepithelial carcinoma lesions and they are characterized by mutations in *TP53* in secretory cells of the distal fallopian tube. As many as 30% of high-grade pelvic serous cancers are associated with somatic or germline *BRCA* mutations, with implications for treatment, prognosis and breast cancer risk.

ENDOMETRIOID, MUCINOUS, CLEAR CELL, BORDERLINE AND LOW-GRADE SEROUS OVARIAN CARCINOMAS

Inclusion cysts of the ovarian surface epithelium and endometriosis give rise to neoplasms that are distinctly ovarian in origin, and can include mucinous, endometrioid, clear cell, borderline and low-grade serous carcinomas. Endometriosis-associated ovarian cancers are usually of an endometrioid or clear cell histological subtype. The origin of these tumours involves driver mutations in *KRAS*, *PTEN*, *BRAF* and *ARID1A*, rather than *TP53*. The clinical distinction between high-grade pelvic serous carcinomas and other histological subtypes is important because of differences in disease progression, response to chemotherapy and prognosis.

BRCA1 and *BRCA2* pathogenic variant carrier status is a risk factor for high-grade serous ovarian cancer. Most ovarian cancers, however, are sporadic and risk relates to reproductive factors that are associated with hormone treatment, contraceptive use, ovulation and pregnancy (Table 14.2). The 'incessant ovulation' theory holds that the repeated damage to the ovarian surface epithelium that occurs at ovulation increases the risk of ovarian cancer. Excess gonadotrophin secretion is also thought to drive tumourigenesis through oestrogen-stimulated epithelial proliferation and subsequent malignant transformation.

Table 14.2 Risk factors in ovarian cancer

Decreased risk of ovarian cancer	Increased risk of ovarian cancer
Multiparity	Nulliparity
Combined oral contraceptive pill (RR reduced by up to 50%)	Intrauterine device (RR 1.76)
Tubal ligation	Endometriosis
Salpingectomy	Cigarette smoking (mucinous tumours only)
Hysterectomy	Hereditary predisposition (e.g. *BRCA* pathogenic variant and Lynch syndrome carriers) Obesity

RR, relative risk.

GENETIC FACTORS IN OVARIAN CANCER

It is estimated that at least 10–15% of patients with epithelial ovarian cancer have a hereditary predisposition. Women with mutations in *BRCA1* or *BRCA2* or with Lynch syndrome have an increased lifetime risk of epithelial ovarian cancer. The lifetime risk in the general population is 1 in 50 (2%). This rises to 1 in 20 (5%) if women have one family member affected by a pathogenic alteration in one of these genes, and it further increases to 40–50% if two first-degree relatives are affected. Hereditary cancers usually occur around 10 years before sporadic cancers and are associated with cancers at other sites (particularly of the breast, colon and rectum).

The most common hereditary predisposition is breast ovarian cancer syndrome, accounting for 90% of hereditary cancers. This syndrome is caused by inherited pathogenic variants affecting the tumour suppressor genes *BRCA1* (80%) and *BRCA2* (15%). *BRCA*-associated ovarian cancers are usually high-grade serous or grade 3 endometrioid tumours that present at an advanced stage and have a poor prognosis. Lynch syndrome is caused by pathogenic variants affecting one of the mismatch repair genes (*MLH1*, *MSH2*, *MSH6* or *PMS2*). It is associated with endometrial cancer and a 10–17% lifetime risk of ovarian cancer, usually of endometrioid or clear cell histological subtypes. Lynch-associated ovarian tumours tend to present at earlier stages than *BRCA*-associated tumours and have a better prognosis.

PREVENTING OVARIAN CANCER

Women who carry a germline pathogenic variant in one of the *BRCA* genes are offered risk-reducing prophylactic BSO when they have completed their families. This can usually be performed laparoscopically. Prophylactic surgery reduces the risk of ovarian cancer (by 90%), although it does not completely eliminate the risk of primary peritoneal cancer. It is important to carry out risk-reducing surgery prior to the age-related surge in ovarian cancer observed in *BRCA* pathogenic variant carriers, which is younger in patients with a variant in *BRCA1* (mid to late 30s) than in those with a *BRCA2* variant (mid to late 40s). Another suggestion for risk reduction builds on the theory that *BRCA*-associated ovarian cancers originate in the fallopian tube; therefore, performing bilateral salpingectomy in carriers in their 30s and early 40s followed by delayed oophorectomy at a later age may offset the morbidity associated with a surgical menopause while reducing their risk of cancer. This strategy has yet to be subjected to rigorous testing and its efficacy is unknown. Recent data indicate that the opportunistic removal of the fallopian tubes during hysterectomy for benign indications reduces ovarian cancer risk in women at average lifetime risk of ovarian cancer. Other procedures associated with ovarian cancer risk reduction include tubal ligation (sterilization) and hysterectomy with ovarian conservation. Chemoprevention using the combined oral contraceptive pill reduces ovarian cancer risk by up to 50% in both *BRCA* pathogenic variant carriers and women at average risk of ovarian cancer.

SCREENING

Screening using transvaginal ultrasound scan (TVUSS) and CA125 measurement has not been shown to improve survival either in the average-risk postmenopausal general population or in women with a familial predisposition to ovarian cancer. This may be because the high-grade serous tumours that are associated with *BRCA* pathogenic variant carrier status (the most lethal ovarian cancers) develop rapidly and most are at an advanced stage before they can be picked up by screening.

CLINICAL FEATURES

Most patients with ovarian cancer have symptoms; however, these symptoms are non-specific and often vague. The difficulty with clinical diagnosis is the main reason that patients with ovarian cancer present with late-stage disease (66% present with stage III disease or greater), and this has a dramatic effect on survival. The most common symptoms are:

- increased abdominal girth/bloating
- persistent pelvic and abdominal pain
- difficulty eating and feeling full quickly

Other symptoms, such as a change in bowel habit, urinary symptoms, backache, irregular bleeding and fatigue, occur frequently and any woman with persistence of these symptoms should be assessed by their general practitioner (GP).

Pelvic and abdominal examination may reveal a fixed, hard mass arising from the pelvis. The differential diagnosis of a pelvic mass includes non-epithelial ovarian cancer, tubo-ovarian abscess, endometriomas or fibroids. In combination with the presence of ascites, a diagnosis of ovarian cancer is highly likely. Early-stage ovarian cancer is difficult to diagnose due to the position of the ovary, but an adnexal mass may be palpable in a slim patient. It should be noted that fewer than 20% of adnexal masses in the premenopausal population are malignant; in the postmenopausal population, this increases to around 50%. Chest examination is important to assess for pleural fluid, and the neck and groin should be examined for enlarged lymph nodes.

DIAGNOSIS AND INVESTIGATIONS

If ovarian cancer is suspected, a TVUSS is the initial imaging modality of choice to check for pelvic pathology. A pelvic mass is characterized in terms of its size and consistency, the presence of solid elements, bilaterality, the presence of ascites and extra-ovarian disease, including peritoneal thickening and omental deposits. The investigation of any pelvic mass includes the measurement of tumour markers (**Table 14.3**). CA125 is a non-specific tumour marker that is elevated in over 80% of epithelial ovarian cancers. It is only raised in approximately 50% of

Table 14.3 Tumour markers used in ovarian cancer diagnosis and follow-up

Tumour marker	Tumour type
CA125	Epithelial ovarian cancer, (serous) borderline ovarian tumours
CA19-9	Epithelial ovarian cancer, (mucinous) borderline ovarian tumours
Inhibin	Granulosa cell tumours
hCG	Dysgerminoma, choriocarcinoma
AFP	Endodermal yolk sac, teratoma

AFP, alpha-fetoprotein; hCG, human chorionic gonadotrophin.

Table 14.4 International Federation of Gynecology and Obstetrics (FIGO) staging of ovarian cancer

Stage	FIGO definition
I	Tumour confined to ovaries
IA	Limited to one ovary, no external tumour, capsule intact, no ascites
IB	Limited to both ovaries, no external tumour, capsule intact, no ascites
IC	Either IA or IB, but tumour on surface of ovary or with capsule ruptured or with ascites positive for tumour cells
II	Tumour confined to pelvis
IIA	Extension and/or metastases to uterus or tubes
IIB	Extension to other pelvic organs
IIC	As IIA or IIB, but tumour on surface of ovary or with capsule ruptured or with ascites positive for tumour cells
III	Tumour confined to abdominal peritoneum or positive retroperitoneal or inguinal lymph nodes
IIIA	Tumour grossly limited to pelvis with negative nodes, but histologically confirmed microscopic peritoneal implants
IIIB	Abdominal implants <2 cm in diameter
IIIC	Abdominal implants >2 cm diameter or positive retroperitoneal or inguinal lymph nodes
IV	Distant metastases. Positive cytology on pleural effusion, liver parenchyma involvement, etc.

early-stage epithelial ovarian cancers and is also commonly raised in benign conditions such as pregnancy, endometriosis and alcoholic liver disease. The risk of malignancy index is calculated from menopausal status, pelvic ultrasound features and CA125 level to triage pelvic masses into those at low, intermediate and high risk of malignancy.

Pelvic pathology at intermediate or high risk of malignancy is further imaged using computed tomography (CT) and/or magnetic resonance imaging (MRI) scans. The CT scan is particularly useful for assessment of extrapelvic disease and for staging. The MRI scan helps define tissue planes and operability. Other investigations required for pre-operative clinical assessment include chest X-ray, electrocardiography, full blood count, urea and electrolytes, and liver function tests.

If the patient presents with gross ascites or pleural effusion, paracentesis or pleural aspiration may be required for symptom relief and/or diagnosis. A sample of the fluid removed is sent for cytological assessment. If primary chemotherapy is being considered (for advanced disease or in patients not fit to undergo surgery), a biopsy is needed before treatment can be given. This is taken laparoscopically or radiologically (ultrasound or CT-guided biopsy) Usually, the omentum is a good site for biopsy.

STAGING

Ovarian cancer staging is based on clinicopathological assessment and, like other gynaecological cancers, uses the International Federation of Gynecology and Obstetrics (FIGO) staging system (**Table 14.4**). Overall, 25% of patients present with stage I disease, 10% present with stage II disease, 50% present with stage III disease and 15% present with stage IV disease. Metastatic spread is by direct spread to peritoneum and other organs and by lymphatic spread to pelvic and para-aortic nodes. A high percentage of patients with advanced disease have evidence of peritoneal disease on the diaphragmatic peritoneum (**Figure 14.1**). Patients with early ovarian cancer

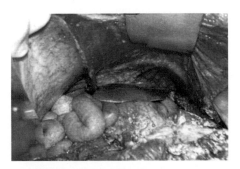

Figure 14.1 Advanced ovarian cancer illustrating diaphragmatic peritoneal disease.

(stages I and II) have up to 20% metastatic spread to lymph nodes and this rises to 60% in advanced disease (stages III and IV).

MANAGEMENT

SURGERY

Provided the patient is fit to undergo anaesthesia, surgery remains necessary for diagnosis, staging and treatment of epithelial ovarian cancer. If the patient is at high risk of ovarian cancer, the surgery should be performed by a gynaecological oncologist at a cancer centre, as this has been shown to improve outcomes. The objective of surgery is to accurately stage the disease and remove all visible tumour. This is vitally important in ovarian cancer, as many studies indicate that the most important prognostic factor is no residual disease following laparotomy.

A vertical incision is required to gain access to all areas of the abdomen. Ascites or peritoneal washings are sampled and a total abdominal hysterectomy and BSO are performed along with an omentectomy. Further debulking may be required, possibly including resection of the bowel, peritoneal stripping or splenectomy in order to remove all tumour deposits. Lymph node resection is important, particularly in early-stage disease, as studies have found occult metastatic disease in nodes in up to 25% of patients with stage I tumours. Complete debulking to no visible disease varies from 40% to 80% of cases. Often in advanced epithelial ovarian cancer, there is diffuse spread of disease throughout the abdominal cavity, making surgical clearance of tumour very difficult.

If a patient has been operated on outside a cancer centre and is found to have ovarian cancer, restaging should be offered, and this may be carried out laparoscopically. Occasionally, young patients who are found to have an early-stage epithelial ovarian cancer wish to have conservative, fertility-sparing surgery. In these cases, when disease is confined to a single ovary, unilateral salpingo-oophorectomy, omentectomy, peritoneal biopsies and pelvic/para-aortic node dissection can be performed with endometrial sampling to exclude a synchronous tumour. Fertility-sparing surgery may also be performed in patients with borderline tumours if fertility is an issue; otherwise, pelvic clearance should be performed. For all other cases, if pre-operative assessment indicates that complete debulking is unlikely to be achievable or if a patient is unfit for surgery, primary chemotherapy may be offered. If the patient responds to the chemotherapy, interval surgery can be carried out after three cycles. Recent studies indicate that this strategy may reduce post-operative morbidity but does not influence survival rates.

Following surgery, all patients with a diagnosis of epithelial ovarian cancer should be discussed at a gynaecological oncology multidisciplinary team (MDT) meeting, where their history, surgical management and histology are reviewed by gynaecological oncologists, oncologists, radiologists, pathologists and nursing staff. If the cancer has been properly staged as stage IA or B and is histologically low grade (well or moderately differentiated), chemotherapy may be withheld. The role of chemotherapy in stage IC disease is uncertain but, in practice, most patients will be offered post-operative chemotherapy as with all other stages of epithelial ovarian cancer. All non-mucinous epithelial high-grade ovarian cancer patients are eligible for germline *BRCA1* and *BRCA2* pathogenic variant testing. A positive result has important implications for the patient's treatment, as well as for the future cancer risk of the patient and their family. Parallel testing for tumour *BRCA1* and *BRCA2* mutations is indicated for advanced high-grade serous or high-grade endometrioid ovarian cancer, as it informs eligibility for systemic treatment with a type of chemotherapy called a poly (ADP-ribose) polymerase (PARP) inhibitor. Testing the tumour for homologous repair deficiency is another method of informing likely response to PARP inhibitors.

CHEMOTHERAPY

Chemotherapy can be given as primary treatment, as an adjunct following surgery or at relapse. It can be used to prolong clinical remission and survival, or for palliation. First-line treatment is usually a combination of a platinum compound with paclitaxel. Most regimes are given on an outpatient basis, 3 weeks apart for six cycles.

BOX 14.1: Surgical management of ovarian cancer

- Surgery combined with platinum-based chemotherapy is the mainstay of treatment for advanced ovarian cancer.
- The aim of surgery is complete or optimal cytoreduction (whereby <1 cm of residual macroscopic disease is left behind).
- Tumour deposits on the bowel, spleen, peritoneal surfaces and diaphragm are usually amenable to resection, while disease involving the porta hepatis and bowel mesentery may not be.
- 'Supraradical ovarian cancer surgery' is appropriate in previously well, fit patients with disseminated disease if complete cytoreduction is achievable; it is associated with perioperative morbidity and mortality, and patients must be carefully counselled.
- Three cycles of neoadjuvant chemotherapy followed by interval debulking surgery is not inferior to upfront surgery and has been shown to be associated with less morbidity.

Platinum compounds are the most effective chemotherapeutic agents in ovarian cancer. They are heavy metal agents that cause cross linkage of deoxyribonucleic acid (DNA) strands, thus arresting cell replication. Carboplatin is now the main platinum compound used, as it is less nephrotoxic and causes less nausea than cisplatin, but is equally effective. The dose of carboplatin is calculated according to the glomerular filtration rate using the area under the curve. *BRCA*-associated ovarian cancers are particularly sensitive to platinum-based chemotherapy in the primary treatment setting.

Paclitaxel is derived from the bark of the Pacific yew and works by causing microtubular damage to the cell. This prevents replication and cell division. Pre-emptive steroids are given due to high-sensitivity reactions; side effects of peripheral neuropathy, neutropenia and myalgia are common and dose-dependent. Paclitaxel causes total loss of all body hair, irrespective of dose.

Following completion of carboplatin and paclitaxel chemotherapy, patients have a further CT scan to assess their response to treatment. This scan can be used for comparison in the future if there is clinical or biochemical evidence of recurrence.

Bevacizumab, a monoclonal antibody against vascular endothelial growth factor, inhibits angiogenesis. It has been shown to be clinically effective at improving progression-free survival when given orally in combination with carboplatin and paclitaxel and for 12–15 months thereafter, as maintenance therapy, in advanced ovarian cancer. The side effect profile of this drug includes hypertension, delayed wound healing, gastrointestinal perforation and arterial thromboembolic events.

Olaparib, a PARP inhibitor, is a targeted treatment for *BRCA*-mutated ovarian cancer. It induces 'synthetic lethality', causing tumour cell death, by blocking the repair of damaged DNA in homologous repair deficiency tumours. Olaparib is given orally as maintenance therapy following successful treatment with carboplatin and paclitaxel, where it reduces the risk of recurrence. PARP inhibitors are generally well tolerated, with some patients experiencing mild side effects such as nausea, loss of appetite and fatigue; serious neutropenia and acute myeloid leukaemia are uncommon toxicities.

The follow-up of patients includes clinical examination and CA125 measurement. Studies have shown that levels of CA125 start to rise prior to the onset of clinical evidence of disease recurrence; however, treating isolated rising CA125 levels does not improve survival. When disease recurs, treatment is largely palliative. If the duration of remission is more than 6 months, carboplatin may be used again; otherwise taxol can be given or other chemotherapy agents, such as topotecan or liposomal doxyrubicin.

PROGNOSIS

Survival depends on stage at presentation, volume of disease following surgery and the histological grade of tumour. The overall 5-year survival from ovarian cancer is 46% in the UK (2010–2011). The figures have improved due to the widespread introduction of centralized MDT care. Survival is stage dependent: overall, 5-year survival for stage I disease is over 90%, while it is 30% for stage III disease. **Table 14.5** shows the 5-year survival rates by stage at diagnosis (see also **Box 14.2** 'Prognostic factors in ovarian cancer').

Table 14.5 Ovarian cancer survival by stage at diagnosis

FIGO stage	5-year survival (%)
I	80–90
II	65–70
III	30–50
IV	15

FIGO, International Federation of Gynecology and Obstetrics.

BOX 14.2: Prognostic factors in ovarian cancer

- Stage of disease
- Volume of residual disease after surgery
- Histological type and grade of tumour
- Age at presentation

PRIMARY PERITONEAL CARCINOMA

Primary peritoneal carcinoma is a high-grade pelvic serous carcinoma. It is histologically indistinct from tumours arising from the fallopian tube or ovary. There are, however, morphological differences between the two groups based on clinical findings at laparotomy. Criteria for diagnosis include:

- normal-sized or slightly bulky ovaries
- more extra-ovarian disease than ovarian disease
- low volume peritoneal disease

The clinical behaviour, prognosis and treatment for this type of carcinoma are the same as for other high-grade pelvic serous carcinomas, although there is a trend towards using primary chemotherapy, as complete surgical debulking is difficult.

SEX CORD STROMAL TUMOURS

These tumours account for approximately 10% of ovarian tumours, but almost 90% of all functional (i.e. hormone-producing) tumours. Generally, they are tumours of low malignant potential with a good long-term prognosis. Some morbidity may arise from the oestrogen (granulosa, theca or Sertoli cell) or androgen production (Sertoli–Leydig or steroid cell) characteristic of these tumours, resulting in precocious puberty, abnormal menstrual bleeding and an increased risk of endometrial cancer. The peak incidence is around the age of the menopause, although juvenile granulosa cell tumour usually presents in those under 10 years of age, causing precocious puberty. Overall, granulosa cell tumours are the most common subtype, accounting for over 70% of sex cord stromal tumours.

CLINICAL FEATURES

A significant percentage of these tumours present with manifestations of their hormone production, typically irregular menstrual bleeding, postmenopausal bleeding or precocious puberty in young people. Granulosa cell tumours may present as a large pelvic mass or with pain due to torsion/haemorrhage.

Sertoli–Leydig cell tumours produce androgens in over 50% of cases. Patients present with a pelvic mass and signs of virilization. Common symptoms are amenorrhoea, deep voice and hirsutism. Occasionally, this group of tumours produce oestrogen and rarely renin, causing hypertension.

Most sex cord stromal tumours present as unilateral ovarian masses, measuring up to 15 cm in diameter. Macroscopically, the tumour is often solid with areas of haemorrhage, and the cut surface may be yellow due to high levels of steroid production.

Granulosa cell tumours produce inhibin, which can be used for follow-up surveillance; levels often rise prior to clinical detection of recurrence.

TREATMENT

Treatment is based on the patient's age and wish to preserve fertility. If the patient is young, unilateral salpingo-oophorectomy, endometrial sampling and staging is sufficient in early-stage disease. In the older group, full surgical staging is recommended. Granulosa cell tumours can recur many years after initial presentation, and long-term follow-up is required. Recurrence is usually well defined and surgery is the mainstay of treatment, as there is no effective chemotherapy regime.

GERM CELL TUMOURS

Malignant germ cell tumours occur mainly in young women and account for approximately 10% of ovarian tumours. They are derived from primordial germ cells within the ovary and, because of this, may contain any cell type. The emphasis of management is based mainly on fertility-preserving surgery and chemotherapy.

The most common presenting symptom is a pelvic mass; 10% present acutely with torsion or haemorrhage and, due to the age incidence, some present during pregnancy. Seventy per cent of germ cell tumours are stage I; spread is by lymphatics or blood.

Dysgerminomas account for 50% of all germ cell tumours. They are bilateral in 20% of cases and occasionally secrete human chorionic gonadotrophin (hCG).

Endodermal sinus yolk sac tumours are the second most common germ cell tumours, accounting for 15% of the total. They are rarely bilateral and secrete alpha-fetoprotein (AFP). They present with a large solid mass that often causes acute symptoms with torsion or rupture. Spread of endodermal sinus tumours is a late event and is usually to the lungs.

Immature teratomas account for 15–20% of malignant germ cell tumours and about 1% of all teratomas. They are classified as mature or immature depending on the grading of neural tissue present. About one-third of teratomas secrete AFP. Mature teratomas are also known as dermoid cysts and are benign. Occasionally, there can be malignant transformation within a mature teratoma; the most common cell type to transform is epithelial, usually squamous cell carcinoma.

Non-gestational choriocarcinomas are very rare, usually presenting in young women with irregular bleeding and very high levels of hCG.

CLINICAL FEATURES

Germ cell tumours should be suspected if a young woman presents with a large solid ovarian mass that is rapidly growing. Tumour markers, as detailed in **Table 14.3**, are measured pre-operatively, as this may influence the need for post-operative chemotherapy. MRI is helpful to assess morphology, particularly within teratomas. CT scanning of the abdomen allows assessment of the liver and lymph nodes. All patients should have a chest X-ray to exclude pulmonary metastases.

TREATMENT

Surgery is tailored to suit the patient. As most women presenting with malignant germ cell tumours are of reproductive age, fertility-sparing treatment may be preferred. An exploratory laparotomy is performed to remove the tumour and assess contralateral spread to the other ovary (20% in dysgerminoma). If there is a cyst present on the other ovary, this should be removed. Careful inspection of the abdominal cavity is required, with peritoneal biopsies and sampling of any enlarged pelvic or para-aortic nodes performed. If metastatic disease is found, it should be debulked at surgery. Intraoperative frozen sections may be required to assess nodal status.

Post-operative chemotherapy depends on the stage of disease. Stage I dysgerminomas and low-grade teratomas are treated by surgery alone and the 5-year survival exceeds 90%. For patients with disease outside the ovary, chemotherapy is given.

🔑 KEY LEARNING POINTS

- Ovarian cancer tends to present late, with advanced disease because symptoms are non-specific.
- Screening has not proven effective using tumour markers or TVUSS.
- Treatment is based on removing all tumour surgically, combined with platinum-based chemotherapy.
- Prognosis is stage-dependent: stage I disease has a 80–90% 5-year survival, whereas stage III disease has a 30% 5-year survival.
- Sex cord stromal tumours usually present with endocrine effects due to excess secretion of oestrogen or androgens.
- Germ cell tumours affect young women and are often cured by fertility-preserving surgery.

The most common regime used is a combination of bleomycin, etoposide and cisplatin, given as a course of three to four treatments 3 weeks apart. This regime gives long-term cure rates of over 90% and also preserves fertility if required.

If the patient has recurrent disease, 90% will usually present in the first year following diagnosis; salvage chemotherapy has very good success rates.

FURTHER READING

Baker-Rand H, Edey K (2021). Nonepithelial ovarian cancers. *Obstetrician & Gynaecologist*, 23: 177–186.

Lheureux S, Gourley C, Vergote I, Oza AM (2019). Epithelial ovarian cancer. *Lancet*, 393(10177): 1240–1253.

SELF-ASSESSMENT

For interactive SBAs and EMQs relating to this chapter, visit www.routledge.com/cw/crosbie.

CASE HISTORY 1

Mrs L is a 62-year-old woman who presents to the gynaecology clinic with non-specific abdominal pain, a change in bowel habit and bloating. Her GP arranged a pelvic ultrasound scan, which found bilateral complex solid/cystic pelvic masses, large volume ascites and omental caking.

A What is the most likely diagnosis?
B What are the key points in the examination and investigation?
C Mrs L is found to have stage III high-grade serous ovarian cancer. How would you manage her?

ANSWERS

A The symptoms associated with ovarian cancer are non-specific, and doctors must maintain a high index of suspicion when faced with persistent symptoms of bloating, irritable bowel and abdominal pain. The scan report shows features suggestive of advanced ovarian cancer (solid/cystic pelvic masses, ascites and extra-ovarian disease).

B Pelvic examination may reveal hard, fixed pelvic masses, and free fluid in the abdomen (ascites) is demonstrated by shifting dullness and/or a fluid thrill. Investigations include serum CA125 levels. If the tumour secretes CA125, this can be used as a non-invasive test to monitor treatment response and subsequently screen for recurrent disease. A CT scan is needed to stage the disease and plan treatment. If there is a pleural effusion, this is generally tapped and a sample sent for cytological assessment. Sometimes there is very large-volume ascites and draining this can improve symptoms in the short term and can facilitate omental biopsy, which is more difficult when there is a lot of fluid around.

C Treatment for most patients with advanced ovarian cancer is determined following discussion at the gynaecological oncology MDT meeting. If Mrs L is fit for surgery and pre-operative investigations suggest that complete tumour debulking is achievable, upfront surgery followed by six cycles of adjuvant carboplatin and paclitaxel chemotherapy is generally preferred. Surgery involves a midline laparotomy, total hysterectomy (removal of uterus and cervix) and BSO (removal of both fallopian tubes and ovaries), omentectomy, pelvic lymphadenectomy and debulking of any extra-ovarian tumour deposits. Sometimes surgery is avoided in the primary setting because the disease is not completely resectable and, in this scenario, three cycles of neoadjuvant chemotherapy are given and a restaging CT scan performed to decide whether surgery is now likely to remove all tumour deposits. If surgery takes place, the patient receives a further three cycles of chemotherapy afterwards.

CASE HISTORY 2

A 58-year-old woman complains of new onset lower abdominal pain. Her GP refers her for a pelvic ultrasound scan to exclude gynaecological pathology. The scan shows a 5 cm simple cyst on her left ovary.

A What is the most likely diagnosis?
B What are the key points in the examination and investigation?
C How would you manage her?

ANSWERS

A A simple ovarian cyst is usually a benign finding. It is inconsequential for most patients but can sometimes rupture, bleed or tort, causing acute pain.

B Examination may reveal a fullness in the left adnexa that is tender to palpation. Sinister features on the ultrasound scan include bilateral ovarian cysts, papillary projections, solid components, free fluid in the pelvis and enlarged pelvic lymph nodes. A CA125 level is measured to further exclude sinister pathology.

C If the ultrasound scan shows no suspicious features and the CA125 level is within normal limits (<35 U/mL), the patient is managed by active surveillance, including a repeat pelvic ultrasound scan and CA125 test in 4 months. If the scan and CA125 level shows no interval change, this is a benign cyst. If the scan shows increasing complexity of the cyst and a rising CA125 level, this may be an indication for surgery to remove the ipsilateral fallopian tube and ovary to exclude early ovarian cancer.

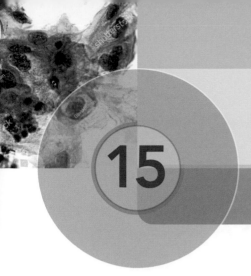

15

Malignant disease of the uterus

EMMA J CROSBIE

Learning Objectives

- Describe the classification of uterine malignancy.
- Learn how malignant disease of the uterus presents.
- Describe which investigations are needed for patients with suspected endometrial cancer.
- Know the International Federation of Gynecology and Obstetrics staging of endometrial cancer.
- Understand how endometrial cancer is managed.

INTRODUCTION

Uterine cancer refers to tumours that arise from the uterine corpus (body of the uterus). By far the most common are endometrial tumours that originate from the lining of the uterine cavity (endometrium). Tumours arising from the myometrium (sarcomas) are rare.

ENDOMETRIAL CANCER

INCIDENCE

Endometrial cancer is the most common gynaecological malignancy in high-income countries with 417,000 new diagnoses globally in 2020. In the UK, the lifetime risk of developing endometrial cancer is approximately 1 in 36. The mean age of diagnosis is 62 years, although cancers can be diagnosed in women throughout their reproductive life. Approximately 15% of endometrial cancers occur

before the menopause. The incidence of endometrial cancer has risen steadily over the past 30 years as a consequence of the ageing population, the trend away from hysterectomy for benign gynaecological disease and the obesity epidemic.

CLASSIFICATION

Endometrial cancer usually arises from the glandular component of the endometrium and stromal tumours are exceedingly rare. Endometrial cancers have historically been classified as type 1 or type 2, depending on their histological subtype (**Figure 15.1**) and grade; grade 1 is low grade and grade 3 is high grade (mostly abnormal cells). Type 1 tumours are low-grade endometrioid adenocarcinomas that are oestrogen driven and arise from a background of endometrial hyperplasia. Type 2 tumours include high-grade serous, clear cell and carcinosarcoma histological subtypes and arise from an atrophic endometrium. A new classification system, based on data from The Cancer Genome Atlas, categorizes endometrial tumours into

10.1201/9781003218036-15

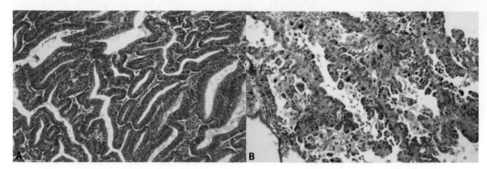

Figure 15.1 Histological comparison of endometrioid adenocarcinoma (**A**) and serous adenocarcinoma (**B**) of the endometrium.

one of four subgroups based on their molecular profile. Molecular classification offers more accurate risk stratification than histological subtype alone and is increasingly being used to guide treatment and discussions about prognosis.

AETIOLOGY

The risk factors for type 1 endometrial cancer are well established (**Table 15.1**). Most of these reflect an increased lifetime exposure to oestrogen. Oestrogen causes endometrial cells to proliferate when it is unopposed by progesterone. Hyperoestrogenic states

Table 15.1 Risk and protective factors for type 1 endometrial cancer

Factors that increase endometrial cancer risk	Factors that protect against endometrial cancer
Obesity	Hysterectomy
Type 2 diabetes	Combined oral contraceptive pill
Nulliparity	Progestin-based contraceptives, including injectables
Late menopause (>52 years)	Intrauterine device, including Cu-IUD and LNG-IUS
Tamoxifen therapy	Pregnancy
Family history of colorectal and endometrial cancer	Healthy bodyweight and regular exercise

Cu-IUD, copper intrauterine device; LNG-IUS, levonorgestrel intrauterine system.

increase endometrial cancer risk, while cyclical or continuous progestin-containing hormone treatments reduce risk. Obesity increases endometrial cancer risk because it is associated with anovulatory menstrual cycles and subfertility. Furthermore, the aromatization of androgens to oestrogen by adipose tissue provides a continuous postmenopausal supply of oestrogen. Besides oestrogen, insulin and insulin-like growth factor stimulate endometrial proliferation, which is why endometrial cancer is more common in those with type 2 diabetes mellitus. Other risk factors include treatment with tamoxifen – a selective oestrogen receptor modulator used to prevent and treat breast cancer, which is antioestrogenic in the breast but stimulatory in the endometrium. Hereditary predisposition to endometrial cancer is increasingly appreciated, as genetic services and tests are being developed. The most common association is with Lynch syndrome, an autosomal dominant condition caused by pathogenic variants affecting one of the mismatch repair genes: *MLH1*, *MSH2*, *MSH6* or, less commonly, *PMS2*. The lifetime risk of endometrial cancer in women with Lynch syndrome is 40–60%, and approximately 3% of endometrial cancers are caused by Lynch syndrome. Other tumour associations in Lynch syndrome include colorectal, ovarian and urothelial tumours. The risk factors for type 2 endometrial cancer are less well understood.

PREVENTION

Maintaining a healthy bodyweight, regular physical exercise, hormonal contraceptives and intrauterine devices reduce endometrial cancer risk (**Table 15.1**). Women with Lynch syndrome are offered prophylactic hysterectomy following completion of childbearing. Aspirin is protective against cancer in Lynch syndrome.

SCREENING

There is currently no evidence to support screening for endometrial cancer in high-risk groups or the general population.

CLINICAL FEATURES

Endometrial cancer usually presents at an early stage following the onset of postmenopausal bleeding (PMB) (see **Chapter 4**). Approximately 5–10% of patients with PMB have an underlying gynaecological malignancy and this 'red flag' symptom should always prompt investigation. Abnormal bleeding is the most common presenting complaint in the premenopausal population too, who variously complain of heavy, irregular or intermenstrual bleeding. Patients at more advanced stages of disease occasionally present with pelvic pain, urinary or bowel dysfunction, or respiratory symptoms.

Sometimes, endometrial cancer is picked up incidentally at cervical screening with 'abnormal glandular cytology'. This opportunity is lost with changes to cervical screening programmes that reserve cytological examination for human papillomavirus (HPV)-positive cervical samples. Signs of endometrial cancer include bleeding from the cervical os on speculum examination and a bulky uterus

BOX 15.1: Postmenopausal bleeding

- PMB is a 'red flag' symptom for gynaecological cancer and should always be taken seriously.
- Careful inspection of the external genitalia followed by speculum examination will exclude vulval, vaginal and cervical cancer as the underlying cause.
- Physical examination may be normal in patients with endometrial cancer, which can only be excluded by transvaginal ultrasound scan (TVUSS), hysteroscopy and/or endometrial biopsy.
- Benign causes of PMB include unscheduled bleeding on hormone replacement therapy and vaginal atrophy.

on bimanual pelvic examination. In most patients with endometrial cancer, however, pelvic examination is completely normal.

DIAGNOSIS AND INVESTIGATION OF POSTMENOPAUSAL BLEEDING

Many hospitals have a one-stop clinic dedicated to the urgent investigation of patients with PMB. The mainstays of diagnosis are TVUSS, hysteroscopy and endometrial biopsy. TVUSS allows a quick and accurate assessment of endometrial thickness (**Figure 15.2**). If the endometrium measures less than 4 mm, cancer is very unlikely and further investigation is not needed. Any measurement greater than this requires further evaluation by hysteroscopy and/or biopsy.

Hysteroscopy is performed in the outpatient setting where possible. A general anaesthetic is required in patients with cervical stenosis, when hysteroscopy is poorly tolerated or upon patient request. A thin scope is passed into the uterine cavity, allowing visualization of the endometrium and directed biopsy of abnormal areas (**Figure 15.3**). In addition, an endometrial sampler is used for histological assessment of the endometrium as described in **Chapter 2**.

The histology report describes the type (endometrioid or other histological subtype) and grade of tumour. Atypical hyperplasia is a premalignant condition that frequently coexists with low-grade endometrioid tumours of the endometrium. The risk of progression to endometrial cancer is 25–50%. Immunohistochemistry (p53 and mismatch repair [MMR]) and next-generation sequencing (for the DNA polymerase epsilon catalytic subunit [*POLE*]

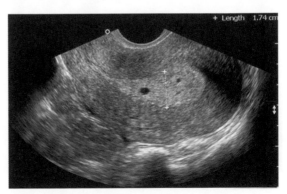

Figure 15.2 Transvaginal ultrasound scan of the uterus showing thickened endometrium.

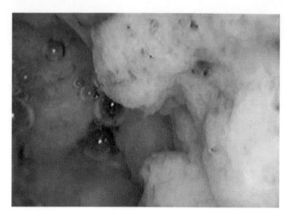

Figure 15.3 Hysteroscopic picture of endometrial carcinoma.

gene) enables the molecular classification of tumours. MMR-deficient tumours are a feature of Lynch syndrome-associated endometrial cancer and prompt genetic counselling. Diagnosing Lynch syndrome enables a woman to protect themselves and their family members from future cancers through colonoscopic surveillance and aspirin chemoprevention.

STAGING

The extent of disease (stage) is determined by magnetic resonance imaging (MRI) scan (**Figure 15.4**),

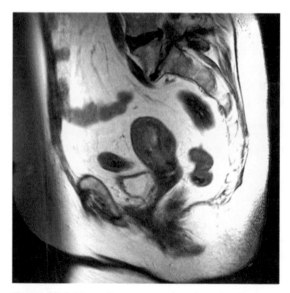

Figure 15.4 Magnetic resonance imaging of stage IB endometrial carcinoma.

Table 15.2 International Federation of Gynecology and Obstetrics (FIGO) staging of carcinoma of the uterus

FIGO stage	Definition
I	Confined to uterus
IA	Less than 50% myometrial invasion
IB	More than 50% myometrial invasion
II	Tumour invading cervical stroma
III	Local and/or regional spread of tumour
IIIA	Invades uterine serosa
IIIB	Invades vagina and/or parametrium
IIIC	Metastases to pelvic and/or para-aortic nodes
IV	Tumour invades bladder and/or bowel and/or distant metastases

and International Federation of Gynecology and Obstetrics staging uses this information (**Table 15.2**). Patients with high-grade tumours undergo a computed tomography scan of the chest, abdomen

---

BOX 15.2: Molecular classification of endometrial cancer into four groups

1. **p53-abnormal.** These tumours have the poorest prognosis and may benefit most from adjuvant chemotherapy. Serous, clear cell and carcinosarcoma histological subtypes are usually p53-abnormal, but endometrioid tumours may also fall into this group.

2. *POLE*-mutant. These tumours have exceedingly good clinical outcomes, with very low recurrence rates and <1% disease-specific mortality.

3. **MMR-deficient.** These tumours are characterized by a defective MMR system; around 10% of MMR-deficient tumours are associated with Lynch syndrome. They have an intermediate, stage-dependent prognosis.

4. **No specific molecular profile.** This is a diagnosis of exclusion and consists mostly of hormone receptor-positive endometrioid tumours with an intermediate to excellent prognosis.

and pelvis to exclude distant metastases. In the UK, patients with low-grade stage IA endometrial tumours are offered surgery at their local hospital. Patients with high-grade tumours or stage IB or above undergo surgery in a cancer centre, as this has been shown to improve outcomes.

MANAGEMENT

SURGERY

Surgery is the mainstay of treatment for endometrial cancer and involves total hysterectomy and removal of both fallopian tubes and ovaries – bilateral sal-pingo-oophorectomy (BSO) (**Figure 15.5**). This can be performed via open or minimally invasive surgery (laparoscopic or robotic), with equivalent oncological outcomes. Minimally invasive surgery offers fewer post-operative complications and a

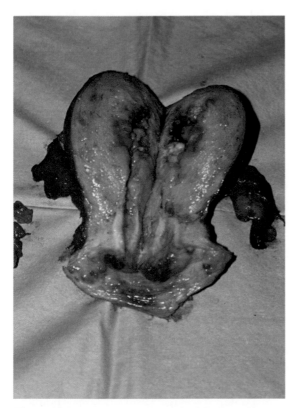

Figure 15.5 Bisected uterus, cervix, fallopian tubes and ovaries removed at hysterectomy for endometrial cancer.

faster return to normal activities than open surgery, and is the preferred approach. If the tumour has high-risk features, many centres perform pelvic and para-aortic node dissection because nodal disease is seen in one-third of patients. Nodal dissection is important for staging but does not improve survival outcomes and its practice increases perioperative morbidity rates. Sentinel lymph node biopsy enables visualization of the 'sentinel' or first node in the lymph node basin to receive lymphatic drainage from a tumour. If the sentinel lymph node is negative for metastatic disease, the other lymph nodes must be negative too. This technique is poised to replace full nodal dissection, as it provides the same staging information but offers far lower perioperative risks.

ADJUVANT TREATMENT

Adjuvant treatment is given after surgery for patients at a high or an intermediate risk of relapse. Post-operative radiotherapy reduces local recurrence but does not improve overall survival. Strategies include radiotherapy delivered directly to the vaginal vault via radioactive inserts (brachytherapy) for local disease, or brachytherapy combined with external beam pelvic radiotherapy for locally advanced disease (stage III). Chemotherapy is given for high-risk tumours and may be particularly beneficial for p53-abnormal tumours, for which the risk of relapse is highest.

HORMONE THERAPY

Some patients are not fit for surgery and others wish to avoid it for fertility-sparing reasons. Treatment with high-dose oral or intrauterine progestin is successful for some patients with atypical hyperplasia and low-grade stage IA endometrial tumours, but relapse rates are high.

ADVANCED DISEASE

Advanced and recurrent disease is treated with surgery, chemotherapy, radiotherapy and/or hormone therapy, depending on its extent, location and various clinico-pathological features, but outcomes are

Table 15.3 5-year survival rate for endometrial cancer

Stage	5-year survival (%)
I	92
II	74
III	48
IV	15

typically poor. New systemic therapies, targeted to the molecular profile of the tumour, offer improved outcomes. Immune checkpoint inhibitors (e.g. dostarlimab), which overcome tumour resistance to T-cell-mediated killing, are licensed for use in advanced or recurrent MMR-deficient endometrial cancers.

PROGNOSIS

The overall 5-year survival rate for endometrial cancer is 76%, although this varies with histological subtype, grade and stage of tumour (**Table 15.3**). Adverse prognostic features include advanced age, grade 3 tumours, non-endometrioid histological subtype, p53-abnormal tumour, deep myometrial invasion, lymphovascular space invasion, nodal involvement and distant metastases.

SARCOMAS OF THE UTERUS

These are rare, accounting for approximately 5% of all uterine cancers. They include pure sarcomas and heterologous sarcomas.

PURE SARCOMAS

These include leiomyosarcomas and endometrial stromal sarcomas. Leiomyosarcomas are rare tumours of the myometrium. Rarely (in 0.75% of cases), they are associated with malignant transformation of benign fibroids and present with a rapidly growing pelvic mass and pain. Pre-operative diagnosis is difficult, but may be aided by MRI, which can delineate areas of necrosis within the fibroid, suggestive of malignant change. The uterus is enlarged and soft on palpation. Surgery is the main treatment and adjuvant treatment may be considered if the mitotic count is high (above 10 mitoses per high-powered field). Metastatic spread is usually vascular to distant sites, such as the lung and brain. Endometrial stromal sarcomas occur in perimenopausal patients presenting with irregular bleeding and a soft, enlarged uterus. The majority are low grade, and surgery is the main treatment.

HETEROLOGOUS SARCOMAS

This rare group of tumours consists of sarcomatous tissue not usually found in the uterus, such as striated muscle, bone or cartilage. The most common is rhabdomyosarcoma, which may present in children as a grape-like mass protruding from the cervix with a watery discharge. Histology reveals primitive rhabdomyoblasts. Recurrence rates are high with distant metastases.

- Endometrial cancer is the most common gynaecological malignancy in the UK.
- Obesity and other hyperoestrogenic states play a major aetiological role.
- The majority of patients present with PMB; however, 15% of cases occur in premenopausal women.
- 5–10% of women with PMB will have an underlying gynaecological malignancy.
- Endometrial biopsy and/or hysteroscopy is the gold standard for diagnosis, while MRI defines the extent of disease.
- Total hysterectomy and BSO is the treatment of choice for most patients.
- The majority of cancers present with stage I disease and the overall 5-year survival is 76%.
- Non-endometrioid histology, p53-abnormal, high-grade and advanced stage disease are predictive of the poorest outcomes.

FURTHER READING

Crosbie EJ, Kitson SJ, McAlpine JN, Mukhopadhyay A, Powell ME, Singh N (2022). Endometrial cancer. *Lancet*, 399: 1412–1428.

Jones E, O'Flynn H, Njoku K, Crosbie EJ (2021). Detecting endometrial cancer. *Obstetrician & Gynaecologist*, 23: 103–112.

Kitson S, Crosbie, EJ (2019). Endometrial cancer and obesity. *Obstetrician & Gynaecologist*, 21: 237–245.

Ryan NA, McMahon RF, Ramchander NC, Seif MW, Evans DG, Crosbie EJ (2021). Lynch syndrome for the gynaecologist. *Obstetrician & Gynaecologist*, 23(1): 9–20.

SELF-ASSESSMENT

For interactive SBAs and EMQs relating to this chapter, visit www.routledge.com/cw/crosbie.

CASE HISTORY 1

Mrs P is a 65-year-old woman who presents to the gynaecology clinic with PMB. She has a body mass index of 40 kg/m² and has type 2 diabetes mellitus. She has no children, has never taken hormone replacement therapy and does not smoke. Her cervical screening results have always been normal.

A What is the most likely diagnosis?
B What are the key points in the examination and investigation?
C Mrs P is found to have a grade 1 stage IA endometrioid adenocarcinoma. How would you manage her?

ANSWERS

A PMB is a red flag symptom for gynaecological cancer. Cancers of the endometrium, cervix, vagina and vulva all present with abnormal bleeding. Mrs P's medical history and risk factor profile make endometrial cancer the most likely malignant diagnosis; however, benign causes of PMB are more common and often no cause can be found.

B Mrs P has several risk factors for endometrial cancer, including obesity, type 2 diabetes and nulliparity. A normal, up-to-date cervical screening history makes cancer of the cervix extremely unlikely. Cancers of the vulva, vagina and cervix should be excluded by careful inspection. Blood coming from the cervical os indicates uterine bleeding. Bimanual pelvic examination may find a bulky uterus or pelvic mass, although a normal examination does not exclude endometrial cancer. Investigation includes TVUSS to measure endometrial thickness, followed by hysteroscopy and/or endometrial biopsy if endometrial thickness exceeds 4 mm in a postmenopausal patient.

C Treatment for most patients with endometrial cancer involves total hysterectomy (removal of uterus and cervix) and BSO (removal of both

(Contd.)

(Contd.)

fallopian tubes and ovaries). It is important to assess fitness for anaesthetic, as many patients with endometrial cancer have comorbidities, including obesity, type 2 diabetes, hypertension, cardiovascular disease, sleep apnoea and poor mobility, which limit their ability to tolerate general anaesthesia. Laparoscopic surgery is now the standard of care for patients with endometrial cancer, but this may be difficult to achieve in individuals with extreme obesity who cannot tolerate the prolonged head-down tilt required or in whom previous abdominal surgery has resulted in adhesions and scarring. All patients with endometrial cancer should be discussed at the central gynaecological oncology multidisciplinary team meeting. Patients with low-grade early-stage disease may undergo surgery in their local hospital, while high-risk cases are referred centrally for care. All women are offered support from gynaecological oncology clinical nurse specialists or Macmillan nurses, who provide a single point of contact for continuity of care as well as written information, contact phone numbers and emotional support. Adjuvant radiotherapy and/or chemotherapy is offered based on high-risk pathological features, including high-grade, non-endometrioid histology, p53-abnormal and advanced stage disease.

CASE HISTORY 2

Ms L is a 35-year-old woman with Lynch syndrome (*MSH2* pathogenic variant carrier). She is worried about her risk of gynaecological cancer and comes to the clinic to discuss her options.

A What is her lifetime risk of endometrial cancer?
B What can she do to reduce her risk of endometrial cancer?
C Can she prevent her children from inheriting her *MSH2* pathogenic variant?

ANSWERS

A A woman with Lynch syndrome has a lifetime risk of endometrial cancer of up to 50% depending on the MMR gene involved. *MSH2* carries the highest risk of endometrial cancer of all of the MMR genes.

B Women with Lynch syndrome can reduce their endometrial cancer risk by undergoing a hysterectomy once their family is complete. Aspirin reduces the risk of cancer in Lynch syndrome. Hormonal contraceptives may be protective, particularly the combined oral contraceptive pill and the LNG-IUS. Maintaining a healthy bodyweight, taking regular exercise and avoiding carcinogens (e.g. smoking and alcohol) may also be protective against endometrial cancer in Lynch syndrome.

C Pre-implantation genetic testing can be used to prevent individuals passing serious inherited disease onto their children. Embryos can be screened for the genetic abnormality and only those that lack the specific MMR pathogenic variant used in a subsequent in vitro fertilization cycle.

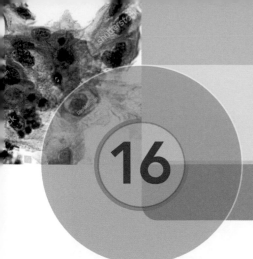

16

Premalignant and malignant disease of the lower genital tract

EMMA J CROSBIE

Learning Objectives
- Understand the pathogenesis of lower genital tract malignancy.
- Understand primary prevention of cervical cancer through human papillomavirus (HPV) vaccination and cervical screening.
- Understand the diagnosis, International Federation of Gynecology and Obstetrics staging, and management of premalignant and malignant disease of the lower genital tract, including the cervix, vagina and vulva.

INTRODUCTION

Cancer of the cervix is relatively uncommon in high-income countries due to screening. Cancers of the vagina and vulva are far less common than cervical cancer. This chapter covers premalignant and malignant disease of the lower genital tract.

PREMALIGNANT DISEASE OF THE CERVIX

Cervical screening reduces diagnoses and deaths from cervical cancer. It has been estimated that cervical screening prevents around 2,000 deaths every year in the UK alone.

EPIDEMIOLOGY AND AETIOLOGY

Cervical cancer is caused by persistent high-risk human papillomavirus (HPV) infection. HPV is a small, double-stranded deoxyribonucleic acid (DNA) virus of which there are more than 100 different types. These are classified as low-risk or high-risk types, depending on their ability to cause cancer. Low-risk HPV 6 and 11 cause benign warts, while 13 high-risk HPV types, including HPV 16, 18, 31, 33 and 45, cause cervical cancer. HPV infection is spread during sexual intercourse. Infection is very common following the onset of sexual activity and up to 80% of adults show serological evidence of previous infection. Infection is usually transient and of no clinical consequence, but a minority of individuals develop a persistent genital infection that predisposes them

10.1201/9781003218036-16

to premalignant and malignant change (see the section 'Natural history of cervical intraepithelial neoplasia' later in this chapter). Smoking reduces the efficiency with which the virus is cleared by the immune system and increases the risk of persistent infection. Patients who are immunocompromised – for example those with human immunodeficiency virus (HIV) and transplant recipients on long-term immunosuppressive therapy – are particularly at risk of premalignant and malignant disease of the cervix.

PATHOPHYSIOLOGY

The tubular cervix is composed of stromal tissue covered by squamous epithelium in the vagina (ecto-cervix) and columnar epithelium within the cervical canal (endocervix). The endocervix contains many deep folds, called crypts, that are lined by columnar epithelium. The meeting of the two types of epithelium is called the squamocolumnar junction (SCJ) and this is usually on the ectocervix (**Figure 16.1**). The position of the SCJ varies throughout life. In children, it lies at the external cervical os; at puberty, it extends outwards onto the ectocervix as the cervix enlarges; and, in adult life, it returns to the external cervical os through the process of metaplasia, which is the physiological transformation of columnar epithelium to squamous epithelium. The so-called transformation zone is defined as the area between the original SCJ and the current SCJ where the epithelium changes from columnar to squamous epithelium over time. Sometimes, the columnar epithelium is covered by squamous epithelium, leading to retention of mucus – this is called a Nabothian follicle (**Figure 16.2**). The transformation zone is the site where premalignancy and malignancy develop.

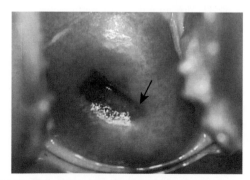

Figure 16.1 Normal cervix with transformation zone.

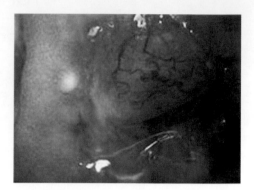

Figure 16.2 Normal cervix with Nabothian follicle.

When HPV infection persists in certain individuals, it triggers an oncogenic process in the region of the transformation zone where metaplasia occurs. Integration of HPV DNA into the basal epithelial cells leads to immortalization and rapid cellular turnover. This disordered immaturity within the epithelium is called cervical intraepithelial neoplasia (CIN) and is truly an intraepithelial condition (cancer is diagnosed when this process breaks the basement membrane). Immature cells are hyperchromatic with large nuclei, minimal cytoplasm and abnormal mitotic figures. CIN is classified as either low-grade (CIN 1) or high-grade disease (CIN 2 and 3), depending on whether the abnormal cells are seen in the bottom third (CIN 1), two-thirds (CIN 2) or full thickness (CIN 3) of the cervical epithelium.

NATURAL HISTORY OF CERVICAL INTRAEPITHELIAL NEOPLASIA

Regression and progression of CIN may occur. Spontaneous regression of low-grade disease is not uncommon and is most likely a consequence of the patient's own cell-mediated immunity. This is the argument for observational follow-up in patients with low-grade abnormalities. High-grade disease is less likely to regress spontaneously and requires treatment, as there is a risk of progression to cancer. If left untreated, around 20% of patients with high-grade abnormalities develop cancer of the cervix. Reasons for progression are not fully understood but include high-risk HPV types, reduced host immunity and smoking. There is a convincing link between CIN and cancer of the cervix, as nearly all microscopic cancers of the cervix coexist with CIN.

DIAGNOSIS AND INVESTIGATIONS

CERVICAL CYTOLOGY

Cells exfoliated from the cervix can be examined under the microscope, and this acts as a good screening test. The 'Pap smear' was originally introduced by Papanicolou, with cells removed from the cervix using a wooden spatula then spread on a glass slide and fixed. The Pap smear has now been superseded by liquid-based cytology, whereby a soft brush is used to sample cells from the transformation zone and then cells from the brush are dislodged into fixative solution. The sample is centrifuged and the cellular aspect of the specimen is examined under the microscope. For more than 95% of women, cervical cytology is normal and normal squamous cells are seen (**Figure 16.3**). Abnormal cervical cytology shows squamous cells at different stages of maturity (dyskaryosis). Like CIN, cervical cytology is classified as low grade (minor cytological abnormalities showing mild dyskaryosis or borderline change) or high grade (moderate and severe dyskaryosis) (**Figure 16.4**). There is some correlation between the grade of cytological abnormality and the extent of CIN found on the cervix, but this is not totally reliable. Cervical cytology triages patients to the colposcopy clinic for further assessment (see the section 'Colposcopy' later in this chapter). The sensitivity of a single cervical smear for high-grade CIN detection is between 40% and 70%; however, as there is slow progression for most patients with CIN to cancer, if a lesion is missed then this should be picked up on a subsequent test. Patients who attend regularly for cervical cytology have a very low risk of developing cervical cancer.

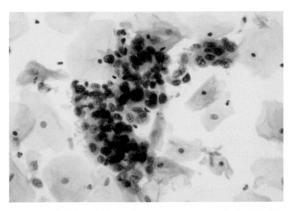
Figure 16.4 Liquid-based cytology – severe dyskaryosis.

HUMAN PAPILLOMAVIRUS TESTING FOR CERVICAL SCREENING

High-risk HPV testing improves the sensitivity of cervical screening. Its value lies in its extremely high negative predictive power, which means that, if an individual tests high-risk HPV negative, their risk of developing cervical cancer over the next 5–10 years is exceptionally low. Many countries, including the UK, have introduced primary HPV screening, that is, testing all cervical specimens for high-risk HPV as the first test and carrying out reflex cytology on those that test positive. This reduces the costs of the screening programme, since HPV testing is automated and achieves a high throughput, while cytological assessment is manual and requires a skilled workforce. The majority of women (around 88–92%) are high-risk HPV negative and are placed on routine recall. High-risk HPV positive samples with cytological abnormalities are referred for colposcopic assessment. Patients with normal cytology are invited for early recall to screening, as they are at significant risk of future neoplastic cervical disease.

NHS CERVICAL SCREENING PROGRAMME

Since 1988, the UK has offered population-based cervical screening. Women aged 25–64 years are invited every 3–5 years to take part in the screening programme. Invitations for cervical screening and the handling of results are coordinated by the NHS Cervical Screening Programme. The coverage in the UK is around 70% of the population. There has been

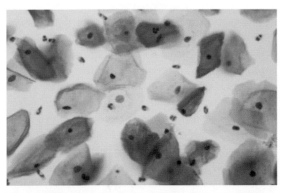
Figure 16.3 Liquid-based cytology – normal cytology.

The main burden of cervical cancer is in low- and middle-income countries, where it is a common killer of women during their reproductive years. This 'hidden' cancer kills young mothers who are the head of their family unit, causing considerable emotional and economic turmoil. Cervical cancer is preventable through screening, vaccination and access to treatment for precancerous lesions. The World Health Organization has set targets for vaccination (90%), screening (70%) and treatment (90%) in every country by 2030 to achieve global elimination of cervical cancer within the next century.

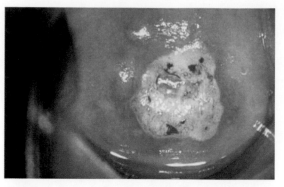

Figure 16.6 Cervix showing acetowhite lesion.

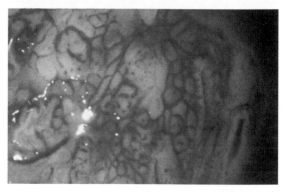

Figure 16.7 Cervix with cervical intraepithelial neoplasia and new vessels.

a recent fall in the uptake of cervical screening and the reasons for this are multiple and varied. Barriers to screening include a fear of intimate examination, embarrassment and inconvenience, and certain groups of women are less likely to be screened than others, specifically those of Black, Asian and mixed ethnicity backgrounds, victims of sexual violence and trans men. Home-based vaginal self-sampling for high-risk HPV is non-inferior to clinician-obtained samples for the detection of high-grade CIN and has the potential to overcome many screening barriers.

COLPOSCOPY

Colposcopy is examination of the magnified cervix using a light source (**Figure 16.5**). It is used for diagnosis and treatment. The patient undresses and places their legs in the semi-lithotomy position. A speculum

is placed in the vagina and the cervix is examined with a light source under magnification (5–20-fold). The application of acetic acid and iodine solutions highlights abnormal areas of the cervix that can be biopsied. Acetic acid causes nuclear proteins to coagulate temporarily; therefore, areas of increased cell turnover, including CIN, appear white (**Figure 16.6**). Areas of CIN lack intracytoplasmic glycogen and fail to stain brown when iodine is applied. CIN is a preneoplastic process and the process of angiogenesis (new blood vessel formation) is apparent in CIN when viewed through the colposcope (**Figure 16.7**). If CIN is present, the colposcopist determines whether the appearances are low or high grade. The latter can be treated in the clinic on the same visit (known as 'see and treat'); the former can be monitored with colposcopy and cervical screening 12 months later. A biopsy usually helps make the decision if unsure ('select and treat'). All doctors and nurses carrying out colposcopy are required to undergo a period of training and examination to ensure high quality and standards

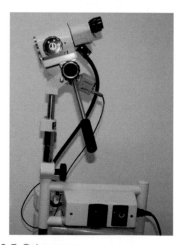

Figure 16.5 Colposcope.

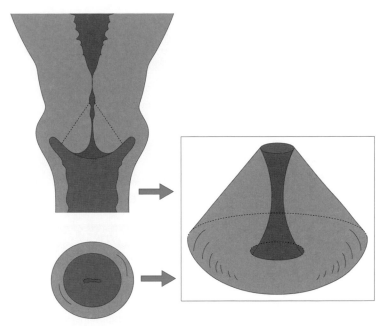

Figure 16.8 Large loop excision of the transformation zone.

TREATMENT

High-grade CIN requires treatment, usually with excision or ablation. Low-grade CIN regresses in up to 60% of cases; therefore, close follow-up is favoured, as this avoids overtreating lesions that may clear spontaneously. In the UK, high-grade CIN is often treated by loop diathermy (large loop excision of the transformation zone). Under local anaesthetic, a diathermy wire loop is used to remove a portion of the cervix that includes the transformation zone with the area of CIN (**Figure 16.8**). CIN can develop within the crypts of the epithelium and therefore excisional techniques need to be at least 7 mm deep. The procedure takes 15 minutes under local anaesthetic. The advantages of this excisional technique are that it is clinically effective (85% of patients have negative cervical screening at 6 months), it is cost-efficient (patients can be treated at the first hospital visit) and it provides a specimen for pathological assessment (1% of loop biopsies have an unsuspected microscopic cancer). The disadvantage relates to its potential impact on obstetric outcomes. Small excisional treatments are unlikely to have obstetric consequences; however, if a large excision or repeat excisions remove a substantial proportion of the cervix, there is an increased risk of mid-trimester miscarriage and preterm delivery in subsequent pregnancies. This concern relates to young women who have not completed their families. Recognizing the potential for overtreatment has been the main reason why women under 25 are not screened, as many lesions in this group of patients are associated with HPV infection and simply regress with observational follow-up.

Other treatment options for high-grade CIN include cold coagulation and cone biopsy. The term 'cold coagulation' is a misnomer, as the treatment involves placing a hot probe on the cervix in outpatients under local anaesthetic. It is a destructive treatment and is effective for both high- and low-grade CIN, but it does not provide a tissue specimen. Cone biopsy involves cutting away a portion of the cervix under general anaesthetic and produces a tissue specimen, like a large loop excision of the transformation zone. Its disadvantage relates to the need for a general anaesthetic, and 5% of patients may develop cervical stenosis or incompetence, which has obstetric implications. It has largely been superseded by loop diathermy.

Patients who have received treatment for CIN undergo a 'test of cure' high-risk HPV test 6 months later. If negative, the patient is returned to routine recall, that is, cervical screening in 3 years' time. If positive, repeat colposcopy is indicated to identify any residual, untreated CIN. A patient with a history of CIN has an increased lifetime risk of recurrent CIN and cervical cancer.

HUMAN PAPILLOMAVIRUS VACCINATION

HPV vaccines are safe and effective at preventing persistent high-risk HPV infection, CIN and cervical cancer. A school-based immunization programme has been active in the UK since 2008. The bivalent vaccine prevents persistent infection with HPV types 16 and 18, which together cause more than 70% of cervical cancers worldwide. In 2011, the bivalent vaccine was replaced in the UK immunization programme by the quadrivalent vaccine, which additionally protects against HPV types 6 and 11, the main perpetrators of genital warts. A nonavalent vaccine was introduced in 2022 that protects against HPV 6, 11, 16, 18, 31, 33, 45, 51 and 58, including seven high-risk types that together are responsible for >85% of cervical cancers globally. The uptake of HPV vaccination has been good (75–85%) among 12- to 13-year-old girls and, since 2018, boys in the UK immunization programme. It is expected that this will result in fewer women being referred for colposcopy when they reach screening age.

KEY LEARNING POINTS

- Cervical cancer is a preventable disease in countries where resources permit.
- Prophylactic HPV vaccination can prevent infection with high-risk HPV types that cause cancers of the cervix and other lower genital tract sites.
- Regular screening by high-risk HPV testing allows premalignant disease to be detected and treated before it undergoes malignant transformation.
- Patients who are treated for high-grade CIN are at an increased risk of cervical cancer compared with other women, but regular cervical screening will pick up residual or recurrent disease that can be treated.

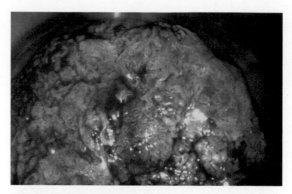

Figure 16.9 Cervical cancer.

MALIGNANT DISEASE OF THE CERVIX

CLINICAL PRESENTATION

Many patients with small-volume microscopic disease are asymptomatic and are picked up incidentally following a loop biopsy of the cervix for preinvasive disease. Most cervical cancers, however, are friable, vascular masses on the cervix, and patients present with abnormal bleeding, typically post-coital bleeding, prolonged intermenstrual or postmenopausal bleeding (**Figure 16.9**). Any patient with these symptoms should undergo pelvic examination, including visualization of the cervix. In advanced disease (stages III–IV), patients may experience distressing symptoms like pain (malignant infiltration of the spinal cord), incontinence (vesicovaginal fistula), anaemia (heavy vaginal bleeding) and renal failure (ureteric compression).

Pelvic and speculum examinations usually clinch the diagnosis with a cervical mass that bleeds on contact and, if advanced disease, a hardness and fixity of the tissues. A biopsy should be taken in the outpatient setting. Very occasionally, the diagnosis can be missed, as some tumours are endophytic rather than exophytic and, therefore, less clinically revealing. The clinician must retain a level of clinical suspicion in the presence of unexplained symptoms and investigate patients with persistent problems.

PATHOPHYSIOLOGY

The majority (70%) of cervical cancers are squamous cell carcinomas, with adenocarcinomas making up most of the remainder. In high-income countries with screening programmes, there has been a relative fall in the proportion of squamous tumours and a concomitant rise in adenocarcinomas. Adenocarcinomas are less likely to be picked up through cervical screening. Precursors of adenocarcinoma, known as cervical glandular intraepithelial neoplasia, can be detected at colposcopy, although lesions reside within the endocervical canal and may be difficult to visualize. Often, cervical glandular intraepithelial neoplasia is found incidentally in loop excision biopsies carried out for high-grade CIN; it is not uncommon for the two precursors to coexist. Cervical tumours are locally infiltrative in the pelvis, but also spread via lymphatics and, in the late stages, via blood. The tumour can invade tissues beyond the cervix to reach the parametria (lateral), bladder (anterior), vagina (inferior) and rectum (posterior). Metastases can affect pelvic (iliac and obturator) or para-aortic nodes and, in the later stages, the liver and lungs.

INVESTIGATION AND THE IMPORTANCE OF STAGING

Assessing the stage of the disease is crucial for planning treatment. Patients are staged according to the International Federation of Gynecology and Obstetrics (FIGO) system, as shown in **Table 16.1**. A biopsy is crucial to confirm malignancy and assess the tumour type. Magnetic resonance imaging (MRI) of the abdomen and pelvis determines the extent of disease and identifies any enlarged lymph nodes in the pelvic and para-aortic lymph node chains. A chest X-ray is vital to exclude lung metastases. An examination under anaesthetic may be helpful when, despite the above tests, the clinician is still unclear if the tumour is operable. Doing a rectovaginal examination under anaesthetic can give crucial information on the tumour, including size, fixity and vaginal involvement, and a cystoscopy can help eliminate bladder involvement. Small mobile tumours favour a surgical approach, whereas larger

Table 16.1 Staging and prognosis of cervical cancer

Stage	Extent of disease	5-year survival rate (%)
I	Tumour confined to the cervix	88
	IA: Microscopic disease. Maximum horizontal dimension is 7 mm and depth of invasion is 5 mm	
	IA1: Maximum horizontal dimension is 7 mm and depth of invasion is 3 mm	
	IA2: Maximum horizontal dimension is 7 mm and depth of invasion is between 3 and 5 mm	
	IB: Clinical lesions confined to the cervix or preclinical lesions greater than IA	
	IB1: Clinical lesions less than 2 cm in size, and depth of invasion less than 5 mm	
	IB2: Clinical lesions less than 4 cm in size, and depth of invasion less than 2 cm	
	IB3: Clinical lesions greater than 4 cm in size	
II	Tumour extends beyond the cervix and involves the vagina (but not the lower third) and/or the parametrium (but not reaching the pelvic side wall)	68
	IIA1: Tumour involves the vagina and is less than 4 cm in size	
	IIA2: Tumour involves the vagina and is more than 4 cm in size	
	IIB: Tumour infiltrates the parametrium	
III	Tumour involves the lower third of the vagina and/or extends to the pelvic side wall	42
	IIIA: Tumour involves the lower third of the vagina	
	IIIB: Tumour extends to the pelvic wall and/or hydronephrosis or non-functioning kidney due to ureteric obstruction caused by tumour	
	IIIC1: Tumour has spread to the pelvic lymph nodes	
	IIIC2: Tumour has spread to the para-aortic lymph nodes	
IV	IVA: Tumour involves the mucosa of the bladder or rectum and/or extends beyond the true pelvis	16
	IVB: Spread to distant organs	

Based on the 2018 International Federation of Gynecology and Obstetrics (FIGO) staging system.

fixed tumours favour primary radiotherapy. FIGO staging includes an intravenous urogram to ensure the integrity of the ureters; however, this is not standard practice in high-income countries, where MRI has superseded such tests. Stage is based on clinical findings, unlike other gynaecological tumours where stage is based on surgical and pathological findings. This is important because radiotherapy, rather than surgery, is favoured in advanced disease and it is still possible to stage patients in low-income countries, where most of the disease burden is seen.

TREATMENT

Treatment for cervical cancer depends on stage, the requirement for future fertility and the patient's performance status. Patients are managed by a multidisciplinary team (MDT) of surgeons, clinical oncologists, radiologists, pathologists and clinical nurse specialists, which ensures that the most appropriate treatment is offered. Surgical fitness must be established before embarking on radical surgery, which may not be appropriate for everyone.

PRECLINICAL LESIONS: STAGE IA

These microscopic tumours are usually picked up as incidental findings after loop excision for precancerous disease. Small lesions must be removed with a clear margin of excision, and the preinvasive disease (CIN) that invariably coexists should also be completely excised, as the cancer is often multifocal. If the preinvasive disease is not completely excised, then a repeat loop biopsy or knife cone biopsy must be carried out. For microscopic lesions (stage IA1), local excision with good clear margins is all that is required. This allows fertility to be preserved and a hysterectomy is not necessary. Stage IA2 disease has an appreciable risk of lymph node metastases, and is managed by local excision and bilateral pelvic lymphadenectomy.

CLINICAL INVASIVE CERVICAL CARCINOMA: STAGES IB–IV

The tumour volumes are much larger in patients with stage IB disease and, therefore, fertility-preserving treatment for this group of patients is more challenging. When disease is confined to the cervix

(stage IB1), radical hysterectomy and bilateral pelvic node dissection (Wertheim hysterectomy) is the standard of care. Open hysterectomy is preferred to minimally invasive surgery, which is associated with significantly poorer long-term survival outcomes, according to the international Laparoscopic Approach to Cervical Cancer (LACC) trial. For young women who have not completed their families, radical trachelectomy (surgical removal of the cervix and upper part of the vagina) and bilateral pelvic node dissection is an alternative (see **Chapter 17**).

It is important to remember that in early stage IB disease, pelvic radiotherapy has similar success rates to surgery and therefore this treatment is considered in patients who are too overweight for radical surgery or who are anaesthetically unfit.

When the disease has spread beyond the cervix (stages II–IV disease), radiotherapy (with or without chemotherapy) becomes the optimal treatment. Surgery in isolation is problematic, as complications can occur (severe haemorrhage) and achieving adequate clearance of the tumour is unlikely. Incomplete excision of cancer by surgery requires adjuvant postoperative radiotherapy, and combined treatments can lead to high complication rates. As an oncological rule, it is not wise to cut through cancer.

SURGERY

The standard surgical operation for stage IB tumours is an open radical hysterectomy and pelvic lymph node dissection. This involves removal of the cervix, the upper third of the vagina, the uterus and the paracervical tissue. Pelvic lymph node removal includes the obturator, internal and external iliac nodes. The ovaries in premenopausal women can be conserved. There is higher morbidity with this procedure than with the standard total abdominal hysterectomy. Bladder dysfunction (atony), sexual dysfunction (due to vaginal shortening) and lymphoedema (due to removal of the pelvic lymph nodes) are not uncommon. An atonic bladder is frequent in the immediate post-operative period due to neuronal damage from the surgery, and intermittent self-catheterization may be required until bladder tone returns.

Lymphoedema is variable and is described by patients as a wooden, heavy feeling to the legs with swelling and reduced mobility. Management includes leg elevation, good skincare (e.g. avoid shaving), massage and occasionally compression stockings. Despite these potential problems, surgery is the preferred treatment, as the cure rate is high, ovarian tissue can be preserved and the patient avoids the complications of radiotherapy (see the next section).

> ## 🔑 KEY LEARNING POINTS
>
> - Cervical cancer affects young women who may not have completed their families.
> - Many cervical tumours are picked up when they are microscopic or very small volume, making fertility-sparing treatment a possibility.
> - Cone biopsy or radical trachelectomy with bilateral pelvic lymphadenectomy allows preservation of the ovaries and uterus, permitting pregnancy in the future.
> - The long-term cure rate of radical trachelectomy is less well established than radical (Wertheim) hysterectomy.

RADIOTHERAPY

The aim of radiotherapy is to deliver a lethal dose of radiation to the tumour and minimize damage to the surrounding tissues. Treatment is overseen by a clinical oncologist and team. Treatment is delivered in two ways: external beam radiotherapy (as teletherapy) and internal radiotherapy (brachytherapy). In external beam radiotherapy, the source of the radiation is from a machine called a linear accelerator, and radiation is delivered to the pelvis a distance from the patient (**Figure 16.10**). The dose of radiotherapy is carefully calculated according to the patient and the tumour, and is usually administered as 45 Gy in total. This is given in several treatments or 'fractions' as an outpatient over 4 weeks. Although this treatment is given daily, the time of each fraction is no more than 5–10 minutes. Brachytherapy is a radiotherapy technique whereby the radiation is delivered internally to the patient. The source of the radiation is usually selenium and patients generally have to undergo an examination under anaesthetic to insert the rods into the uterus. These rods are then attached to the radiotherapy source; the patient receives this internal treatment in isolation to protect staff. Brachytherapy delivers a high dose of radiation to the tumour and its harmful effects on the bladder and bowel are minimized, as its effects are targeted only 5 mm from the rod.

Patients frequently suffer lethargy with treatment and may experience both bowel and bladder urgency, which is due to the initial inflammatory effects of the radiation. Skin erythema, like sunburn, is not uncommon after external beam radiotherapy. Symptomatic treatment is usually required, such as anti-inflammatory creams for the skin. Around 5% of patients experience a serious side effect that might interrupt treatment, for example bowel perforation. There are many long-term complications of radiotherapy that affect only a minority of patients but do have a significant impact on patients' quality of life. The initial inflammatory process is replaced by fibrosis in the long term. Vaginal stenosis can cause sexual pain, bladder damage can lead to cystitis-like symptoms, and haematuria and bowel damage leads to malabsorption and mucous diarrhoea. None of these complications can be managed easily. Patients who are premenopausal will undergo a radiotherapy-induced menopause, as the ovaries are very sensitive to small doses of irradiation.

Chemotherapy (cisplatin) is ideally given in conjunction with the radiotherapy, as this combination increases cure rates more than when radiotherapy is used in isolation. It probably works by enhancing the effects of radiotherapy and might also address micrometastases that are outside the radiotherapy field.

PALLIATIVE TREATMENT

When it is not possible to offer curative treatment, palliation of symptoms becomes important and early involvement of the palliative care team is essential

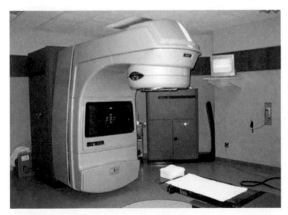

Figure 16.10 Linear accelerator.

233

for symptom control. The disease can be hidden from family and friends even in the late stages of the disease; patients may experience several unpleasant symptoms from local infiltration of the pelvis by the cancer. Malignant pain, recto- and/or vesicovaginal fistulae and bleeding may occur. Distant spread is a very late event. Radiotherapy may be considered with a palliative intent; for example, a one-off treatment may be used for symptomatic bone metastases.

MALIGNANT DISEASE OF THE VAGINA

EPIDEMIOLOGY AND AETIOLOGY

Vaginal cancer is rare, accounting for just 1–2% of gynaecological malignancies. Most vaginal tumours arise from metastatic spread from the endometrium or cervix. Primary cancers of the vagina are usually squamous cell carcinomas, although clear cell adenocarcinomas and malignant melanomas can occur. The peak age of incidence is 60–70 years of age. Sarcoma botryoides is a rare vaginal tumour affecting young girls, with a peak incidence at 8 years of age.

More than 60% of primary vaginal tumours are HPV associated, and risk factors for the disease include previous malignant and premalignant disease of the cervix and vaginal intraepithelial neoplasia – a premalignant disease with a 10% risk of progression to invasive disease. Vaginal cancer is also sometimes seen in women with a history of pelvic radiotherapy.

CLINICAL PRESENTATION AND DIAGNOSIS

Abnormal bleeding or blood-stained vaginal discharge is the most common presenting complaint. Speculum examination reveals a mass or an ulcer, usually at the top of the vagina. Advanced disease presents with haematuria, constipation, pelvic pain or tenesmus (a feeling of incomplete emptying of the rectum). Diagnosis is confirmed by biopsy. Staging of vaginal cancer uses the FIGO system (**Table 16.2**). An examination under anaesthetic, cystoscopy and sigmoidoscopy defines local spread. An MRI scan of the pelvis confirms clinical findings and a computed tomography (CT) scan of the thorax and abdomen establishes whether distant metastases are present.

Table 16.2 Staging and prognosis of vaginal cancer

Stage	Extent of disease	5-year survival rate (%)
I	Tumour confined to the vagina	75
II	Tumour invades the subvaginal tissue	40
III	Tumour invades the pelvic side wall	30
IV	Tumour involves the bladder or bowel mucosa or extends beyond the true pelvis	0–20

Based on the International Federation of Gynecology and Obstetrics (FIGO) staging system.

TREATMENT

Most vaginal cancer is treated by primary radiotherapy, although early-stage tumours may be managed surgically. Prognosis depends on stage.

MALIGNANT DISEASE OF THE VULVA

EPIDEMIOLOGY AND AETIOLOGY

Vulval cancer is uncommon, with just 1,000 new diagnoses every year in the UK. It was previously a disease that exclusively affected older women, but recent years have witnessed rising incidence rates among young women in their fourth, fifth and sixth decades of life.

Almost 90% of vulval cancers are squamous cell carcinomas, with malignant melanoma, basal cell carcinoma and adenocarcinoma of the Bartholin gland making up the remainder. It is generally accepted that squamous cell carcinoma of the vulva is a disease of two separate aetiologies: (1) high-risk HPV-associated cancers, which arise on a background of multifocal high-grade vulval intraepithelial neoplasia, often in younger patients and (2) non-HPV-associated tumours, affecting older patients and associated with the premalignant vulval condition lichen sclerosus (**Table 16.3**).

CLINICAL PRESENTATION

Vulval cancer presents as a lump or ulcer associated with bleeding or discharge that may be painful or painless. Patients may present late due to embarrassment

Table 16.3 Premalignant conditions of the vulva

Condition	Aetiology	Characteristics	Symptoms	Treatment	Risk of malignancy
VIN	High-risk HPV	Multifocal leukoplakic, erythematous or pigmented lesions	Itch, irritation, asymptomatic	Imiquimod cream, surgical excision, LASER (Light Amplification by Stimulated Emission of Radiation) treatment	10% – may be higher in immunocompromised individuals (e.g. HIV, renal transplant recipients of immunosuppressive treatments)
Lichen sclerosus	Unknown	Leukoplakia of the vulval skin in a 'figure of 8' distribution, with loss of vulval architecture	Itch, irritation, asymptomatic	Superpotent steroid cream if symptomatic	10%
Extramammary Paget disease of the vulva	Unknown	Well-demarcated erythematous lesion affecting the vulva with 'cake icing' effect	Itch, irritation, asymptomatic	Surgical excision aiming for wide margin of healthy skin to reduce risk of recurrence	10% risk of invasive vulval disease at presentation; 30% risk of associated internal malignancy (of urethra, bladder, uterus, vagina or bowel)

HIV, human immunodeficiency virus; HPV, human papillomavirus; VIN, vulval intraepithelial neoplasia.

and reluctance to be examined. Clinical assessment should include an evaluation of the patient's performance status and general fitness for anaesthetic.

On examination, a well-demarcated raised or ulcerated lesion that is hard and craggy and bleeds on touch is highly suspicious of vulval cancer (**Figure 16.11**). There is often associated premalignant change, specifically vulval intraepithelial neoplasia in younger patients and lichen sclerosus in older patients. Examination includes an assessment of the size of the lesion, its position on the vulva and its proximity to important midline structures, particularly the urethra and anus. Vulval tumours spread locally and metastasize first via the inguinofemoral lymph nodes, before involving pelvic lymph nodes. It is therefore important to examine the groins for lymph node metastases, which are palpable as hard, craggy and fixed subcutaneous lymph node swellings. Haematogenous spread to the liver and lungs is a late event.

INVESTIGATION

Patients with vulval cancer are managed by specialist gynaecological oncology MDTs in cancer centres, where there is sufficient experience and expertise in the management of this relatively rare condition. The team includes gynaecological cancer surgeons, clinical oncologists, specialist radiologists, histopathologists and clinical nurse specialists who guide the investigation and treatment of the patient according to nationally agreed guidelines.

A biopsy is needed to confirm the diagnosis. For large tumours, this should incorporate the edge of the lesion with the transition to normal epithelium, as this aids histological assessment. For smaller tumours, for which biopsy would effectively excise the lesion, it is

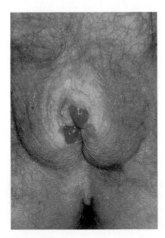

Figure 16.11 Vulval cancer.

235

important to take a clinical photograph first. The vulva heals well and it can be difficult to locate the scar if further excision is necessary. Alternatively, the patient may be referred prior to biopsy if there is a small but clinically suspicious lesion. An examination under anaesthetic is sometimes useful to assess the suitability of the tumour to resection, particularly if the tumour is very large and involving midline structures.

Most patients do not require pre-operative imaging, apart from a chest X-ray to confirm suitability for surgery. Imaging of the groins is unreliable in the detection of groin node metastases, although the high negative predictive power of an MRI scan of the groins can sometimes spare very unfit, elderly patients from the morbidity associated with full groin lymphadenectomy. A staging CT scan of the thorax, abdomen and pelvis is necessary for large vulval tumours or those with obvious groin node disease, to exclude distant metastases. Staging is according to FIGO (**Table 16.4**).

TREATMENT

VULVAL EXCISION

Radical surgical excision aiming for a clear surgical margin of at least 10 mm is the standard of care. Margins less than 2 mm are associated with high recurrence rates and may necessitate further excision or radiotherapy. When lesions impinge on the urethra or anus, achieving good surgical clearance is more challenging. Sometimes it is appropriate to shrink very large or midline tumours with neoadjuvant radiotherapy, often given in combination with chemotherapy, prior to surgery. This allows better preservation of urinary or bowel function than upfront radical surgical excision. For small lesions, primary closure is straightforward, but larger lesions necessitate vulval reconstruction using 'flaps' of skin, subcutaneous tissue and blood vessels, usually from the buttock crease or inner thigh.

SENTINEL LYMPH NODE BIOPSY AND GROIN LYMPHADENECTOMY

Untreated groin lymph node metastases are invariably fatal, but it is not possible to predict whether groin nodes are involved using current radiological techniques. The standard approach until recently has been to carry out full inguinofemoral lymphadenectomy, that is, to remove all the lymph nodes in the groin for all patients where the tumour depth of invasion exceeds 1 mm. Tumours with a depth of invasion of less than 1 mm are extremely unlikely to have groin node metastases (less than 5%). Lymph drainage for lateral vulval tumours is to the ipsilateral

Table 16.4 Staging and prognosis of vulval cancer

Stage	Extent of disease	5-year survival rate (%)
I	Tumour confined to the vulva	80
IA	≤2 cm in size, stromal invasion ≤1 mm, no nodes	
IB	>2 cm in size or stromal invasion >1 mm, no nodes	
II	Tumour extending to the lower third of the urethra or vagina, or anus	50
III	Positive inguinofemoral lymph nodes	30
IIIA1	One lymph node metastasis ≥5 mm	
IIIA2	One or two lymph node metastases <5 mm	
IIIB1	Two or more lymph node metastases ≥5 mm	
IIIB2	Three or more lymph node metastases <5 mm	
IIIC	Extracapsular spread	
IV	Tumour invading regional or distant sites	0–15
IVA1	Upper urethra/vaginal mucosa, bladder or rectal mucosa, fixed to pelvic bone	
IVA2	Fixed or ulcerated inguinofemoral lymph nodes	
IVB	Distant metastases including pelvic lymph nodes	

Based on the International Federation of Gynecology and Obstetrics (FIGO) staging system.

groin nodes, but lesions within 10 mm of the midline drain to nodes on either side of the groin, necessitating bilateral groin lymphadenectomy. Groin lymphadenectomy is a highly morbid procedure, associated with significant post-operative and long-term complications, including wound healing problems, infection, venous thromboembolism, prolonged hospital stay, lymphocyst and chronic lymphoedema. Since groin node metastases affect just 15% of patients undergoing surgery for vulval cancer, many patients are exposed to the unnecessary risks and long-term sequelae of groin lymphadenectomy without receiving any direct benefit from it.

Sentinel lymph node biopsy is an attempt to address this issue. The sentinel node is the first node in the lymph node basin to receive lymphatic drainage from a tumour. The theory states that if the sentinel lymph node is negative, then the rest of the lymph node basin must be negative for metastatic disease too. Therefore, if the sentinel lymph node can be identified and carefully checked for metastatic disease, full groin lymphadenectomy can be reserved for those patients who really need it. Removing the sentinel lymph node is a far less morbid procedure than full groin lymphadenectomy. The sentinel lymph node principle has been established in tumours originating from other anatomical sites, including breast cancer and malignant melanoma, and is now the standard of care for selected cases of vulval cancer.

Small vulval tumours (<4 cm) with greater than 1 mm depth of invasion are injected with radioactive nucleotide on the day before surgery. Intraoperative identification of the sentinel node is by gamma probe detection. This is facilitated by injection of blue dye into the tumour immediately pre-operatively. The sentinel node is the 'hot' blue node or nodes. It is important to identify bilateral sentinel lymph nodes in which tumours impinge on the midline. Careful assessment ('ultrastaging') of the sentinel node(s) identifies the presence or absence of metastatic disease; if the sentinel node is positive for metastatic disease, full groin lymphadenectomy is indicated as a secondary procedure. False-positive nodes are unlikely, but false-negative nodes have been described in the literature and threaten the safety of the procedure; it is essential that high standards are achieved through strict adherence to sentinel node protocols to reduce this risk.

RADIOTHERAPY

Adjuvant radiotherapy, given after surgery with curative intent, is indicated when vulval excision margins are close or involved, in the presence of two or more groin node metastases, or with extracapsular spread. Adjuvant radiotherapy is given to reduce the risk of recurrence. Neoadjuvant radiotherapy, given before surgery to shrink the tumour and render it operable, is used for very large vulval tumours, particularly those that involve the urethra or anus and when adequate surgical effort would have functional urinary or bowel implications. Occasionally, radical radiotherapy is given instead of surgery in patients who are not fit for an anaesthetic due to severe medical comorbidities (see previous section). Chemoradiotherapy is associated with improved cure rates compared with radiotherapy alone. Treatment of recurrent disease and palliative treatment follows the same principles as for cervical malignancy, as discussed in the previous section.

KEY LEARNING POINTS

- Cervical cancer is a disease that commonly affects women in low- and middle-income countries. Most affected individuals never see a healthcare professional and die from their disease in the community.
- Population-based cervical screening has prevented 70% of deaths from cervical cancer in the UK. HPV vaccination of adolescents in schools is likely to reduce rates further, but this will take several years to show benefit.
- All patients with abnormal bleeding should undergo speculum and pelvic examinations to exclude malignant disease.
- Early-stage malignant disease of the lower genital tract is treated by surgical excision. The principle of surgery in this context is to remove all of the tumour with adequate surgical margins.
- Fertility-sparing treatment is possible in early-stage cervical tumours in young women who have not completed their families.
- Most lower genital tract tumours are radiosensitive, but surgery is preferred as the first-line treatment due to a lower toxicity profile.
- Chemotherapy is used alongside radiotherapy to improve response rates and in the case of metastatic disease.

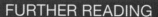

FURTHER READING

BouvardV, Wentzensen N, Mackie A, et al. (2021). The IARC perspective on cervical cancer screening. *New England Journal of Medicine*, 385(20): 1908–1918.

Crosbie EJ, Einstein MH, Franceschi S, Kitchener HC (2013). Human papillomavirus and cervical cancer. *Lancet*, 382: 889–899.

Davies-Oliveira JC, Smith MA, Grover S, Canfell K, Crosbie EJ (2021). Eliminating cervical cancer: Progress and challenges for high-income countries. *Clinical Oncology*, 33(9): 550–559.

SELF-ASSESSMENT

For interactive SBAs and EMQs relating to this chapter, visit www.routledge.com/cw/crosbie.

CASE HISTORY 1

Mrs S is an 88-year-old woman who presents to the gynaecology clinic with a vulval lump. It has been bleeding intermittently. It is very sore and she is finding it difficult to sit down. She is frail and lives in sheltered accommodation.

A What is the most likely diagnosis?

B What are the key points in the examination and investigation?

C Mrs S is found to have a 6 cm vulval tumour involving the clitoris, right labium majorum and the introital margin. It extends to a few millimetres away from the external urethral meatus. Her staging CT scan excludes distant metastases. How would you manage her?

ANSWERS

A A new vulval lump in an elderly woman is vulval cancer until proven otherwise. It is not unusual for elderly women to put off consulting their general practitioner because of embarrassment and a reluctance to be examined.

B It is important to inspect the vulva, noting the size of the lesion, its position on the vulva and its proximity to the urethra and anus. A biopsy in the outpatient setting will expedite diagnosis but may be difficult if the lesion is exquisitely tender, as the history suggests. An examination under anaesthetic including biopsy may be necessary. Assessment of the groin is important, as enlarged, hard, fixed nodal masses may not be resectable. If distant metastases are suspected, a CT scan of the thorax, abdomen and pelvis is important for treatment planning.

C It is important to establish up front what treatment the patient wants and whether she is fit for general anaesthetic and the morbidity of radical vulval cancer surgery. From an oncological point of view, the best treatment is radical vulval excision with flap reconstruction of the vulva and bilateral groin lymphadenectomy. This may be followed by adjuvant radiotherapy if surgical margins are close or two or more groin nodes are positive. If the proximity of the tumour to the urethra prohibits good surgical clearance without rendering Mrs S incontinent, it may be appropriate to consider neoadjuvant (chemo)radiotherapy to shrink the tumour prior to surgery. Radical vulval surgery and placement of a permanent suprapubic catheter is another option. If Mrs S is not fit or does not wish to have surgery, radical radiotherapy with/without chemotherapy is the treatment of choice. All decisions are made following full consultation with the patient and her family and after discussion with the specialist gynaecological oncology MDT.

CASE HISTORY 2

Miss M is a 70-year-old woman who attends the gynaecology clinic with a history of vulval itch and soreness. She has tried several creams for thrush but nothing has helped. She has noticed that her vulval skin is very thin and scratching causes bleeding.

A What is the most likely diagnosis?

B What are the key points in the examination?

C Miss M is found to have whitened skin around her vagina and anus in a figure of eight distribution. There is a loss of vulval architecture and a narrowed introitus. There are no suspicious lumps or ulcers concerning for malignancy. How would you manage her?

ANSWERS

A Lichen sclerosus is a common vulval skin condition that causes itch and vulval discomfort. It is a condition most frequently seen in postmenopausal women and its diagnosis is usually made clinically following vulval inspection.

B Lichen sclerosus causes vulval atrophy, a loss of vulval features and a whitened discolouration affecting the vulva and perianal skin. The important thing is to exclude vulval cancer, which may coexist and is more common in women with lichen sclerosus.

C Empirical management with a strong steroid cream, self-applied daily initially and with decreasing frequency over a 6-week period, should bring symptoms under control. If not, a biopsy should be taken to exclude an alternative diagnosis. Women are encouraged to self-manage their lichen sclerosus with steroid creams and to examine themselves regularly to look for sinister skin changes.

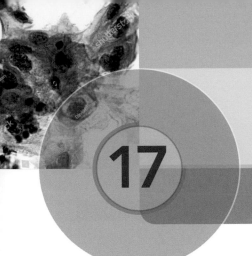

Gynaecological surgery and therapeutics

17

TIMOTHY HILLARD

Learning Objectives

- Revise the key points of surgical anatomy applied to gynaecology.
- Understand general surgical principles as they apply to gynaecology.
- Recognize the importance of fully informed consent.
- Understand the purpose of careful pre-assessment and post-operative care.
- Understand the advantages and disadvantages of different surgical approaches.
- Be aware of how to minimize surgical risk during and immediately after surgery.
- Understand the advantages and principles of minimal access surgery.
- Be aware of the common gynaecological procedures and their risks.
- Describe the common hormonal and non-hormonal drugs used in gynaecology, and understand the principles of safe prescribing.

INTRODUCTION

In this chapter, we discuss the principles of good surgical practice and therapeutics as they relate to gynaecology. Although there is an increasing focus within gynaecology on ambulatory and medical interventions, gynaecology is still largely a surgical specialty; before obstetrics and gynaecology was recognized as a speciality in its own right, most gynaecological procedures were performed by surgeons.

GYNAECOLOGICAL SURGERY

KEY SURGICAL ANATOMY

A thorough knowledge of pelvic anatomy is essential for safe surgical practice (see **Chapter 1**). The major vessels supplying the uterus and adnexa are the ovarian vessels (arising in the abdomen from the aorta and renal artery), which enter the pelvis over the sacroiliac joints in the infundibulopelvic ligament (a fold of peritoneum), and the uterine vessels

10.1201/9781003218036-17

(see **Chapter 1**: **Figure 1.7**). The uterine arteries are branches from the anterior trunk of the internal iliac artery and run medially in the base of the broad ligament to turn upwards and course along the lateral border of the uterus on each side. At the base of the broad ligament, the uterine artery runs 1 cm above and 1 cm lateral to the ureter, where it is at risk of injury during surgery if care is not taken. This is more likely if the anatomy is distorted by scarring from endometriosis, by previous infection or surgery, or by malignancy, uterine fibroids or ovarian cysts.

The ureter runs from the kidney over the psoas muscle in line with the lateral processes of the lumbar vertebrae and enters the pelvis over the sacroiliac joint. It runs in the posterior leaf of the broad ligament to the level of the ischial spine, where it turns inwards and forwards to enter the bladder. To safely dissect the uterine arteries away from the ureter, the bladder is reflected downwards at an abdominal or laparoscopic hysterectomy or upwards at a vaginal hysterectomy. The bladder is emptied before open and laparoscopic surgery to protect it from injury. The bladder is intimately associated with the anterior vaginal wall and the front of the uterine cervix and isthmus. The vesicouterine fold of peritoneum must be opened to allow the bladder to be reflected before clamping the uterine arteries during hysterectomy. It is for these reasons that bladder and ureteric injuries may occur during gynaecological surgery. If there is any doubt as to the position of the ureter, the broad ligament can be opened by dividing the round ligament, and the ureter can always be seen on the reflected peritoneum.

The sigmoid colon runs along the left side wall of the abdomen and pelvis and becomes retroperitoneal midway along its passage through the pelvis. In a healthy pelvis, the rectum falls away when the uterus is lifted to allow clear identification of the rectum and posterior vagina in the pouch of Douglas. Scarring (particularly from endometriosis) can obliterate the pouch of Douglas and increase the risk of rectal injury considerably. In addition, after hysterectomy, the anatomical planes between the vagina and rectum are less easily seen and so rectal injury can occur at the time of operations deep in the pelvis, such as sacrocolpopexy. For a discussion of the anatomy of the ligaments and fascial supports relevant to prolapse, see **Chapters 1** and **10**.

Before considering individual gynaecological procedures, it is necessary to be familiar with the general surgical principles that apply for any proposed intervention, as outlined in the following sections.

BOX 17.1: General surgical principles

- Indication for surgery and decision-making
- Pre-assessment
- Consent
- Surgical safety
- Good surgical practice
- Post-operative care and recovery

INDICATION FOR SURGERY AND DECISION-MAKING

Safe surgical practice and careful decision-making begins in the outpatient clinic. With the exception of cancer, most gynaecology conditions affect quality of life and are not life-threatening. It is important, therefore, to work with the patient to ensure that all available conservative and non-medical interventions have been tried or at least discussed before considering surgery. Although modern anaesthesia and surgery are safe, any surgical procedure does carry risks and complications, some of which, although rare, can be life-threatening or cause significant physical morbidity. It is our professional duty to ensure that patients are made aware of all the issues and the alternative options available. Many patients have unrealistic expectations about the likely outcome of surgery and haven't always considered the possibility of complications. The best way to avoid surgical complications is not to operate!

Having arrived at the decision to perform a surgical procedure for a particular condition, it is then necessary to select the most appropriate operation for that particular patient. For instance, abdominal surgery requires a longer recovery than vaginal surgery and involves an abdominal incision, while laparoscopic surgery requires a patient to endure a longer anaesthetic (often) while in a steep Trendelenburg position (head down). Therefore, in a frail elderly patient with comorbidities, it might be more appropriate to avoid an abdominal approach in favour of a laparoscopic or vaginal approach. Similarly, in a patient who has had several previous procedures for extensive endometriosis and intra-abdominal adhesions, very careful consideration should be given about any further abdominal or laparoscopic intervention. In complex cases, it is now considered best practice to seek the views of colleagues, which is now usually done through a multidisciplinary team (MDT). MDTs have existed for some time in oncology but have now also evolved in urogynaecology, endometriosis and other benign gynaecology areas. At the MDT meeting, the patient's case is discussed and the views and collective expertise of gynaecologists, specialist nurses and other relevant specialists (e.g. physiotherapists, oncologists, radiologists, pathologists, urologists and colorectal surgeons) can be shared to decide on the safest and most effective treatment plan. The results of the MDT discussions should be clearly documented and communicated to the patient.

PRE-ASSESSMENT

Once the decision to operate has been made, the process begins to optimize the patient's pathway through the system to make sure it is as safe, short and trouble-free as possible. Some of this is logistical, and appropriate processes have evolved to facilitate this that will vary in detail between hospitals.

The first decision is whether or not the procedure can be done as outpatient (ambulatory) care, should be done as day-case surgery or requires inpatient admission and an overnight stay. Generally, if a procedure such as a hysteroscopy or cystoscopy can be done in the ambulatory setting, this is the preferred option, but any potential risks and the patient's wishes need to be taken into consideration. Not all patients want to have procedures done under local anaesthetic. Anyone coming into hospital for a procedure (as a day case or requiring inpatient admission) needs appropriate assessment to make sure they are operated on in the appropriate setting with relevant anaesthetic support. Pre-surgical preparation of patients is usually performed in a pre-assessment clinic (PAC) a few weeks before the planned date of surgery. At pre-assessment, a clinical review is undertaken, usually by a specialist nurse, to confirm the proposed procedure and to identify any medical comorbidities that may affect the risks of anaesthesia or increase the risk of intra- or post-operative complications. Investigations such as a full blood count and 'group and save' will be taken, as appropriate for the procedure. Additional tests such as serum biochemistry (urea, electrolytes, renal function and hepatic function), chest X-ray and electrocardiography will be organized depending on age and known cardiac, renal or respiratory problems. In the event of any concerns, the case will be discussed further with the anaesthetist prior to admission, and additional investigations such as echocardiography or lung function tests may be required. Most PACs have a lead consultant anaesthetist who will provide expert review of high-risk patients and make detailed plans for the care of very high-risk patients, including the provision of a high dependency or intensive care bed in the immediate post-operative period.

Thromboembolism remains one of the biggest preventable risks of any surgical procedure, and it is mandatory for a formal assessment of a patient's individual risk prior to surgery (**Figure 17.1**). This is best assessed at the PAC so that plans can be made for peri- and post-operative thromboprophylaxis. For major procedures, thrombogenic medication such as the combined oral contraceptive pill should be stopped 4 weeks prior to surgery and alternative contraception used. All patients are given thromboembolic deterrent (TED) stockings and advised about the importance of keeping well hydrated and early mobilization after surgery. Low molecular weight heparin (LMWH) is given according to the standard risk assessment. Patients with known coagulation disorders or those taking long-term anticoagulants, such as apixaban, can be discussed with the haematologist and a detailed bridging plan prepared.

PACs are an opportunity for patients to discuss any remaining concerns or questions they may have about their impending surgery. The surgical teams are often not directly involved in the PAC, so, if concerns or queries about the procedure do arise, the PAC may need to contact the specialist again. This is particularly pertinent if there has been a long gap between the initial listing for the procedure and the proposed surgery date, as the patient's condition may have changed in the interim.

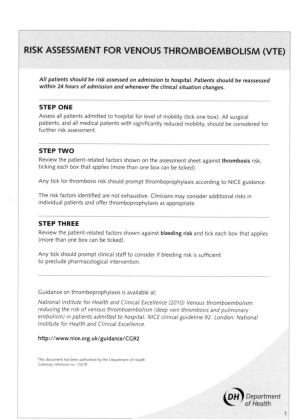

RISK ASSESSMENT FOR VENOUS THROMBOEMBOLISM (VTE)

All patients should be risk assessed on admission to hospital. Patients should be reassessed within 24 hours of admission and whenever the clinical situation changes.

STEP ONE
Assess all patients admitted to hospital for level of mobility (tick one box). All surgical patients, and all medical patients with significantly reduced mobility, should be considered for further risk assessment.

STEP TWO
Review the patient-related factors shown on the assessment sheet against **thrombosis** risk, ticking each box that applies (more than one box can be ticked).

Any tick for thrombosis risk should prompt thromboprophylaxis according to NICE guidance.

The risk factors identified are not exhaustive. Clinicians may consider additional risks in individual patients and offer thromboprophylaxis as appropriate.

STEP THREE
Review the patient-related factors shown against **bleeding risk** and tick each box that applies (more than one box can be ticked).

Any tick should prompt clinical staff to consider if bleeding risk is sufficient to preclude pharmacological intervention.

Guidance on thromboprophylaxis is available at:
National Institute for Health and Clinical Excellence (2010) Venous thromboembolism: reducing the risk of venous thromboembolism (deep vein thrombosis and pulmonary embolism) in patients admitted to hospital. NICE clinical guideline 92. London: National Institute for Health and Clinical Excellence.

http://www.nice.org.uk/guidance/CG92

This document has been authorised by the Department of Health
Gateway reference no. 10278

DH Department of Health

1

DH Department of Health

RISK ASSESSMENT FOR VENOUS THROMBOEMBOLISM (VTE)

Mobility – all patients (tick one box)	Tick		Tick		Tick
Surgical patient		Medical patient expected to have ongoing reduced mobility relative to normal state		Medical patient NOT expected to have significantly reduced mobility relative to normal state	
Assess for thrombosis and bleeding risk below				Risk assessment now complete	

Thrombosis risk

Patient related	Tick	Admission related	Tick
Active cancer or cancer treatment		Significantly reduced mobility for 3 days or more	
Age > 60		Hip or knee replacement	
Dehydration		Hip fracture	
Known thrombophilias		Total anaesthetic + surgical time > 90 minutes	
Obesity (BMI >30 kg/m²)		Surgery involving pelvis or lower limb with a total anaesthetic + surgical time > 60 minutes	
One or more significant medical comorbidities (eg heart disease;metabolic,endocrine or respiratory pathologies;acute infectious diseases; inflammatory conditions)		Acute surgical admission with inflammatory or intra-abdominal condition	
Personal history or first-degree relative with a history of VTE		Critical care admission	
Use of hormone replacement therapy		Surgery with significant reduction in mobility	
Use of oestrogen-containing contraceptive therapy			
Varicose veins with phlebitis			
Pregnancy or < 6 weeks post partum (see NICE guidance for specific risk factors)			

Bleeding risk

Patient related	Tick	Admission related	Tick
Active bleeding		Neurosurgery, spinal surgery or eye surgery	
Acquired bleeding disorders (such as acute liver failure)		Other procedure with high bleeding risk	
Concurrent use of anticoagulants known to increase the risk of bleeding (such as warfarin with INR >2)		Lumbar puncture/epidural/spinal anaesthesia expected within the next 12 hours	
Acute stroke		Lumbar puncture/epidural/spinal anaesthesia within the previous 4 hours	
Thrombocytopaenia (platelets< 75x10⁹/l)			
Uncontrolled systolic hypertension (230/120 mmHg or higher)			
Untreated inherited bleeding disorders (such as haemophilia and von Willebrand's disease)			

© Crown copyright 2010
301292 1p March 10

2

Figure 17.1 Thromboembolism risk assessment tool.

BOX 17.2: Thromboprophylaxis in surgery

- *Low risk*: surgery less than 30 minutes without risk factors – no specific thromboprophylaxis needed
- *Moderate risk*: surgery more than 30 minutes, age >60 years, body mass index (BMI) >30, significant family history, varicose veins, sepsis, comorbidity or pregnancy – use TED stockings and LMWH
- *High risk*: cancer, prolonged surgery, immobility, previous thromboembolic event, thrombophilia or three or more of the moderate risk factors – use TED stockings and LMWH for 7 days or 28 days (known cancer) or until mobile

CONSENT

Obtaining valid consent prior to surgery is an integral step in the care of the patient. This is a continuous process that begins in the outpatient clinic, rather than a single event when the patient signs the form. It is essential that all discussions are clearly documented in the case notes and that the patient is fully informed. Patients must be provided with all of the relevant information about their planned procedure, including the likely success rate or outcome, alternative options available to them, the usual recovery time and any particular measures to be observed during recovery. They should also be made aware of all of the potential complications of surgery, how likely they are and how these might have an impact on their recovery and eventual outcome (**Table 17.1**).

While written consent is obtained, the process is much more than just completing a form. The physician has a duty to ensure that the patient has been provided with all of the relevant information in a way that they can understand, and the patient should be able to demonstrate understanding of this information. It is good practice to ask the patient to repeat back their understanding of what they have been told. The person obtaining consent should be

Table 17.1 Presenting information on risk

Term	Numerical value	Colloquial phrase
Very common	Up to 1:10	Person in family
Common	1:10–1:100	Person in street
Uncommon	1:100–1:1,000	Person in village/ locality
Rare	1:1,000– 1:10,000	Person in small town
Very rare	Less than 1:10,000	Person in large town

someone competent to undertake the procedure, who understands what is involved and the risks. Where possible, the patient should be given site- or surgeon-specific success and complication rates. All discussions should be clearly documented. Although it is natural to want to avoid creating unnecessary anxiety by discussing serious complications, it is important to be as comprehensive as possible, explaining the rarity and context of any complications. Ultimately, it is up to the patient to consider what is important to them.

When obtaining consent, one should be aware of the patient's mental capacity. Mental capacity is the ability of a person to make decisions for themselves about things that influence their lives, from simple to complex decisions, including the decision to undergo medical or surgical treatment.

From a legal perspective, a person lacks capacity when, at the time of decision-making, they are unable to make or communicate that decision due to an 'impairment of, or a disturbance in the function of the mind or brain'. Assessing capacity has two stages. First, is there an impairment or disturbance to the mind or brain? Second, is this sufficient to render the person unable to make a decision? It should be remembered that capacity is task- and time-specific. Thus, a person with dementia, for example, may have the capacity to make simple decisions (e.g. to have a cup of tea), but not complex decisions, and their capacity might vary from day to day. The key issue for health professionals is to ensure that capacity has been assessed. When capacity is in doubt, the responsibility to ascertain capacity lies with the healthcare professional, and sometimes it may be necessary to seek the opinion of more than one practitioner. Many hospitals have a formal process whereby a panel will make the decision. When capacity is absent or unclear, clinical decisions have to be made on the basis of what is in the patient's best interests. This can be difficult to establish and will often require discussion with family members or friends who can advise on what the patient would usually wish or any previous expressions or views made when the patient had capacity. An individual will be protected by law when making a clinical decision when they have 'reasonable belief' that the person lacks consent and that the course of action is in the person's best interest. This is limited by certain things, including any advance decision by the individual (e.g. a 'living will') or by a legal judgement. In many cases, the issue of capacity is easy to determine, but sometimes it can be difficult, and identifying the patient's 'best interests' can also be difficult. If in doubt, clinicians should seek advice from their employer's legal team. Occasionally, decisions on care need to be made by court ruling.

SURGICAL SAFETY

On the day of surgery, the surgical and theatre team must work together to ensure that the whole procedure occurs efficiently without complications or

---

⚷ KEY LEARNING POINTS

- Consent for surgery is a continuous process and should be fully documented.
- All alternative options and potential complications should be explained to the patient in a format and language they can understand.
- Where possible, site- or surgeon-specific figures for success and complications should be used.
- Mental capacity is required to give consent.
- Assessing mental capacity when doubt exists is a formal process and must be carefully documented. Formal legal advice may be necessary.
- When capacity is lacking, treatment decisions can be made only if they can be shown to be in the patient's best interests.

adverse events. Communication within the team is of paramount importance. Worldwide, the crude mortality rate after surgery is between 0.5% and 5%, and post-operative complications occur in up to 25% of cases. In higher income countries, nearly half of adverse events in hospital relate to surgical care, half of which are considered to have been avoidable. To help combat this, the World Health Organization (WHO) has developed a safe surgery checklist, which is now in routine use in most hospitals. The checklist is a validated and tested tool to reduce these risks, and it includes specific tasks to be undertaken before, during and after surgery to ensure that the whole team is aware of issues relating to the specific case (**Figure 17.2**). It includes elements to ensure anaesthesia safety, identification of the correct surgical site and confirmation of the procedure planned, discussion of any specific or non-standard elements to the procedure and attention to careful postoperative care in the immediate recovery period.

The three main components are: (1) An initial team brief before the list starts. During this brief all team members (surgical, anaesthetic and theatre) should be present and introduce themselves. The operating list is reviewed to check the order and each case discussed in detail with regard to the procedure, likely problems and any special requests for equipment or additional support. (2) Before the start of each individual procedure the patient details are again checked, and specific issues for that patient are discussed such as the need for blood products, antibiotics and thromboprophylaxis. (3) At the end of the procedure there is a sign out check to make sure that all swabs/instruments are accounted for and to document any specific concerns or instructions for the recovery staff. Finally at the end of the list there is a debrief to review how the list went and any issues that arose that need further attention. It is a written checklist developed to minimize surgical adverse events.

GOOD SURGICAL PRACTICE

During surgery, careful tissue handling is a prerequisite. Careful dissection of tissues and gentle handling of other organs and the abdominal wall will both minimize the risk of surgical trauma and reduce

the release of acute phase proteins and inflammatory mediators. This is very likely to aid the patient's recovery in the immediate post-operative period. Careful and methodical surgery is the key to successful outcomes, particularly when faced with difficult surgery and distorted anatomy. Where necessary, normal anatomy should be restored by dividing adhesions and mobilizing adjacent organs before doing the proposed procedure. Every surgeon should be aware of their limitations and, if the procedure is more complex than anticipated or unexpected difficulties are encountered, it is sound practice to call an experienced colleague to assist you. Increasingly, more complex surgery is done by two consultants working together.

ROUTE OF SURGERY AND COMMON INCISIONS

In gynaecology, there are three potential surgical routes: transvaginal, laparoscopic and open abdominal. The decision about which of these to use is usually dictated by the procedure. For instance, a hysteroscopy is done transvaginally, whereas a diagnostic laparoscopy is clearly done laparoscopically. However, for some procedures, such as a hysterectomy, there is a choice. The decision-making process around this is discussed in more detail later in this chapter (see the section 'Hysterectomy'). However, in general terms, the vaginal or laparoscopic approach is preferred to open abdominal surgery. When an abdominal approach is deemed necessary, the laparoscopic approach is usually preferred to open abdominal, except when there are specific contraindications to minimal access surgery.

For vaginal prolapse surgery, the surgical incision is usually a midline incision in whichever vaginal wall (anterior or posterior) is affected. This allows the skin to be reflected and to gain access to the fascia and underlying tissues. For vaginal hysterectomy, the vaginal mucosa around the cervix is excised to gain access to the uterosacral ligaments and vesico-uterine space and pouch of Douglas. The morbidity associated with vaginal incisions is very low and many patients experience little or no pain after vaginal surgery.

Before induction of anaesthesia

(With at least nurse and anaesthetist)

Has the patient confirmed his/her identity, site, procedure, and consent?

☐ Yes

Is the site marked?

☐ Yes
☐ Not applicable

Is the anaesthesia machine and medication check complete?

☐ Yes

Is the pulse oximeter on the patient and functioning?

☐ Yes

Does the patient have a:

Known allergy?

☐ No
☐ Yes

Difficult airway or aspiration risk?

☐ No
☐ Yes, and equipment/assistance available

Risk of >500 ml blood loss (7 ml/kg in children)?

☐ No
☐ Yes, and two IVs/central access and fluids planned

Before skin incision

(With nurse, anaesthetist and surgeon)

☐ **Confirm all team members have introduced themselves by name and role.**

☐ **Confirm the patient's name, procedure, and where the incision will be made.**

Has antibiotic prophylaxis been given within the last 60 minutes?

☐ Yes
☐ Not applicable

Anticipated critical events

To surgeon:

☐ What are the critical or non-routine steps?
☐ How long will the case take?
☐ What is the anticipated blood loss?

To anaesthetist:

☐ Are there any patient-specific concerns?

To nursing team:

☐ Has sterility (including indicator results) been confirmed?
☐ Are there equipment issues or any concerns?

Is essential imaging displayed?

☐ Yes
☐ Not applicable

Before patient leaves operating room

(With nurse, anaesthetist and surgeon)

Nurse verbally confirms:

☐ The name of the procedure
☐ Completion of instrument, sponge and needle counts
☐ Specimen labelling (read specimen labels aloud, including patient's name)
☐ Whether there are any equipment problems to be addressed

To surgeon, anaesthetist and nurse:

☐ What are the key concerns for recovery and management of this patient?

Note: This checklist is not intended to be comprehensive. Additions and modifications to fit local practice are encouraged.

Figure 17.2 WHO surgical checklist used in the NHS. (IV, intravenous line.)

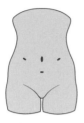
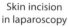

Skin incision
in laparoscopy

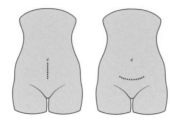

Traditional skin incisions

Figure 17.3 Incisions used in gynaecological surgery.

BOX 17.4: Midline incision

- Vertically from pubic symphysis up to (or beyond) umbilicus
- Less strong; prone to herniation or dehiscence
- More painful (involves several dermatomes)
- Cosmetically unattractive
- Can easily be extended around umbilicus up to the xiphisternum
- Gives excellent surgical access

For open abdominal gynaecological surgery, the choice of incision is usually between a transverse lower abdominal incision (Pfannenstiel incision) and a sub-umbilical midline incision (**Figure 17.3**). Pfannenstiel incisions are ideal for uncomplicated gynaecological procedures. The incision is quick to make and open, as there is no posterior rectus sheath at the level of the incision, it being below the arcuate line. It is a strong incision that is not prone to herniation and is cosmetically attractive. The major drawback with the Pfannenstiel incision is that it cannot easily be extended, so, in situations in which the anatomy is unexpectedly distorted or some unanticipated pathology is encountered, the surgeon is forced to make an inverted T incision to improve access, which is neither strong in repair nor attractive.

A midline (or paramedian) incision is often favoured by oncologists and also when significant surgical difficulty is anticipated (e.g. from adhesions, large fibroids or ovarian cysts). Although less strong than a Pfannenstiel incision, the major advantage of the midline incision is that it can easily be extended

BOX 17.3: Pfannenstiel incision

- Transversely, two finger breadths above the pubic symphysis
- Strong when repaired, with a low risk of herniation or dehiscence
- Not very painful (limited to one or two dermatomes)
- Cosmetically attractive (lower than the 'underwear line')
- Cannot easily be extended or made larger
- Surgical access limited to pelvic organs

to provide excellent surgical access. A large incision will of course cause more post-operative pain, which can increase the risk of respiratory infection by limiting breathing and coughing efforts. A vertical incision is often recommended in emergency cases (laparotomy) when the exact underlying diagnosis is not entirely clear (e.g. a pelvic mass in a pyrexial patient) to allow flexibility of access should the findings be unexpected. Where possible, the potential for a midline incision should be discussed with the patient in advance.

Laparoscopic surgery holds several advantages over open abdominal surgery. Laparoscopic entry wounds are no more than 1 cm in length and thus cause much less post-operative pain than an open wound. The risk of herniation is very low. The lack of pain and extensive external wounds means that patients become mobile after surgery very quickly, and most laparoscopic procedures (even hysterectomy) allow for hospital discharge within 2 hours. The laparoscopic approach allows enhanced visibility for some pelvic procedures, especially those deep in the pelvis, such as excision of infiltrating endometriosis or performing the mesh attachment at a laparoscopic sacrocolpopexy. Although the operating time may be longer than with open surgery, the more rapid discharge from hospital makes laparoscopic surgery more cost-effective in general; there are also limited data suggesting laparoscopic surgery leads to better surgical outcomes. Ultimately, any decision regarding surgical entry should be patient- and surgeon-specific.

Robotic surgery is currently limited to a relatively small number of hospitals, but its use in gynaecological surgery is increasing. The robotic approach has all the potential benefits of the minimal access (laparoscopic) approach, with the additional benefits of very clear tissue visualization and manoeuvrability of instruments, which is particularly valuable in tight spaces. It also allows the surgeon to sit at the console during surgery, which aids surgeon comfort during long procedures and enables easier teaching on a parallel console. Currently, robots are still very expensive and have yet to be shown to be cost-effective with longer operating times. However, with rapidly advancing technology (including the incorporation of artificial intelligence) and falling costs, it is likely the use of robotic surgery will become more widespread, particularly in more complex cases such as oncology, severe endometriosis and pelvic floor reconstruction.

BOX 17.5: Laparoscopic approach

Advantages

- Small incision and reduced scarring
- Enhanced view of pelvic organs
- Less post-operative pain
- Quicker recovery and mobilization

Disadvantages

- Open surgery offers better oncological outcomes in stage IB cervical cancer
- Large pelvic masses may rupture or be too large to remove intact, spilling malignant cells in the event of unsuspected ovarian cancer or uterine sarcoma

KEY LEARNING POINTS

- Surgical pre-assessment allows personalized plans of care to be made for those with comorbidities.
- Multidisciplinary review of planned cases can be helpful in deciding on the safest approach to complex or medically unfit patients.
- Surgical incisions should be made after consideration of the requirements for surgical access and the potential difficulties, but also the strength and recovery time for each type of incision.
- Many gynaecological procedures are performed by minimal access techniques, thereby minimizing incisional pain and recovery.

SUTURES

Surgical suture materials are essential elements for surgical practice; they are necessary for tying off vascular pedicles, closing the vaginal vault at hysterectomy and repairing abdominal and vaginal incisions. The ideal suture material is one that allows secure knot tying without slippage, provokes little tissue reaction, does not increase the risk of infection, retains enough tensile strength until the healing process has laid down enough collagen and connective tissue to restore integrity of the tissues, and can be wholly reabsorbed by the body. Such a material does not exist! The choice of suture for any particular purpose will depend on which of the above characteristics are considered most important. Broadly, sutures can be characterized by two properties: absorbable versus non-absorbable and monofilament versus multifilament (Table 17.2).

Multifilament sutures are generally more secure in knot tying than monofilament sutures, due to greater friction from the braided filaments, and so will require fewer throws to secure the knot and thus reduce the amount of suture material used. Suture volume is relevant to the risk of surgical site infection, as more foreign material increases this risk. Conversely, multifilament sutures carry a greater risk of infection than monofilament sutures, because the spaces between the filaments retain bacteria. Monofilament sutures will generally cause less tissue reaction.

Table 17.2 Examples of sutures used in gynaecology

	Absorbable (>50% strength retention)	Non-absorbable
Multifilament	Polyglactin (Vicryl®) (21 days)	Silk Braided nylon Braided polyester/ dacron (Ethibond®)
Monofilament	Poliglecaprone (Monocryl®) (7 days) Polydioxanone (PDS®) (28 days)	Nylon Polypropylene (Prolene®)

For most indications in gynaecology, absorbable sutures will be preferred to non-absorbable sutures. Most modern sutures are polymers of synthetic material that can be broken down by tissue enzymes and macrophages over time. The time taken to degrade is material-dependent but is also influenced by inflammation, infection and the general health of the patient. The choice of which material is used depends on the length of time for which tensile strength is required.

Non-absorbable 'permanent' sutures are not absorbed so retain their strength indefinitely, but carry a risk of erosion through the skin or vaginal epithelium in the long term. Non-absorbable sutures are reserved for specific situations in which long-term strength is required. In gynaecology, this is most often for the closure of midline abdominal incisions, incisions in cases of malignancy or in a patient with major chronic illness compromising healing (e.g. chronic kidney disease or diabetes), or in a patient in whom the same incision has been opened more than once before.

POST-OPERATIVE CARE AND RECOVERY

The increasing focus on day surgery and the utilization of the Enhanced Recovery After Surgery® pathway means that, for many procedures (even major gynaecological surgery such as pelvic floor repair or laparoscopic hysterectomy), most patients are discharged within 24 hours. To achieve this, the patient's condition should be optimized pre-operatively (see the earlier section 'Pre-assessment' in this chapter) and the patient should be encouraged to mobilize and start eating and drinking normally soon after surgery. The first 12–24 hours after surgery are when the patient is most at risk of immediate surgical complications. Thus, initial nursing and medical care is focused on identifying early warning signs of sepsis or haemorrhage: temperature, pulse and blood pressure will be monitored in the first 12–24 hours to identify any clinical signs of infection or hypovolaemic collapse. Following more major surgery, some patients will require intravenous fluids for the first 12–24 hours. Thromboprophylaxis measures will be continued as per previous risk assessment.

> **BOX 17.6: Key principles of the Enhanced Recovery After Surgery® pathway**
>
> **Pre-operative**
> - Counselling
> - Optimization of health
> - Avoid overnight fasting and dehydration
> - Carbohydrate loading
>
> **Perioperative**
> - Venous thromboembolism prophylaxis
> - Minimally invasive surgery where possible
> - Antibiotic prophylaxis (certain procedures only)
> - Prevention of hypothermia
> - Avoid unnecessary tubes/drains
> - Short-acting anaesthetics
>
> **Post-operative**
> - Good analgesia (avoid opiates)
> - Early mobilization
> - Early resumption of fluids and normal diet
> - Nurse-led discharge pathway where possible
> - Constant audit of service

Post-operative management and the decision to discharge is increasingly a nurse-led process based on regular observations and following strict pathways. Surgical post-operative ward rounds should occur at least once daily, but more frequent review may be required if there are concerns. Post-operative review should include a debrief for the patient of the surgical procedure and how it went. If any complications occurred, the patient should be informed at the earliest opportunity and given the chance to ask questions (duty of candor). Blood sampling for full blood count should be done if there are concerns about post-operative bleeding or if there was significant blood loss at the time of surgery. Urea and electrolytes may need to be checked for those patients who remain on intravenous fluids.

Single-dose antibiotic prophylaxis is given intra-operatively for most major gynaecological surgery, but empirical prescription of antibiotics in the post-operative period should be avoided. Intravenous cannulae should be removed as soon as possible, as they can be uncomfortable and sometimes can be a source of infection.

Most wounds are now closed with dissolvable sutures, but any non-absorbable abdominal wound sutures are usually removed 7–10 days after surgery. This can be arranged in the community. Thromboprophylaxis should continue until discharge and, in high-risk cases, may need to be continued for up to 6 weeks. Before discharge, the patient should have the opportunity to address any remaining concerns about their recovery, resumption of normal activities, intercourse and the need (or not) for hormone replacement therapy (HRT). It takes around 6–8 weeks for scar tissue to regain full strength, so, after major abdominal or vaginal surgery, patients are usually advised to wait this long before gradual resumption of normal activities. However, there is little evidence supporting this recommendation and a lot depends on the individual patient and the procedure. For those undergoing laparoscopic surgery, a gradual resumption of activity from about 7–10 days after surgery is acceptable. For those recovering from major pelvic floor reconstruction, a longer recovery period may be advised.

FOLLOW-UP

Good surgical practice should normally include a post-operative review with the surgical team at some point after surgery to review recovery, assess the outcomes and address any ongoing concerns. In some clinical scenarios, this may not be necessary (e.g. following a normal hysteroscopy for postmenopausal bleeding), but the patient should be informed of the results of any investigations. Traditionally, surgical follow-up has been around 6 weeks after surgery. Some hospitals discourage follow-up appointments after routine surgery, expecting it to be done in primary care. As practice changes, the place and timing of any post-operative follow-up may well vary, but it is still the responsibility of the operating surgeon to clearly state what follow-up is anticipated and with whom and to communicate that clearly to the patient and their general practitioner.

HYSTERECTOMY

Hysterectomy is one of the most common surgical procedures in gynaecology and is therefore given special mention here, as it illustrates many of the surgical principles and much of the decision-making that takes place in gynaecology. Other routine gynaecological operations are described more briefly later. Hysterectomy is performed for a variety of benign indication reasons, such as heavy and/or painful or irregular periods when medical treatment or less invasive surgery has failed, vaginal prolapse, large fibroids, pelvic pain and as part of the management of various cancers (see relevant chapters). After the decision has been made to perform a hysterectomy, there are two subsequent questions that must be asked. First, which route is most appropriate? Second, should the ovaries and fallopian tubes be removed at the same time?

The choice of route has to balance the benefits and risks of each approach (**Table 17.3**). Generally, the laparoscopic approach is now considered the default for most gynaecologists. If the uterus is very enlarged by fibroids or if significant intra-abdominal adhesions are expected, then an open abdominal approach may be preferred, although the threshold for this will very much depend on the individual surgeon. Ovarian cancer surgery and radical hysterectomy for cervical cancer are mostly open procedures to ensure the best oncological outcomes. The vaginal route is preferred if there is significant uterine prolapse or if the procedure is being done as part of a transvaginal prolapse repair. Depending on their training, some surgeons are more comfortable operating vaginally than laparoscopically. The vaginal route has many of the advantages of the laparoscopic route, so is a suitable alternative.

Removal of the ovaries and fallopian tubes is not essential if hysterectomy is being performed for benign indications, and the decision about whether to do so should be made in discussion with the patient

> ### BOX 17.7: Types of laparoscopic hysterectomy
>
> - *Laparoscopically assisted vaginal hysterectomy*: the first two pedicles are completed laparoscopically and the third is completed vaginally
> - *Total laparoscopic hysterectomy*: the whole procedure is completed laparoscopically and the uterus is removed vaginally
> - *Subtotal laparoscopic hysterectomy*: the cervix is preserved and the uterus is removed either laparoscopically via morcellation or through culdotomy (posterior vaginal fornix incision)

Table 17.3 Hysterectomy routes

Procedure	Key points	Advantages	Disadvantages
Abdominal hysterectomy	Abdominal incision Cervix and uterus removed Ovaries and fallopian tubes can be easily removed	Allows full inspection of abdominal cavity and pelvis Can remove large fibroid uterus and deal with difficult anatomy May offer best oncological outcomes in ovarian and cervical cancer surgery	Abdominal incision More pain Longer recovery period
Vaginal hysterectomy	Vaginal incision Cervix and uterus removed Ovaries and fallopian tubes not normally removed but can be done with laparoscopically assisted vaginal hysterectomy Can be combined with vaginal prolapse surgery	No abdominal incision Rapid recovery Suitable for spinal anaesthesia More appropriate for those who are frail/elderly	Ovaries not removed Surgical access can be limited Not suitable for large fibroid uterus or if intra-abdominal pathology is suspected
Laparoscopic hysterectomy	Laparoscopic entry Cervix and uterus removed Fallopian tubes and ovaries can be removed Most procedures can be done this way Allows inspection of abdomen and pelvis	Rapid recovery Less pain Quick return to normal activity	May take longer Appropriate skills required May not be feasible if there are dense adhesions or in the case of a large uterus May compromise oncological outcomes if there is intraoperative spillage of tumour or smaller excision margins
Robotic hysterectomy	Same as for laparoscopic surgery Enhanced vision and access to deep pelvic structures Operator seated at console	Quick recovery Ergonomically favourable for surgeon Dual control allows training Potential for interaction with artificial intelligence	Expensive and time consuming Specific training required Limited availability

in advance of surgery. In the absence of any suspected ovarian pathology, the decision is primarily to do with eliminating the subsequent risk of ovarian cancer. Although an uncommon cancer, it classically presents late with poor outcomes (see **Chapter 14**) and many people feel that removal of the ovaries and fallopian tubes is the best way to prevent it. This is often advised if there is a strong family history of ovarian cancer. However, the advantage of this has to be balanced against the potential impact of a sudden menopause, which results from the ovaries being removed.

The current thinking that high-grade serous ovarian cancer actually originates in the fallopian tube has led to some gynaecologists offering opportunistic bilateral salpingectomy with ovarian conservation at the time of hysterectomy as a risk-reducing measure. In a patient who is already postmenopausal, oophorectomy may be a sensible option because it removes the risk of later ovarian cancer without any likely hormonal consequences. For a patient who is still menstruating regularly, it is usually advisable to leave the ovaries in situ to preserve endogenous ovarian function and prevent the early onset of menopausal symptoms and osteoporosis. For patients in the perimenopausal years who may have some early menopausal symptoms and a degree of menstrual irregularity, the decision about removing the ovaries should be individualized in relation to personal preferences regarding taking HRT (this is discussed in **Chapter 8**). In some situations, it may be necessary to remove both ovaries in a young person, such as severe endometriosis, severe premenstrual dysphoric disorder or those with a strong family history of ovarian cancer. This should be done only after appropriate counselling about the impact of early menopause and the recommendation to take systemic HRT at least until the age of 50.

A hysterectomy operation involves taking three pedicles, which, in laparoscopic or abdominal hysterectomy, are taken top down:

1. the infundibulopelvic ligament, which contains the ovarian vessels
2. the uterine vessels

BOX 17.8: Complications of hysterectomy

Intraoperative

- Haemorrhage requiring blood products (common)
- Bladder injury (uncommon)
- Ureteric injury (rare)
- Rectal injury (rare)

Immediate post-operative

- Immediate onset of menopausal symptoms (if ovaries are removed in a premenopausal person) (common)
- Wound infection (common)
- Pelvic infection (uncommon)
- Secondary haemorrhage (uncommon)
- Deep vein thrombosis or thromboembolism (pelvic surgery/cancer) (uncommon)
- Vesicovaginal or rectovaginal fistula (consequence of injury) (very rare)

Longer-term post-operative

- New bladder symptoms (both overactive bladder and stress incontinence) (common)
- Vaginal prolapse after hysterectomy for any cause (common)
- Long-term consequences of menopause if oestrogen not adequately replaced (common)
- Persistent scar pain (abdominal) (uncommon)

---

3. the angles of the vault of the vagina, which contain vessels ascending from the vagina; the ligaments to support the uterus can be taken with this pedicle or separately

In vaginal hysterectomy, the same steps are taken but in the reverse order.

Hysterectomy by any route carries specific complications that can be minimized by careful surgical planning and pre-operative preparation. Any situation in which there is distortion of the normal anatomy (e.g. fibroids or malignancy) or significant inflammation (e.g. previous pelvic infection or endometriosis) will increase the potential for serious complications and patients should be advised accordingly.

OTHER GYNAECOLOGICAL PROCEDURES

Full details of each procedure are beyond the scope of this book, but a brief summary of the most common procedures, indications and complications is presented in **Table 17.4**.

🔑 KEY LEARNING POINTS

- The bladder and ureters are closely related to the uterus, cervix and uterine vessels and are at risk of injury during hysterectomy.
- Laparoscopic hysterectomy is the route of choice for benign indications.
- Abdominal hysterectomy has a longer recovery time than laparoscopic or vaginal hysterectomy, but may be necessary if there is a large uterus or malignancy.
- Robotic hysterectomy is increasingly being used in oncology, but the benefits have yet to be clearly established.
- Hysterectomy by any route increases the risk of new urinary and prolapse symptoms.
- The decision of whether or not to remove the ovaries should consider the patient's age, the presence of menopausal symptoms, pain, the individual risk of later ovarian cancer and the patient's suitability for HRT.
- If the ovaries are conserved, the fallopian tubes are usually removed, as this can reduce subsequent ovarian cancer risk and they have no endocrine role.

Table 17.4 Common gynaecological surgeries

Reason	Procedure	Key points	Short description	Complications
For prolapse	Anterior vaginal repair (colporrhaphy)	For symptomatic anterior vaginal prolapse Not a procedure for stress incontinence	Sutures to reinforce fascia between vagina and bladder	Risk of bladder injury and urinary retention Relatively high recurrence rate
	Posterior vaginal repair (colporrhaphy)	For posterior vaginal prolapse Can improve obstructed defaecation	Sutures to reinforce fascia between vaginal and rectum	Risk of rectal injury Associated with post-operative dyspareunia
For incontinence	Transvaginal tape or transobturator tape	For stress incontinence	Tape made of mesh inserted running either through both obturator fossae under bladder neck or through retropubic space	Mesh erosion Bladder damage Pain Voiding problems Currently not used in the UK due to high mesh complication rate
	Colposuspension	For stress incontinence	Bladder neck elevated and replaced intra-abdominally Can be open or laparoscopic	Haemorrhage Infection Bladder damage Voiding dysfunction Long-term rectocele development
For assessment of uterine cavity	Hysteroscopy	Uterus distended with saline or glycine to view cavity Performed as day-case or outpatient surgery	Cervix is dilated to enable introduction of hysteroscope. Cavity and ostia are viewed Can be used for surgical removal of polyps, septum and submucous fibroids Can be used for directed endometrial biopsy	Bleeding Perforation Infection Pain (local)
For miscarriage	Evacuation of retained products of conception	To remove pregnancy tissue retained after miscarriage The procedure for the termination of pregnancy is identical	Cervix is dilated Suction curette used to evacuate uterus	Bleeding Perforation Infection Need for further procedure
For heavy menstrual bleeding	Endometrial ablation	Variety of energy devices that are deployed into the uterine cavity to ablate the endometrium	Usually performed after a hysteroscopy and biopsy Procedures only take 3–10 minutes and can be done in the outpatient setting under local anaesthetic	Bleeding Perforation Infection Incomplete ablation (80% success)

Reason	Procedure	Key points	Short description	Complications
For cervical abnormality	LLETZ and cone biopsy	To remove transformation zone of cervix when cervical intraepithelial neoplasia is present	Transformation zone removed under local anaesthetic (LLETZ) using diathermy or cut away under general anaesthetic with the benefit of histological confirmation of excision	Haemorrhage and secondary haemorrhage from infection Preterm delivery
For assessment of pelvis	Laparoscopy	Minimal access surgery through umbilical port to view and treat pelvic organs Can be diagnostic or route of surgery for oophorectomy, division of adhesions, ligation or clipping or removal of fallopian tubes, removal of ovarian cysts, treatment of endometriosis Route of preference for most benign abdominal gynaecological procedures	Carbon dioxide is insufflated through a Veress needle to expand the abdominal cavity, and instruments are then introduced	Haemorrhage Infection Damage to pelvic organs Perforation of uterus
For fibroids	Myomectomy	Abdominal or laparoscopic operation to remove uterine fibroids	Individual fibroids are 'shelled' out of the myometrium of the exposed uterus, which is sutured closed	Haemorrhage and haematomas requiring transfusion Adhesion formation

LLETZ, large loop excision of transformation zone.

HYSTEROSCOPY

Hysteroscopy involves passing a small-diameter telescope, either flexible or rigid, through the cervix to directly inspect the uterine cavity (**Figures 17.4** and **17.5**). Excellent images can be obtained. A flexible hysteroscope may be used in the outpatient setting. Rigid instruments employ circulating fluids and therefore can be used to visualize the uterine cavity even if the patient is bleeding and to carry out procedures such as polypectomy.

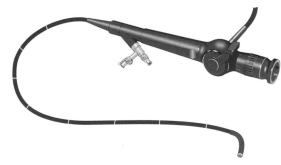

Figure 17.4 Flexible fibre-optic hysteroscope.

255

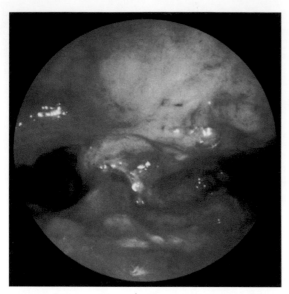

Figure 17.5 View of endometrial cavity demonstrating Asherman adhesions.

INDICATIONS

- Any abnormal bleeding from the uterus:
  - postmenopausal bleeding
  - irregular menstruation, intermenstrual bleeding and post-coital bleeding
  - persistent heavy menstrual bleeding

- Persistent discharge
- Suspected uterine malformations
- Suspected Asherman syndrome

COMPLICATIONS

- Perforation of the uterus
- Cervical damage – if cervical dilatation is necessary
- If there is infection present, hysteroscopy can cause ascending infection

An operating hysteroscope can also be used to resect endometrial pathology such as fibroids, polyps and uterine septae.

LAPAROSCOPY

Laparoscopy allows visualization of the peritoneal cavity (**Figures 17.6**, **17.7** and **17.8**). This involves insertion of a Veress needle umbilically. This allows insufflation of the peritoneal cavity with carbon dioxide so that a larger instrument can be inserted. The majority of instruments used for diagnostic laparoscopy are 5 mm in diameter, and 10 mm instruments are used for operative laparoscopy. A 2 mm laparoscope is available for diagnostic procedures.

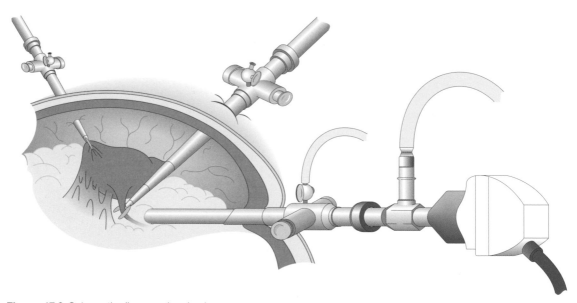

Figure 17.6 Schematic diagram showing laparoscope.

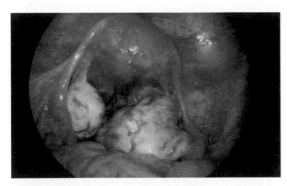

Figure 17.7 Laparoscopic view of bilateral endometriomas.

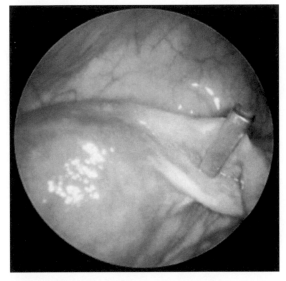

Figure 17.8 Laparoscopic view showing Filshie clip on the right fallopian tube.

INDICATIONS

- Suspected ectopic pregnancy
- Ovarian cyst accident and acute pelvic pain
- Undiagnosed pelvic pain
- Tubal patency testing
- Sterilization

Operative laparoscopy can be performed for a wide range of procedures, including complex benign, oncological and pelvic floor surgery.

COMPLICATIONS

Complications are uncommon but include port site infection and hernia and, rarely, damage to any of the intra-abdominal structures, such as the bowel and major blood vessels. The bladder is always emptied prior to the procedure to avoid bladder injury. Safe entry techniques are essential.

CYSTOSCOPY

Cystoscopy involves passing a small-diameter telescope, either flexible or rigid, through the urethra into the bladder. Excellent images of both of these structures can be obtained. A cystoscope with an operative channel can be used to biopsy any abnormality, perform bladder neck injection, retrieve stones and resect bladder tumours (**Figures 17.9** and **17.10**).

INDICATIONS

- Haematuria
- Recurrent urinary tract infection

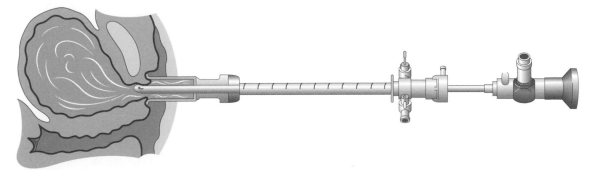

Figure 17.9 Diagram showing the cystoscopic procedure.

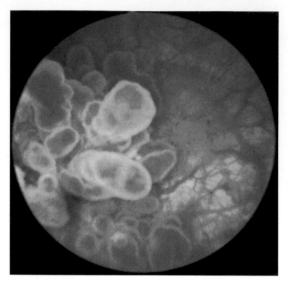

Figure 17.10 Cystoscopic view of bladder papilloma.

- Sterile pyuria
- Persistent irritative symptoms
- Suspected bladder abnormality (e.g. diverticulum, stones, fistula)

- As part of operative procedures, such as bladder neck injections for stress incontinence or botulinum toxin injections for overactive bladder

COMPLICATIONS

- Urinary tract infection
- Bleeding (if biopsy)
- Rarely, bladder perforation

THERAPEUTICS

The drugs used in gynaecology have been described in the relevant chapters, but the key ones are summarized in **Table 17.5**. The British National Formulary (BNF) should be consulted for further information and contraindications.

The key principles of prescribing should always be applied on an individual basis. These include weighing up the potential advantages and disadvantages, correct dosing and the duration of treatment, clear advice about possible side effects and appropriate review.

Table 17.5 Common gynaecological therapeutic agents

Agent	Action	Use
Antifibrinolytics (tranexamic acid)	Reduce blood loss through antifibrinolysis in small capillaries of endometrium	HMB, reducing blood loss by up to 50% Surgical haemorrhage
Non-steroidal anti-inflammatory drugs (e.g. mefenamic acid)	Inhibit prostaglandin synthesis Anti-inflammatory and analgesic	HMB, reducing blood loss by 30% Dysmenorrhoea
GnRHs (e.g. Zoladex®)	Block receptors in the pituitary gland and cause ovarian suppression via hypogonadotrophism	Suppression of the menstrual cycle in endometriosis or other cyclical conditions To reduce the size of fibroids prior to surgery
Synthetic oestrogens (ethinyl oestradiol, which is used in most oral contraceptive pills) Natural oestrogens (oestradiol)	Contraception: inhibit the pituitary feedback loop, thus stopping ovulation HRT: stimulate oestrogenic activity on end-organs of bone, endometrium and many others, such as skin Relieve menopausal symptoms	Usually oral but can be delivered transdermally Can also be delivered vaginally in low doses for urogenital atrophy

Agent	Action	Use
Progestogens (different types with varying androgenic activity)	Suppress endometrium and ovulation in some cases Can be given cyclically or continuously Side effects are common	For HMB, contraception and HRT Levonorgestrel can be delivered by intrauterine system for contraception, HMB or as part of HRT
Tibolone (a synthetic steroid converted in vivo to have activity of all three steroid groups)	Relieves menopausal symptoms Conserves bone mass and improves libido	Used as HRT or with long-term GnRH suppression to preserve bone strength
Clomiphene citrate	Ovulation induction	Antioestrogen at level of the hypothalamus and pituitary gland, leading to increased release of follicle-stimulating hormone and luteinizing hormone, hence initiating folliculogenesis

GnRH, gonadotrophin-releasing hormone; HMB, heavy menstrual bleeding; HRT, hormone replacement therapy.

FURTHER READING

British Medical Association (BMA) (2023). BMA guidance: Mental Capacity Act toolkit. https://www.bma.org.uk/advice-and-support/ethics/adults-who-lack-capacity/mental-capacity-act-toolkit.

BNF. https://bnf.nice.org.uk.

NHS (2021). Mental Capacity Act. https://www.nhs.uk/conditions/social-care-and-support-guide/making-decisions-for-someone-else/mental-capacity-act/.

Royal College of Obstetricians and Gynaecologists (RCOG) (2015). Clinical governance advice No. 6: Obtaining valid consent. https://www.rcog.org.uk/guidance/browse-all-guidance/clinical-governance-advice/obtaining-valid-consent-clinical-governance-advice-no-6/.

WHO (n.d.). WHO safe surgery checklist. https://www.who.int/teams/integrated-health-services/patient-safety/research/safe-surgery/tool-and-resources.

SELF-ASSESSMENT

For interactive SBAs and EMQs relating to this chapter, visit www.routledge.com/cw/crosbie.

CASE HISTORY 1

A 34-year-old asthmatic woman has been seen in the clinic with severe dysmenorrhoea and pelvic pain and a possible diagnosis of endometriosis. She would also like to become pregnant. An ultrasound has shown a normal uterus and 'kissing ovaries', with a 6 cm endometrioma on the right ovary. She would like to undergo a laparoscopy for diagnosis and treatment.

A What additional points in the history should be sought?
B What pre-operative checks and tests should be made for this woman?
C What consent process should take place?

ANSWERS

A The gynaecological history should cover the length of symptoms, their severity, interference with normal function and her expectations of surgery. In particular, symptoms of dyschexia are important to assess the likelihood of rectovaginal nodes.

The length of time trying for a pregnancy, any treatments tried and assessment of her partner's fertility are vital here, as they may affect a decision to treat tubal or ovarian disease. The balance of fertility issues and symptomatology are crucial in surgery for endometriosis (e.g. if she is about to undergo in vitro fertilization, then minimal intervention is advised beyond draining large endometriomas if they will affect egg collection).

As in all surgery, past medical history is important; for example, previous surgery on the abdomen may make laparoscopic surgery more hazardous.
The woman reveals that she has not yet tried for a pregnancy but has just come off the pill and is awaiting a period. She has been tricycling this for 2 years, as endometriosis was suspected from symptoms. Initially she felt better, but her pain is returning. She has developed new abdominal swelling over the last year, and attributes this to the endometrioma. She does not have dyspareunia or dyschexia. At the moment, her symptoms are of greatest importance.

She reveals that she has asthma, although she rarely takes an inhaler. However, she was once hospitalized after contracting the flu, requiring nebulizers.

B She requires referral for anaesthetic assessment for her asthma. A pregnancy test is very important, and she must use contraception in the cycle in which her surgery will fall.

C Before agreeing to do the procedure, she should be informed of all the alternative options, the details of the procedure and the risks associated with it. This should all be clearly documented and backed up with written information or signposting to suitable online resources. Common potential complications are listed on the consent form, including perforation of uterus, damage to bladder, bowel or viscera, procedures to repair damage and laparotomy.

Potential additional procedures should also be discussed, including insertion of a levonorgestrel intrauterine system (not appropriate if she wishes to conceive). Potential scenarios that may occur should be discussed; for instance, if the pelvic anatomy is very stuck with adhesions, the procedure may have to be abandoned and the patient subsequently referred to a specialist endometriosis centre. On the day of the procedure, confirmation of consent will be completed and further questions answered.

CASE HISTORY 2

A 43-year-old woman is offered a hysterectomy as treatment for her painful heavy periods. She has tried other conservative measures without success and has completed her family. She has a BMI of 34, has had two previous caesarean sections and is known to have fibroids.

A Which type of hysterectomy should she be offered?
B What additional investigations should be done pre-operatively?
C The patient asks for her ovaries to be removed, as a cousin had ovarian cancer. What would you advise?

ANSWERS

A The laparoscopic approach is usually the default procedure for benign hysterectomy. A vaginal approach might be preferable if there was significant prolapse or a planned concomitant pelvic floor repair, but that is not the case here. The choice is really between laparoscopic or open abdominal. The key determining factor here is her fibroids. If these are large (>10 cm) or multiple, then an open approach may be preferred. However, there is no absolute size at which the procedures change – it is down to the individual surgeon's decision based on their experience and competence. In some situations, the fibroids can be reduced in size by up to 30% with 3 months of a gonadotrophin-releasing hormone analogue prior to surgery. Other factors that may influence decision-making are her BMI and history of two previous caesarean sections. The latter increases the risk of bladder adhesions and injury.

B An up-to-date pelvic ultrasound of the uterus would help determine the size and number of any fibroids. Further clarification on exact size could be determined from magnetic resonance imaging if there were particular concerns. Hysterectomy carries a risk of haemorrhage, so a full blood count is required together with a 'group and save' sample in case blood is required. Transfusion policies require a second sample before blood is issued, but the first one prior to surgery is necessary to check the blood group and exclude unusual antibodies.

C The main advantage of removing ovaries is to eradicate the risk of ovarian cancer. Her family history is not sufficient to increase her own risk significantly and overall ovarian cancer is quite uncommon. On the other hand, removing her ovaries will render her menopausal, with all of the potential attendant problems and risks. Although she could take HRT (oestrogen-only), it is not suitable for all, and she would need to take it for a number of years. Ultimately, it is a joint decision but, in a premenopausal woman, most surgeons would favour conserving the ovaries. The fallopian tubes, on the other hand, have no endocrine function and may play a role in the development of ovarian cancer, so bilateral salpingectomy should be offered.

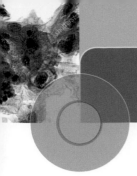

Index